Instructor's Resource Manual to accompa

Community Health Nursing

Promoting Health of Aggregates, Families, and Individuals

Marcia Stanhope, RN, DSN, FAAN
Professor and Director
Division of Community Health Nursing and Administration
College of Nursing
University of Kentucky
Lexington, Kentucky

Jeanette Lancaster, RN, MSN, PhD, FAAN
Dean and Sadie Heath Cabaniss Professor
School of Nursing
University of Virginia
Charlottesville, Virginia

Testbank prepared by:

Susan A. Heady, PhD, RN
Associate Professor
Nursing Department
Webster University
St. Louis, Missouri

FOURTH EDITION

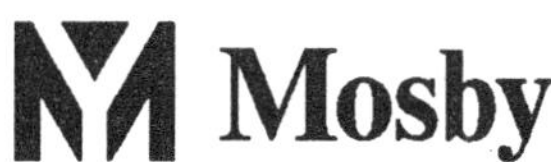

St. Louis Baltimore Boston Carlsbad Chicago Naples New York Philadelphia Portland
London Madrid Mexico City Singapore Sydney Tokyo Toronto Wiesbaden

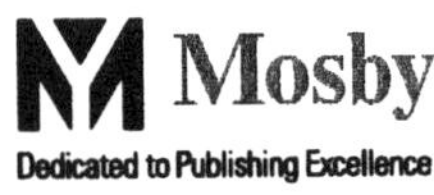

A Times Mirror Company

Printed in the United States of America
Composition by Wordbench

International Standard Book Number 0-8151-8513-8

28457

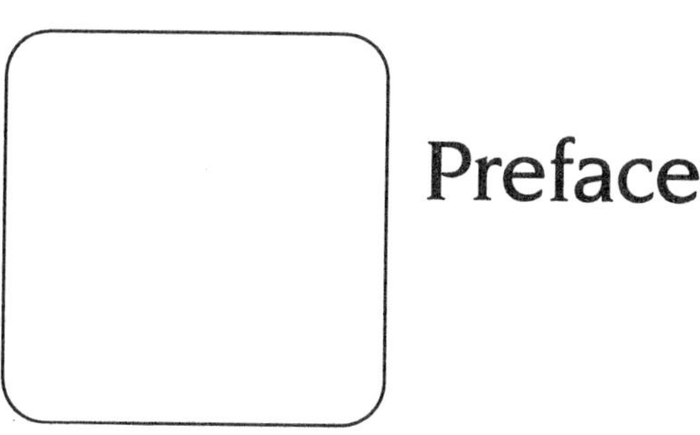

Preface

This Instructor's Resource Manual to accompany *Community Health Nursing: Promoting Health of Aggregates, Families, and Individuals*, fourth edition, has been designed as a guide for the instructor to be used in the development of class presentations, clinical experiences, or evaluations of student learning. The Manual may also be used to help create modules for self-directed learning of students.

Each chapter of the Manual corresponds with a chapter in *Community Health Nursing*. A consistent format is used in each chapter of the Manual and includes a chapter summary, annotated outline, additional critical thinking activities, and critical analysis questions with answers.

A separate Testbank includes over 600 multiple choice questions with Answers. Instructors may use these questions, as well as the critical analysis questions, to test student knowledge and comprehension.

New to this edition are 75 Transparency Masters which consist of figures, tables, and boxes from *Community Health Nursing*. Instructors may use these transparencies to explain and clarify important community health nursing concepts presented in the text.

A number of other resources have been developed to assist instructors teaching from *Community Health Nursing*:

- A *Quick Reference to Community Health Nursing* comes with each copy of the text and makes an ideal clinical companion.
- Computerized versions of the Testbank from this Manual are available in both Windows and Macintosh formats.
- Canadian users of the text will find information on issues unique to the Canadian context in *Introduction to Community Health Nursing in Canada* by Janet Ross Kerr and Jannetta MacPhail.
- The *Handbook of Community and Home Health Nursing* by Marcia Stanhope and Ruth N. Knollmueller provides an abundance of tools and guides useful to nurses as they apply the principles learned from the text to clinical situations.
- *Mosby's Community Health Nursing Video Series* offers eight videos on important topics in community health nursing, giving students a direct, visual picture of the practice of community health nursing.

We thank our text contributors for their contributions to this Manual. We also thank Susan A. Heady for the preparation of the Testbank.

Marcia Stanhope
Jeanette Lancaster

Contents

1 The History of Community Health and Community Health Nursing

Chapter Summary

The roles of the community health nurse are varied and challenging. Many of the current roles can be traced to the early nineteenth century, when public health efforts focused on environmental conditions such as sanitation, control of communicable diseases, education in personal hygiene, disease prevention, and care of the sick in their homes. While health threats from communicable diseases, the environment, chronic illnesses, and the aging process have changed over time, the foundational principles and goals of community health nursing have not changed. Many diseases such as diphtheria, cholera, and typhoid fever have been controlled in developed countries; however, they have been replaced by hepatitis, AIDS, and a resurgence of diseases such as measles and tuberculosis. Similarly, the environment in industrialized countries is no longer polluted with garbage in the streets but now is threatened by overcrowded garbage dumps; seepage of garbage into the waters that feed crops; and toxins in the air, water, and soil. In addition, instead of experiencing illnesses related to the physical toll of manual labor on their bodies, individuals now experience debilitating diseases that are often stress related. Finally, as the population of the United States ages and desires to remain at home in spite of decreased family and community resources, different community health care needs emerge.

Throughout history, the roles of the community health nurse have changed to respond effectively to the prevailing public health problems of the times. The roles have been dynamic and multifaceted and have relied heavily on the science of public health. Part of the appeal of community health nursing is due to the autonomy of the practice and the use of problem solving and decision making skills in the role.

This chapter describes the contemporary role of the community health nurse in the United States. To do this, it is necessary to briefly trace the history of Western health care from Pre-Hellenistic times to the present.

Annotated Outline

I. Historical review of health care practices: A review of the dominant cultural ideas and practices of each era is useful in understanding the current community health care system because the patterns of health care in previous eras are reflected in current practice.
   A. Pre-Hellenistic Period: The Babylonians, Egyptians, and Hebrews emphasized hygiene, had some medical skills, and were concerned about systematizing their health care practices.
   B. Hellenistic Period: The early Greeks saw health care delivery as a responsibility of a civilized society; therefore, they established a code of medical ethics and emphasized cleanliness, exercise, diet, and sanitation.
   C. Roman Empire: The Roman Empire was similar in focus yet more pragmatic in application than the Greeks and was quite advanced in administrative and engineering skills, including the regulation of medical practice, punishment for negligence, drainage of swamps, provision of pure water, establishment of sewage systems, and supervision of both street cleaning and public food preparation.
   D. Middle Ages: The period between 500 and 1500 AD was a heterogeneous phase in history during which superstitions dominated thinking; however, advances such as the development of health care facilities originated during this time period.
   E. Renaissance: The Renaissance ushered in a new period of history during which community health as it is currently known began, sanitation was emphasized, and technological advances in health care blossomed.
   F. Industrial Revolution: During the Industrial Revolution, the population grew, thus experiencing an increase in such problems as the following: a high infant mortality rate, neglect and often murder of illegitimate infants, poor working conditions, diseases of certain occupations, and mental illnesses.
   G. Colonial Period: During the Colonial Period, many epidemics occurred; however, public health efforts aimed at fighting these epidemics included the collection of vital statistics, im-

proved sanitation, and avoidance of exotic diseases.

II. Nursing developed by Nightingale: Although concern about the health care of individuals in the community has existed throughout the centuries, the organized discipline of nursing was not developed until the mid-1800s in England by Florence Nightingale.

   A. Need for nurses: During the Crimean War, conditions for injured soldiers were appalling; therefore, Florence Nightingale was asked to go to Scutari to improve conditions for the sick and injured soldiers.

   B. Origins of organized nursing: The roots of organized nursing were grounded in the provision of health care to poor, discriminated against, and powerless individuals. Similar to Nightingale, community health nurses typically identify health care needs that affect the entire population, mobilize resources, and organize themselves and the community to meet these needs.

   C. Principles of nursing: Nightingale identified principles that continue to guide the practice of community health nursing, such as the essential nature of proper nutrition, rest, sanitation, and hygiene in health promotion. Community health nurses continue to focus on the role of health promotion, disease prevention, and environment as they deliver care to their patients.

III. Community health nursing in the United States in the nineteenth century: Community health nursing developed in the United States in the nineteenth century.

   A. Need for community health nursing: Although the United States grew tremendously between 1800 and 1850, community health efforts did not keep pace. During this period, threats to health escalated as epidemics of smallpox, yellow fever, cholera, typhoid, and typhus entered the country along with the influx of migrants from many parts of the world.

   B. Origins of organized nursing: Nurses became active in establishing visiting nursing services and community-based settlement houses. The first visiting nurse society began in Philadelphia in 1886 in order to provide home health for the sick. In 1893, Lillian Wald and her friend Mary Brewster organized a visiting nursing service and established a settlement house for the poor of New York City, which became known as the Henry Street Settlement.

   C. Community health organizations: In 1893, Isabel Hampton Robb led the effort to establish the Society of Superintendents of Training Schools of Nurses in the United States and Canada. The society, which later became the National League for Nursing (NLN), established training standards and promoted collegial relationships among nurses. Two years later, the Associated Alumnae of Training Schools for Nurses, which later became the American Nurses' Association (ANA), was organized to strengthen the union of nursing organizations, improve nursing education, and promote ethical standards in nursing.

IV. Community health nursing in the United States in the twentieth century: In the twentieth century, community health nursing in the United States has continued to evolve and adapt in order to meet the health care needs of the nation.

   A. 1900 to WWI: In 1912, the National Organization for Public Health Nursing (NOPHN) came into existence, with Lillian Wald as its first president. They sought to standardize public health nursing activities and community health nursing education. During the early portion of the twentieth century, the scope of community health nursing included disease prevention, health promotion, and family-oriented services.

   B. WWI to WWII: The large numbers of nurses involved in WWI left few nurses to practice in the community setting. However, after WWI, many federally funded relief projects utilized nurses. For example, in 1934 Pearl McIver became the first nurse employed by the U.S. Public Health Service to provide consultation services to state health departments. In addition, the Frontier Nursing Service (FNS) was developed by Mary Breckenridge to provide community health programs geared towards improving the health care of a rural and often inaccessible population in the Appalachian sections of Kentucky.

   C. WWII to 1960: The onset of WWII in 1941 accelerated the need for nurses; thus, many nurses joined the Army and Navy Nurse Corps, and community health nursing expanded its scope of practice. Changes after WWII subsequently affected community health nursing and included increased funding for specific health problems such as venereal disease, cancer, tuberculosis, and mental illness. In addition, the number of local health departments increased. During the 1950s, there was considerable interest in nurse-midwifery, equality and advancement of black nurses in community health nursing, cost analysis methods and studies, inclusion of nursing services in health insurance programs, and better coordination of organized nursing.

   D. 1960 to the present: Two major factors influenced community health nursing during the 1960s: (a) the development of the nurse practitioner movement and (b) the call for the evaluation of the effectiveness of community health programs. The nurse practitioner movement began in 1965 at the University of Colorado and opened a new era for nursing's involvement in primary health care. The individual orientation of health care in the 1960s gave way in the 1970s to the following: (a) a review of health care systems aimed at providing comprehensive community-based services and (b) the evaluation of the effectiveness of community care. The 1980s saw an increase in the presence of community health nurses in many states. Also, the establishment in 1985 of the National Center for Nursing Research within the National Institutes of Health in Washington, D.C., has been a major tool in promoting the work of nurses.

V. Summary: Over the years, community health nursing in the United States has evolved from a home care service delivered by caring women who ministered to both the health and spiritual needs of individuals and families to a broadly based, population-focused discipline that considers individuals, families, groups, and communities as its scope of practice.

Additional Critical Thinking Activities

1. Write a summary of what you believe were Lillian Wald's greatest contributions to community health nursing.
2. If you were Lillian Wald and chose to devote your energy to critical forces affecting the health of Americans, what would be your highest priority efforts?
3. Telephone or visit one voluntary agency in your community and describe its purpose, source of funding, major programs or services, and eligibility of recipients of services.
4. Interview three nurses employed in community health nursing to determine how they currently define their role.
5. Analyze nursing organizations in your state and assess which have the greatest potential for furthering the cause of community health nurses.
6. Review the programs sponsored by your state's chapter of ANA and NLN, and note how many have applicability for community health nurses.
7. Assess the number of home health care agencies in your community to determine how many exist, the type of clients they serve, and how they receive funds.
8. Identify the types of community health nursing projects that you feel should be funded by the National Center for Nursing Research.

Critical Analysis Questions

1. Identify five of the seven time periods that are important to consider in the historical development of community health nursing.
2. What was Florence Nightingale's role in the development of nursing?
3. True or False? Because of the influx of immigrants into the United States during the nineteenth century, crowding and communicable diseases were problematic.
4. What were the two types of community-based nursing practices that existed in the nineteenth century?
5. List three of the five accomplishments of Lillian Wald mentioned in this chapter that have influenced the current scope of community health nursing.
6. Differentiate between the early functions of what became the NLN and the ANA.
7. True or False? The name of the organization established in 1912 to standardize public health nursing and community health nursing education was called the National Organization for Public Health Nursing.
8. What was the name of the community health program that Mary Breckenridge established to improve the health care of rural sections of Kentucky?
9. True or False? After WWII, the number of local health departments dramatically declined.
10. True or False? The nurse practitioner movement began as a way to promote advance practice nursing in the hospital setting.
11. True or False? In the future, community health nurses will be less involved in the delivery of primary health care, health maintenance, and health promotion.
12. True or False? Community health nursing is focused on providing health care and promoting the health of individuals, families, groups, and the community.

Answer Key

1. 1. Pre-Hellenistic, 2. Hellenistic, 3. Roman Empire, 4. Middle Ages, 5. Renaissance, 6. Industrial Revolution, and 7. Colonial Period.
2. She organized care for the wounded soldiers in the Crimean War, developed hospital nursing, coined the phrase "health nursing," and established the basic principles upon which nursing is founded.
3. True
4. 1. Visiting Nursing and 2. Settlement Houses

5. 1. Established the Henry Street Settlement, 2. Established the first nursing service provided by an insurance company, 3. Established rural health services through the Red Cross, 4. Established Children's Bureau, and 5. Fought for many social and health improvements
6. NLN: Established training standards and promoted collegial relationships among nurses
   ANA: Strengthened the union of nursing organizations and promoted ethical standards
7. True
8. Frontier Nursing Service
9. False
10. False
11. False
12. True

2 Community-Based Population-Focused Practice

Chapter Summary

A basic definition of a population is a collection of individuals who share in common one or more personal or environmental characteristics. Thus those who are members of a community defined either in terms of geography or special interest can be seen as constituting a population. The basic notion in population-focused practice is that problems are defined (diagnoses) and solutions proposed (interventions) for defined populations or subpopulations as opposed to diagnosis and intervention/treatment at the patient or client level.

As America looks toward the twenty-first century, its citizens and health professionals are experiencing major changes in health care delivery. Despite the failure of the Clinton administration's efforts to reform health care, other federal, state, and private market forces are transforming the health care system. Questions about access to care, the ability to maintain insurance coverage, quality, and health care costs represent key forces for reform at the federal and state levels as well as in the private sector. In this context a community-based, population-focused approach to planning, delivering, and evaluating nursing care has never been more important. This is a crucial time for public health nursing and community health nursing, a time of opportunity and challenge.

The main points made in this chapter are these: (1) In the last years of the twentieth century and the beginning of the twenty-first century, strong public health-minded leadership will be needed to provide the direction for the development of a health care system in which prevention of dysfunction and disease are primary concerns, and (2) the specialties of public health nursing and community health nursing can and should have major roles in bringing about this new order. The argument to be presented is that although there are problems with the present status of the health care system and the roles that public health nursing and community health nursing currently play, there is a great potential for a new flowering of the respective specializations. It is further suggested that whether or not this potential is realized depends on the extent to which the leadership in public health nursing is able to prepare and support nurses who have the knowledge and skills to design, manage, monitor, and evaluate systems of care (prevention included) that address the high importance and high-impact problems experienced by populations. It is argued that nursing's future in community-based practice will be determined by the extent to which the profession takes seriously and adopts a population-focused approach to practice.

Annotated Outline

I. The key role of public health practice: It is very important to put forward the key role which public health practice plays in influencing the health of the population.
   A. As stated in the U.S. Public Health Services Report on the Core Functions of Public Health, reform of the medical insurance system is necessary, but it is not a sufficient condition for improving the health of Americans. "Historically, gains in the health of populations have derived largely from changes in the safety and adequacy of food supplies, in the provision of safe water, in sewage disposal, and in personal behavior, including reproductive behavior. . . . The dramatic gain in life expectancy for Americans over the course of this century, from less than 50 years in 1900 to more than 75 years in 1990, is attributed primarily to improvements in sanitation, the control of infectious diseases through immunizations, and other public health activities" (p. 2).
   B. The U.S. Public Health Service estimates that medical treatment can prevent only about 10% of all early deaths in the United States. Yet, "population-wide public health approaches have the potential to help prevent some 70% of early deaths in America through measures targeted to the factors that contribute to those deaths. Many of these contributing factors are behavioral such as tobacco use and diet and sedentary lifestyles; others are environmental in nature" (Prevention Report, p. 2).
   C. In 1988, the Institute of Medicine published a report on the future of Public Health. In that report Public Health was defined as "what we, as a society, do collectively to assure the conditions in which people can be healthy" (p. 1). The committee stated that the aim of public health was "to generate organized community

effort to address the public interest in health by applying scientific and technical knowledge to prevent disease and promote health" (p. 7).

D. The report also stated that assessment, policy development, and assurance are the core functions at all levels of government. Assessment refers to systematic data collection on the population, monitoring of the population's health status, and making information available on the health of the community. Policy development refers to the need to provide leadership in developing policies which support the health of the population, including the use of the scientific knowledge base in decision-making about policy. Assurance refers to the role of public health in making sure that essential community-wide health services are available, which may include providing essential personal health services for those who would otherwise not receive them. Assurance also refers to making sure that a competent public health and personal health care workforce is available.

E. Public health practice is a great buy! The U.S. Public Health Service estimated in 1993 that only 0.9% of all national health expenditures support population-based public health functions, yet as described above, the impact is enormous. Unfortunately, much of the public is unaware of the contributions of public health practice, and the proportion of expenditures for public health activities has actually declined by approximately 25% over the last ten years!

F. Because of its importance in influencing the health of the population and in providing a strong foundation for the health care system, the U.S. Public Health Service and other groups are vigorously advocating a renewed emphasis on the population-wide essential functions and services of public health that have made the greatest impact on improving the health of the entire population.

The list of essential services presented in Figure 2-1 represents a specification and illustration of the fundamental obligations of public health for the core functions of assessment, assurance, and policy development discussed above. The Health Services Pyramid (See Figure 2-2) shows that population-based public health programs, focused on disease prevention, health protection, and health promotion, provide a foundation upon which primary, secondary, and tertiary health care services rest.

II. The relationship between public health nursing and community health nursing: Diverse opinions abound as to what public health nursing and community health nursing are and how they relate to each other. Many individuals use the terms as though they were completely interchangeable, wishing to minimize the differences.

A. Much of the material in current community health textbooks presents the view that the focus of community health nursing is on providing services to people in community settings. This emphasis is also the predominant focus of the American Nurses' Association's statement, A Conceptual Model of Community Health Nursing, developed by the Division of Community Health Nursing (1980). First, the statement identifies two categories of nurses in community health—generalists prepared at the baccalaureate level, who practice in community health settings, and specialists in community health nursing, who have a master's level preparation or beyond. In describing scope of practice for community health nursing, the major objectives of the community health nurse are stated as "the preservation and improvement of the health of community" (ANA, 1980, p. 11).

B. One way to look at the relationship between public health nursing and community health nursing is to view public health nursing as a specialized field of practice with certain attributes within the broad arena of community health nursing. This view is consistent with recommendations developed at a Consensus Conference on the Essentials of Public Health Nursing Practice and Education, sponsored by the Division of Nursing and held in Washington in September 1984.

III. Problems inherent in defining nursing specialties by setting: If one takes seriously the 1984 consensus conference's definitions of the community health nurse and the public health nurse, it is clear that the setting in which one practices is viewed as the single feature distinguishing community health nurses from other nurses. Yet setting is not used to set apart public health nurses; here, type of preparation is the distinguishing feature! Using setting as a distinguishing feature for community health nursing is problematic for several reasons.

A. First, the way community is equated with "noninstitutionalization" leads to further confusion. According to this statement, an individual who has received preparation in any clinical or subclinical area and who practices in a noninstitutional setting can be seen as a community health nursing specialist.

B. Another problem with the use of setting as a distinguishing feature is that there is so much shifting and reorganization occurring in the health care system, that the institutional/noninstitutional distinction made in the consensus statement is outdated.

IV. Public health nursing as a field of practice, an area of specialization: It is then reasonable to ask, "Is community health nursing really a specialty area?" It was suggested by those participating in the consensus conference mentioned above that "the term 'community health nursing' came into broad use when the American Nurses' Association sought to create a unit within the organization to which nurses working in scattered community settings could belong." The consensus conference report went on to elaborate that "the term 'community health nurse' is simply an umbrella term used for all nurses who work in the community, including those who have format preparation in community health nursing."

   A. "Public health nursing requires specific educational preparation, and community health nursing denotes a setting for the practice of nursing" (p. 4). Thus, rather than calling nurses with graduate preparation who simply work in community settings community health nurse specialists, it might be appropriate to refer to them in a manner that is more in keeping with their area of practice specialization.
   B. In contrast, a case can be made that public health nursing clearly is an area of specialization. What makes it so? The focus of practice, described as follows, and the specialized knowledge supporting the practice. Multifoci of public health nursing include the following: populations that are free-living in the community as opposed to those that are institutionalized; the predominant emphasis on strategies for health promotion, health maintenance, and disease prevention; the concern for the interface between health status of the population and the living environment; and the use of political processes to affect public policy as a major intervention strategy for achieving goals.
   C. In 1981, the Public Health Nursing Section of the American Public Health Association put forth a statement on the Definition and Role of Public Health Nursing in the Delivery of Health Care, which clearly describes the field of specialization.

V. Population-focused practice versus practice focused on individual: It is proposed that the fundamental factors that should distinguish public health nursing from other areas of specialization in nursing are the following: a focus on populations that are free-living in the community as opposed to those institutionalized for episodes of care; a focus on strategies for health promotion, health maintenance, and disease prevention; and the use of strategies which take into account the broad social political context in which community problems occur and are resolved. Such practice is built upon, but different from, basic clinical nursing practice.

   A. Basic professional education in nursing, medicine, and other clinical disciplines focuses primarily on the individual. Population-level decision making is different from decision making in clinical care and demands the specialized preparation described previously.
   B. It is important to recognize that those who specialize in public health nursing frequently are concerned with more than one subpopulation. Those concerned with the health of a given community must ultimately consider the health of multiple and sometimes overlapping populations. In addition, a population focus requires consideration of those who may need particular services but have not entered the health care system.

VI. The arenas for specialization in public health nursing and community health nursing: A very broad understanding of public health should include some concern for all populations within the community, both free-living and institutionalized. Further, a very broad understanding of public health should also consider the match between the health needs of the population and the health care resources in the community, including services offered in institutional settings.

   A. What roles in the care system would public health nursing specialists have? Options include Director of Nursing for a health department, Director of the Health Department, State Commissioner for Health, or Director of Maternal and Child Health services for a state health department or a local health department. While it may not be generally known, nurses have occupied and continue to occupy all of these roles, but they are in the minority.
   B. Where does the staff public health nurse fit into the scheme? It is suggested that the staff public health nurse is not a public health nurse specialist.
   C. It is suggested that there is a need and place for specialization in community health nursing that is more focused than the definition put forth in the consensus conference discussed earlier in the chapter. Such specialization would include some responsibilities for providing direct care services and some responsibilities for dealing with subpopulations in the community, and preparation for such specialization would include master's preparation in a direct-care clinical area and some work in the public health sciences.

VII. The need to think broadly about roles in public health nursing: Within public health and community nursing circles there has been a tendency to talk about public health nursing and community health nursing from the point of view of a role, such as the public health nursing role or the community health nursing specialist. This is limiting. In discussing such provider orientation, rarely is attention given to how nurse administrators in public health (public health nursing specialists) might reorient their practice to be concerned with a population focus, which is more critical, useful, and possible for an administrator than for the staff nurse.

A. With regard to public health nursing administrators, those who are prepared to practice in a population-focused manner should be more effective than those who are not prepared. Another problem with thinking in terms of nursing roles is that present role conceptualizations are frequently too limited to allow for population-focused practice.

B. If population-focused public health nursing is to be taken seriously and strategies for its implementation (assessment, intervention, and evaluation) at the population level are to be applied, more consideration must be given to organized systems for assessing population needs and managing care.

C. Rather than focusing on defining roles for the immediate future, it may be more useful to concentrate on the identification of skills and knowledge necessary for the type of decision making suggested as being inherent in population-focused practice.

VIII. Challenges: There are several challenges to the full development of specialization in public health nursing, and our challenge is to address them. One of the most serious is the "mind set" of many nurses that the only role for a nurse is at the bedside or at the client's side, the direct care role. Another barrier to the type of practice implied in population-focused public health nursing is the structures within which nurses work and the process of role socialization that occurs within those structures. There is also the barrier of relatively few nurses receiving graduate level preparation in the concepts and strategies of disciplines basic to public health.

A. The massive organizational changes that are occurring in the delivery system present a unique opportunity to establish new opportunities for nurse leaders who are prepared to think in population terms. Individuals will be needed who can span in-patient and community-based settings and who can focus on providing a wide range of services to the population served by the system. An example of such an opportunity is the director of patient care services for a health care system. In addition to those who will have the administrative responsibility for a large programmatic area, there will be a demand for individuals who can design programs of preventive and clinical services to be offered to targeted subpopulations within the system.

B. Perhaps it is time to forge a creative synthesis between specialization in public health nursing and nursing administration (Williams, 1985). One basis for suggesting this is that regardless of how the population is defined, there will be a growing need for nurses with population level assessment, management, and evaluation skills. Another way of looking at the future is to accept the prediction that community-based strategies for health promotion and disease prevention, primary care, and much of secondary care will be the primary focus of the health care system of the future. The field must also be ready to direct more attention to developing the specialty of public health nursing as a way of providing nursing leadership. To prepare for such population-focused decision making will entail more attention on master's and doctoral level programs with a strong basis in the public health sciences and health services research.

C. Because of pressures in the health care system to cut costs and not shift costs, there is now a growing concern that the problem of access to basic primary care will get worse before it gets better, particularly for special, vulnerable populations (the homeless, the frail elderly, and persons with HIV).

The history of public health nursing shows that a common feature of those considered leaders are individuals who moved forward to deal with unresolved problems in a positive, proactive way. This is the legacy of Lillian Wald at the Henry Street Settlement and many others who have met need with innovation. Within the context of the core public health function of assurance, there clearly is an opportunity for public health nursing in population-based outreach programs directed to "the matching of the needs of vulnerable groups in the community with the services that hold promise for helping them" (Aiken and Salmon, p. 328). As a specialty, public health nursing can have a positive impact on the health status of populations, but to do so "it will be necessary to have broad vision; to prepare nurses for leadership roles in policy making and in the design, development, management, monitoring, and evaluation of population-focused health care systems; and to develop strategies to support nurses in these roles" (Williams, 1992).

Additional Critical Thinking Activities

1. Observe two community health nurses who are functioning in two different community settings. If possible, review their job descriptions. From your observations state the following:
   A. Which concept of community health nursing does their practice reflect?
   B. Which concept is emphasized in their job description?
   C. Is there a correlation between their job description and their practice?
   D. Are the nurses involved in policy formulation that affects client services?
   E. In the settings you have observed, which concept (in your opinion) is the most effective for implementation? What is your rationale?

Critical Analysis Questions

1. State the mission, core functions, and essential services of public health.
2. Define the population-focused public health nurse practitioner.
3. State the goal of public health nursing as described by the Public Health Nursing Section of APHA (1981).
4. State the major difference between clinically-focused community health nursing practice and population-focused practice.
5. Is the arena for community health nursing practice the total population of the community, including institutionalized populations, or is the arena for community health nursing practice limited to noninstitutionalized populations in the community? Give the rationale for your answer.
6. Name three major factors contributing to the confusion about population-focused practice.

Answer Key

1. See Section on The Importance of Public Health.
2. See section on The Relationship of Public Health and Community Health Nursing.
3. To improve the health of the entire community
4. Clinical nursing provides direct personal care services to clients and encourages health-promoting behavior. Population-focused nursing identifies subgroups within the population who are at risk and directs resources toward these groups as the most effective approach for accomplishing the goal of public health nursing.
5. See section on The Arenas for Specialization in Public Health Nursing and Community Health Nursing.
6. Perplexity about community health nursing specialty and its distinction from other nursing practice; Lack of clarity about meaning of population-focused practice; Nurses' ambivalence to move from provision of direct care services to population-focused practice

3 The Public Health and Primary Health Care Systems and Health Care Reform

Chapter Summary

The American health care system has done a remarkable job in many ways in providing health care to the American people, particularly in technology development and skilled provider training. Today's health care facilities would defy the imagination of our predecessors. While public and private health insurance programs protect most Americans from the financial ravages of illness, the system has some serious liabilities. Major concerns include cost, access to care, and quality of care.

This chapter describes the current primary care and public health systems in the United States and the trends that affect these systems. The systems are compared and contrasted both to each other and to the concept of primary health care. Current concepts of health care reform are outlined in order to discuss what an emerging health care system might look like. This chapter describes a reformed health care system as one that weaves primary care and public health into a single integrated system. The role of the community health nurse is presented in all of the systems, current and future.

Annotated Outline

I. Definitions
   A. Managed care is health care that manages or controls the amount and type of care a person receives for a set fee. Examples of managed care are health maintenance organizations and preferred provider organizations.
   B. A health maintenance organization (HMO) is an organized system of health care that, for a fixed fee, provides primary care services, emergency and preventive treatment, and hospital care to people who have agreed to obtain their medical care from the HMO for a specified period of time.
   C. A preferred provider organization (PPO) is an organization of providers that contracts on a fee-for-service basis with third-party payers to provide comprehensive medical services to subscribers. The agreement between the PPO and the third-party payer allows subscribers to receive medical services at lower than usual rates.
   D. Primary care is personal health care services that provide for first contact, continuous, comprehensive, and coordinated care. Care is directed primarily at an individual's pathophysiological process.
   E. Primary health care is essential care made universally accessible to individuals and families within a community and made available to them through their full participation, and provided at a cost that the community and country can afford.
   F. Primary care generalists include family physicians, general internists, general pediatricians, nurse practitioners, physician assistants, and nurse midwives. Some physicians with special training in preventive medicine/public health and obstetrics/gynecology also deliver primary care.
   G. Community-oriented primary care (COPC) is a community-responsive model of health care delivery that integrates aspects of both primary care and public health. It combines the care of individuals and families in the community with a focus on the community and its subgroups when services are planned, provided, and evaluated.
   H. Cost shifting is the process of making up for lost revenue by charging more to those who are able to pay (usually through insurance).
   I. The National Health Service Corps is a commissioned corps of health care professionals that serve residents of medically underserved areas and populations.

II. Cost, quality, and access to care: The current health care system does a good job of providing health care to the American people, particularly in technology development and skilled provider training. It is also a system plagued by its liabilities of cost, quality, and access to care.
   A. The cost of health care in this country is 40% higher than in Canada, the country that spends the next largest amount on health care. By the year 2003, United States health care costs are predicted to rise to $2.1 trillion, or 20% of the GDP. Current cost containment efforts are

curbing costs, but doing little to solve the overall crisis.

B. Access to care is a problem for those without insurance, especially the working poor, illegal immigrants, and those who are sick or at risk for getting sick with an illness that insurance companies consider too costly to cover. In 1994, 39 million Americans or 14.7% of the total population were uninsured. In addition, the access problem has been compounded by the gradual erosion of public health services. Funding to clinics in rural and heavily populated urban areas has been reduced, which means that many uninsured people seek care at the emergency room. Cost shifting occurs when this happens.

C. Quality often depends on location (suburban, urban, rural), insurance status, and employment status. However, even those individuals who do have insurance, as well as easy access to medical care, lack adequate preventive care.

III. Trends affecting the health care system: Because of the national concern for the cost, access to, and quality of health care, significant change is expected in the next decade. Several trends will affect how these changes will evolve.

A. Demographic trends that will affect health care include size and characteristics of the population. The population increased by 22 million between 1980 and 1990. It is predicted that immigration (legal and illegal) will constitute almost half of all population growth in the United States in the next generation. The population is also aging. There is a prediction of a 74% increase in the number of people aged 50 or older by the year 2020, while the number of people under 50 will only grow by 1%. By 2050 the over 85 year group will comprise approximately 24% of the elderly population. Blacks are currently the largest minority group, but will be surpassed by Hispanics by the year 2015. Asian-Americans, although the smallest minority group, will wield the largest influence due to their rapid acculturation. Three out of ten families are headed by single parents, usually the mother. Single-parent families constitute 24.5% of all white families with children, while 35% of Hispanic families with children and 63% of black families with children reside with only one parent. Mortality rates are declining predominantly due to the decline in infectious diseases.

B. Social trends that influence health care include changing lifestyles, a growing appreciation of the quality of life, changing composition of families and living patterns, rising household incomes, and a revised definition of quality health care. There is a growing emphasis on the belief that people are responsible for their own health and an awareness that health is a valuable asset and efforts should be taken to improve it.

C. Economic trends show that household income has risen and is more evenly distributed. There continues to be disparity between whites and minority groups. A sizable proportion of low-income Americans will continue to rely on public support to maintain a minimum standard of living.

D. Health workforce trends are emphasizing primary care as a way to cut costs. This includes increasing the number of primary care physicians and advanced practice nurses, such as nurse practitioners and certified nurse midwives. The trend is toward community-based care with a downsizing of acute care facilities. Increasing minority representation within the health professions is a priority.

E. Technological trends are having both positive and negative effects. Although technological advances promise improved health care services and many times reduce costs, the up-front costs are very high. Efforts will continue to focus on devising simpler, cheaper, and more mobile tests and procedures that are less oriented to tertiary care and can be used in nonhospital settings.

IV. Components of the current health system: Organization of the health care system, although made up of many entities, can generally be divided into two distinct components: a private or personal care component and a public health component, with some overlap.

A. The primary health care (PHC) system includes a comprehensive range of services including public health, preventive, diagnostic, therapeutic, and rehabilitative services, provided by a multidisciplinary team of health care providers. PHC encourages self-care and self-management in health and social welfare aspects of daily life. The PHC movement began when the 30th World Health Organization Health Assembly adopted a resolution accepting the goal of attaining a level of health that permitted all citizens of the world to live socially and economically productive lives. The resolution became known by the slogan "Health for All by the Year 2000." The Alma Mata declaration is the basis for PHC and the global evolvement of this strategy over the past 10 to 15 years. PHC is not the primary strategy for health care in America.

B. The primary care system is the strategy of choice for delivering care in the United States. It is a personal health care system that provides for first-contact, continuous, comprehensive, and coordinated care. It addresses the most common needs of patients within a community by providing preventive, curative, and rehabilitative services to maximize their health and well-being. The focus is on the pathophysiological process. Providers include primary care physicians, physician assistants, and advanced practice nurses, including nurse practitioners and certified nurse midwives. The primary care delivery system is comprised of a variety of accessible community settings and emphasizes cost containment. Health maintenance organizations and preferred provider organizations are two systems that strive to contain costs.

C. The public health system is mandated through laws that are developed at the national, state, or local levels that work to ensure health protection, promotion, and restoration for the people. The public health system provides some overlap with the personal care system. The overlap comes not only from the personal care system providing health promotion and disease prevention, but also through the public health system providing personal care.

D. The federal system is comprised of the Department of Health and Human Services (DHHS), with the U.S. Public Health Service, the largest public health program in the world, coming under its auspices. The Public Health Service is headed by the Assistant Secretary for Health and is organized into eight functional units. The Division of Nursing lies within the U.S. Public Health Service within the Health Resources and Services Agency. The National Institute of Nursing Research is also part of the U.S. Public Health Services, as part of the National Institutes of Health. There are several other federal departments that have responsibility for functions related to health. They include the Department of Commerce; the Department of Defense; the Department of Labor; the Department of Agriculture; and the Department of Justice.

E. The state systems provide a wide array of services including health care financing (Medicaid), mental health and professional education, establishing health codes, licensing facilities and personnel, and regulating the insurance industry. They also have a substantial role in direct assistance to local health departments. States also have control over the board of examiners of nurses, which generally has responsibility for licensing and examination of registered nurses and licensed practical nurses; approval of schools of nursing; revocation, suspension, or denial of licenses; and writing of regulations about nursing practice and education.

F. The local system has direct responsibility to the citizens in their community or jurisdiction. Services and programs offered by local health departments vary greatly depending on the state and local health codes that must be followed, the needs of the community, and available funding and other resources.

V. Reform efforts: Health care reform efforts have centered on cost-containment, quality, and access to care. Nothing definitive, especially at the federal level, is expected in this century. States and especially health care systems, such as academic health centers and managed care organizations, have made changes on their own. Some common ground issues among the legislative health care proposals that might see reform in the future include health care alliances, guaranteed coverage, increase in managed care, cost-control mechanisms, and an increased interest in primary and preventive care. The Pew Health Professions Commission has outlined other characteristics of an emerging health care system. They include an orientation toward health with an emphasis on the population as a whole, a consumer focus, a balance between the benefits and burdens of technology, and care that is more effective and efficient with the increased use of coordinated services and health provider teams.

VI. Community-oriented primary care (COPC): Public health and primary care can be integrated into a community responsive model of care—community-oriented primary care (COPC). COPC combines the care of individuals and families in the community with a focus on the community and its subgroups when services are planned, provided, and evaluated. COPC utilizes a planning process that targets resources to high priority needs and empowers communities to encourage individual responsibility. COPC attempts to invite and maintain community participation within a community-based primary care practice. Steps for using COPC are similar to the nursing process. Community health nurses are ideally suited to a COPC practice due to their comfort with working in the community and their knowledge of prevention, health promotion, assessment, and case-management skills.

VII. Summary: The health care delivery system in America is complex. There is a primary care or personal care system, and a public health system, both of which overlap each other. The overall system provides high quality, technologically proficient care to many, yet for over 14% of our population the care is not accessible and, because of a lack of insurance, is not affordable. Lack of adequate federal legislation has created movement on the part of the state and local government, as well as private industry, to create accessible and cost-effective systems of care. Managed care systems, including health maintenance and preferred provider organizations, have been established for this purpose.

A model of care, community-oriented primary care (COPC), is introduced that emphasizes important aspects of both primary care and public health. Strategies for using COPC are similar to those used in the nursing process. Community participation is an important component in this model. Community health nurses are viewed as key participants in this model of care due to their skills in assessment, health promotion, and disease and injury prevention, and due to their knowledge of community resources and their ability to develop relationships with community members/leaders.

Additional Critical Thinking Activities

1. Think carefully about the program that provides health care to you and members of your family. What kind of program is it? Discuss the advantages and disadvantages of your own health care program to you and to the insurer who underwrites your health coverage.
2. Interview ten people of varying backgrounds, educational levels, careers or occupations. Ask each person to list three ways in which health care costs might be cut. Evaluate the validity of each suggestion and determine whether you think it would work in your community.
3. Identify four organizations in your community that deliver primary health care. Based on the objective material that you can obtain, determine whom they serve; what services they provide; where their funding comes from; and evaluate the relative value to the individuals and families in the community of their services.
4. Divide the class into groups of six each. Have each group debate the following health care issues:
   A. The American system of health care delivery is the best in the world.
   B. Compared to several other industrialized nations, the quality of health care provided in terms of its cost is inferior.
   C. People, not the health care system, are responsible for their own health. That is, good health is a matter of personal responsibility.
   D. Primary health care is (is not) effectively practiced in the United States.
   E. The policy makers who determine the local, state, and federal regulations related to health care are concerned more about their popularity than about truly developing a better health care system.

Critical Analysis Questions

1. True or False? The primary care system can be differentiated from the primary health care system by its distinct focus on the pathophysiological process.
2. True or False? Primary care is essential care made universally accessible to individuals and families in a community, and is made available to them through their full participation, and is provided at a cost that the community can afford.
3. The system that refers to organized community efforts designed to prevent disease and promote health is the:
   a. public health system.
   b. primary health care system.
   c. managed care system.
   d. primary care system.
4. True or False? Immigration (both legal and illegal) will constitute almost half of all population growth in the United States in the next generation.
5. Health care reform efforts generally focus on:
   a. quality.
   b. access to care.
   c. cost containment.
   d. b and c only.
   e. all of the above.
6. The community-oriented model of care emphasizes important aspects of which of the following?
   a. public health
   b. managed care
   c. primary care
   d. a and c only
   e. all of the above
7. True or False? The specialty of family practice and the arrival of nurse practitioners and physician assistants emerged in this country in response to the need to provide primary care.
8. The difference between nurse practitioners (NPs) and physician assistants (PAs) is:
   a. NPs usually receive training at the master's level, while PAs usually receive training at the baccalaureate level.
   b. NPs operate under their own license, while PAs operate under the license of a physician.
   c. NPs are licensed to prescribe medication, while PAs are not licensed to do so.
   d. a and b only
   e. all of the above.

Answer Key

1. True
2. False
3. a
4. True
5. e
6. d
7. True
8. d

4 International Health Care

Chapter Summary

It is important that community health nurses obtain knowledge of health problems that exist outside of the United States because many of these problems have an impact on health care delivery in this country.

Annotated Outline

I. Overview of international health: The goal of Health for All by the Year 2000 was first proclaimed at the World Health Assembly in 1977. The idea has been supported by many international health organizations and countries since then. It's more difficult for the lesser developed countries to achieve the goals of health for all of their population. Developed countries are those with a stable economy and advanced industrial and technological development. Lesser developed countries do not exhibit these characteristics. By proportion, the population of the lesser developed countries experience more difficulty with control and eradication of communicable diseases, diseases related to environment, national-related diseases, and illnesses associated with maternal, child, and women's health.

II. International health and the role of primary health care: The concept of primary health care arose from the conferences which proclaimed Health for All by the Year 2000. The central ideas involving primary health care reflect (1) multidisiplinary participation; (2) involvement of communities in both planning and implementation of all health intervention projects; the use of advanced technology and up-to-date medical practices; (3) accessibility and affordability; (4) availability of chemotherapeutics; (5) focus on health promotion and prevention; (6) nutrition education; (7) collaboration with traditional practitioners; and (8) development of maternal and child health programs.

III. Major international health organizations: These include:
   A. Private voluntary - Religious and secular groups.
   B. Philanthropic - W.K. Kellogg, Mibank, Memorial Fund, Pathfinder Fund, Hewlett Foundation, Ford Foundation, Rockefeller Foundation, Carnegie Foundation.
   C. Professional and technological - Institut Pasteur.
   D. Private and commercial - Pharmaceutical and trade organizations.
   E. Government organizations - Many of the more economically advantaged governments enter into agreements with other, lesser developed countries.
   F. Intergovernmental organizations - World Bank, World Health Organization, United Nations Children's Fund, Pan American Health Organization.

IV. International health and economic development: There is a relationship between the health of a country's population and its economic development. The poorer countries tend to have sicker populations and more complex and endemic health problems. The healthier a country's population, the more it can help contribute to its country's economic growth and development. A continuing problem among lesser developed countries is lack of funding for health programs. Instead, monies are often used to build up the military and for risky, and often unsafe, economic ventures.

V. Health care systems: Most health care systems in the world can be described by the following characteristics: (1) usership; (2) benefits; (3) acceptable providers; (4) facilities; and (5) who controls access and provision.

VI. Major world health problems and the burden of disease: Present indications of the status of the world's health indicate that there are still many critical health care needs throughout the world. The global burden of disease (GBD) combines losses from premature death and losses of healthy life that result from disability. Premature death is the difference between the actual age at death and life expectancy at that age in a low-mortality population. The Daly is a measure of the GBD or disability-adjusted life years.
   A. Communicable disease: The eradication of smallpox worldwide is an indication of the long-term benefits of immunization programs.
      1. Tuberculosis (TB): TB, especially the varieties that are associated with AIDS and those

that are drug resistant, is of growing worldwide concern. A third of the world's population currently harbors the tuberculosis pathogen, and this number is expected to grow in the next 20 years, especially in the lesser developed countries.

2. AIDS: AIDS is rapidly becoming a major cause of morbidity and mortality throughout the world. Present worldwide efforts at AIDS eradication are aimed at prevention programs.
3. Malaria: Malaria remains one of the most prevalent communicable diseases in the world. Malaria is most endemic in countries that lie in tropical areas.

B. Maternal and women's health: Deaths related to pregnancy and women's health problems remain problematic throughout the world but are of special concern in the lesser developed countries. Access to family planning, good nutrition, prenatal care, and safe birthing practices are very limited, if nonexistent, in many of the lesser developed countries. Disease conditions that contribute to poor pregnancy outcomes are highest in Sub-Sahara Africa, Bangladesh, Pakistan, and India. Several agencies, including WHO and UNFPA (World Health and Development), have initiated strategies and programs for safe motherhood initiatives and women's health programs.

C. Diarrhea disease: Diarrhea disease is one of the leading causes of death and illness in children under five years of age worldwide. Causes range from nutritional deficits to viruses, bacteria, environmental toxins, and parasites.

D. Nutrition and world health: A large portion of the world's burden of disease may be attributable to poor nutrition by itself or that which accompanies disease. Poor nutrition is associated with poverty. Protein, iron, vitamin A, and calcium deficiencies are among the leading nutrient deficiencies. Women and children are those most affected by poor nutrition.

Additional Critical Thinking Activities

1. Review recent research studies that have been conducted on some of the major world health problems. Include those articles that address health policy and that describe the relationship of development to health care.
2. You have been asked to address a group of recent immigrants from Southeast Asia to discuss health care in the United States. What kinds of health-related interventions would you expect that they might be most interested in? As a community health nurse, what kinds of questions might you ask them to determine what their health needs are? Go to the library and research the country that they come from. What are the major health problems in that country, and will those problems affect any interventions that you might have planned?

Critical Analysis Questions

1. True or False? The Pan American Health Organization is an example of a professional organization.
2. Provide a definition of the GBD.
3. List five health problems that are still considered critical throughout the world.
4. Differentiate between "developed" vs "lesser developed" countries.
5. Give examples of why an understanding of international health is important to nurses who work in community setting.
6. Name the organization whose primary aim is to foster the kind of economic development needed to enhance good health outcomes.
7. Describe ways in which the good health of a population contributes to the economic, industrial, and technological growth of a country.
8. Name the fundamental elements of all health care systems throughout the world.
9. True or False? The most widespread form of tuberculosis is "pulmonary tuberculosis."
10. True or False? Malaria is most endemic in the tropical areas of Asia, Africa, and Latin America.

Answer Key

1. False
2. The Global Burden of Disease combines losses from premature death and losses that result from disability.
3. AIDS, drug resistant tuberculosis, diarrhea disease, malaria, nutritional deficits, maternal and women's health, various communicable diseases such as measles, mumps, rubella, and polio.
4. Developed countries are those that exhibit advanced technology and industrial development with stable economics. Those countries that are lesser developed do not exhibit these characteristics.
5. Examples might include (1) interaction with clients who are new immigrants; (2) exposure of clients to potential health hazards in other areas of the world; (3) identification of potential risks with opening of United States border areas; (4) awareness of health concerns worldwide has an impact on health.
6. World Bank

7. (1) reduces production loss by workers due to illness; (2) increases use of natural resources that might have been unavailable because of presence of disease; e.g., malaria, yellow fever, schistosomiases; (3) children attend school and eventually contribute to the workforce; (4) money allocations needed for disease control can be used for economic development.
8. (1) usership; (2) benefits; (3) providers; (4) facilities; (5) power
9. True
10. True

5 Economics of Health Care Delivery and Nursing

Chapter Summary

The contemporary health care delivery system, characterized by limited resources, regulatory restrictions, and increased technological advances, is unlike the health care delivery system of the 1960s and 1970s. Because of the present system characteristics, the concerns of the twenty-first century will have to focus on the economics of health care delivery. Nursing will, of necessity, be concerned with justifying its contribution to the health of the nation and its economic viability in the market structure.

The purpose of this chapter is to provide an overview of the economic issues of the health care delivery system. Discussion focuses on factors influencing health care, schema for financing health care, economics of primary prevention, poverty and health care financing, and health care reform.

Annotated Outline

I. Definitions

A. Economics is defined as the social science concerned with the problems of using or administering scarce resources in the most efficient way to attain maximum fulfillment of society's unlimited wants.

B. Health economics is concerned with the problems of producing and distributing the health care resources of the nation in a way that will provide maximum benefit to the most people. The goal of health economics is maximum benefit, or quality care, from the goods produced and supplied by health providers. The goods are then demanded and purchased by consumers.

C. Gross national product is the total value of all goods and services produced in the economy in one year.

The consumer price index is a shopping basket approach that compares prices of all consumed goods and services on a monthly or quarterly basis.

D. Gross domestic product is a statistical measure used to compare health spending between countries.

II. Economic theories: Two basic theories applicable to understanding economics are microeconomic theory and macroeconomic theory.

III. Health services components: The developmental stages of the United States health care delivery system can be described using the health services component framework: labor, facilities, technology, and service intensity.

IV. Factors influencing the economics of health care: Inflation, technology, intensity, and changes in population demography have been instrumental in influencing the growth of the health care system throughout history.

A. Inflation: Health care costs have grown approximately twice as fast as the overall inflation rate from 1990 to 1993. New technology and third-party payers have contributed most to the inflationary nature of health care.

B. Technology and intensity: The development of new technology, the use of technology, consumer demands for use of sophisticated technology and increased services, regulation, reimbursement mechanisms, and lack of program incentives have contributed to rising health care costs.

C. Changes in population demography: Data indicate that the increases in health care expenditures have been influenced by population changes, such as increases in the elderly population.

V. Financing of health care

A. Third-party payers: Private third-party payers emerged in 1847. The purpose of the first insurance was to provide protection and to defray financial losses against disability attributable to accidents. The system began as a major industry in the 1930s with the Blue Cross system.

B. Consumer payments: Direct out-of-pocket payment by the consumer has declined. The future may bring an increase in this method of payment for service. The private third-party payers and the government's contributions are two factors that have affected declining consumer payments. Consumer demands for third-party payment have contributed to health care inflation and are causing a financial drain on the economic potential of the individual.

C. Government: Health care financing has evolved through the twentieth century from a system primarily financed by the consumer to a system primarily financed by the government. The federal government first became involved in health care financing of a population segment in 1798. Today the federal government pays a major portion of the nation's health care bill. The federal government underwrites five major health insurance programs, some of which include the offering of direct services. These programs are Medicare, Medicaid, CHAMPUS, the Military Medical Care System, and the Veterans Administration Health Care System.

VI. Poverty and health care financing: In 1992, 73% of the United States population had health insurance through employment arrangements, 10% had insurance through public programs, and 17% were uninsured. Children and the elderly comprised a large number of the uninsured and underinsured.

VII. Health care trends: Managed care, health care rationing, health care financing, and payments for nursing service are current trends affecting the economics of the health care system.

A. Managed care: This concept provides for organized services that are coordinated by a designated agency to provide the type of care needed by a client. With the federal government's interest in providing an integrated comprehensive health care system for the United States population, the development of integrated health alliances and health maintenance organizations has been encouraged. HMO systems are affecting health care costs.

B. Health care rationing: Rationing is not new to health care. Whenever a client is denied a program or service due to restrictive eligibility criteria, rationing has occurred. Several states have introduced models for rationing health care services.

C. Health care financing plans: A two-tiered health care system has been suggested as a way to provide health care for all.

D. Health care reform: In October 1993, President Clinton introduced the Health Security Act. While national health care reform is occurring only in programs such as Medicare and Medicaid, eight states have passed legislation introducing managed competition into health care systems.

E. Cost of nursing care delivery: Nurses and professional organizations continue to work toward direct reimbursement for nursing services. Studies are beginning to show the cost effectiveness of nursing services. In 1990, Medicare amendments included select direct reimbursement of nurse practitioners and clinical nurse specialists.

VIII. Primary prevention: An area in the health care delivery system that needs to show cost effectiveness is the area of primary prevention. Although estimates indicate that 97% of the health care dollars are spent on treatment and cure, the major causes of morbidity and mortality in our adult population have shown little net decline. Emphasis on primary prevention may reduce the burden of avoidable illness and disability, thereby reducing the human and economic costs imposed on the United States population in the future.

The value of human life: A major goal of the health care delivery system is to preserve and maximize human capital by offering health-preserving and social practices that result in disease avoidance, and diagnosis, treatment, and rehabilitative services for existing disease. The outcome of health care goals should be the provision of a quality of life that will promote happiness, productivity, efficiency, and the capacity to engage in and to enjoy life.

IX. Factors affecting health levels: Four major factors affect the health of an individual. They are the health care system, personal behavior, the environment, and biological influences.

Additional Critical Thinking Activities

1. Preview Chapter 6, Ethics in Community Health Nursing Practice. Debate this topic in class: The ethical implications of the goal of health economics. Focus your debate on the implications for community health nursing practice.
2. Read the first three pages of a regional or state newspaper for three days. Select an article that is concerned with the costs of health care. Write a paragraph on the significance of this article and how it relates to what you have learned in Chapter 5.
3. In discussions with a nurse administrator, ask about sources of reimbursement for client services at a community agency.
   A. Inquire about methods of agency reimbursement to providers.
   B. Explore reimbursement schemes used to establish agency budgets; that is, prospective versus retrospective reimbursement for payment of health goods and services delivered by the agency.
   C. Inquire about the contributions of national health insurance and direct care programs to the agency budget.
   D. Discuss the impact of block grants on agency services (past, present, and future).

4. Interview two of the following consumers of health care:
   A. An elderly person over 65 years of age.
   B. A young mother (under 25 years of age).
   C. A married man or woman, middle to late twenties.
   D. A single man or woman, middle to late thirties. Include the following points for discussion in your interview:
      (1) How the person pays for major health care (Medicare, Medicaid, insurance, direct, etc.).
      (2) If the person is insured, what out-of-pocket expenses he or she has to pay.
      (3) How much each individual or family spends on nonreimbursable health care each month, including over-the-counter and self-treatment products.
      (4) How adequate each person feels his or her health care is at meeting his or her needs.

   Compare and contrast the responses.
5. Soon you will be graduating from your nursing program and will become a wage earner. Consider the proposed two-tiered health plan.
   A. Explain how this system will function. What services are likely to be provided in each tier?
   B. Explore the implications of this type of system to specific population groups.
6. Debate the merits of a primary versus a secondary and tertiary prevention goal for the health care delivery program for nursing.
   A. How do the factors that affect health levels influence your decision about the health care goal for the nation?
   B. How does your philosophy about the value of human life influence your decision?

Critical Analysis Questions

1. True or False? Health economics is concerned with problems of producing and distributing the health care resources of the nation in a way that will provide maximum benefit to the most people.
2. True or False? Inflationary health costs are directly attributable to the increase in nursing salaries.
3. True or False? The major portion of health care bills are directly paid out-of-pocket by the consumer.
4. True or False? The federal government does not directly provide health care services.
5. True or False? The prospective cost reimbursement method encourages health care agencies to stay within budget limits.
6. True or False? The prospective payment approach to health care financing will require the consumer to pay a larger portion of the health bill.
7. True or False? A health care delivery system with primary prevention as the major focus could possibly reduce human and economic costs by decreasing avoidable illness and disability.

Answer Key

1. True
2. False
3. False
4. False
5. True
6. True
7. True

6 Ethics In Community Health Nursing Practice

Chapter Summary

Community health nurses experience many ethical conflicts in today's health care delivery system. The nursing profession has traditionally upheld the rights and human needs of the individual client. Yet in today's community health care system, this traditional focus is difficult to maintain when nursing services have the additional goal of maximizing the health of aggregate populations at risk. The traditional focus is also difficult to maintain in systems in which nursing resources are influenced by legislation and funding for specific population groups. One result of this latter difficulty is that other identified populations at risk are not adequately served by community health nursing efforts because of the lack of funds to meet their needs. Nurses who experience this conflict between the individualistic focus of the professional ethic and the aggregate focus of community health may recognize the dilemma of professional nursing in community health settings.

Annotated Outline

I. Clients' rights and professional responsibilities in community health care
   A. Clients' rights: Clients' rights to assert themselves and be recognized in the health care delivery system date back to 1793 during the French Revolution. Clients' rights to informed consent, to refuse treatment, and to privacy have been aided by consumerism and organizations of health providers.
      1. Right to health: The individual's right to health has evolved through the centuries as a result of the passage of public health laws. The right to health is becoming comparable to the rights to life, liberty, and the pursuit of happiness.
      2. Right to health care: The right to health and the right to health care, often used synonymously, are two separate concepts. The right to health is a negative right not to have one's health interfered with by others. The right to health care is a positive right to the health care system's resources to improve or maintain one's health.
      3. Other rights: The 1970s brought widespread attention to clients' rights. A commission of the DHEW, in its final report of medical malpractice, recommended the distribution of patients' rights statements by all health care facilities. In 1972, The American Hospital Association issued "The Patients' Bill of Rights" to highlight the basic human rights of clients involved with the health care delivery system. In 1991, the Omnibus Budget Reconciliation Act of 1990 became effective, requiring all health care institutions receiving Medicare or Medicaid funds to inform clients that they have the right to refuse medical treatments and the right to initiate written *advance directives.*
   B. Societal obligations: The President's Commission studied differences in the availability of health services in 1983 and concluded that society has an ethical obligation to ensure equitable access to health care for all citizens. The Commission recommended that costs for health care should be equitably shared at the national level and that the federal government assume responsibility for ensuring that equitable access to health care by all is achieved.
   C. Professional responsibilities
      1. Code duties: Professional codes of ethics have evolved to illustrate the relationship between clients' rights and health care professionals' duties and responsibilities. Two questions are usually asked about the importance of codes of ethics: (1) are they universal moral principles, and (2) are they legal requirements for professional practice? The professional code of ethics for nurses prescribes moral behavior and actions based on moral principles. Some of the rules in this code are also related to legal requirements.
      2. Veracity: The duty of veracity specifically mentioned in the ANA *Code for Nurses* is the duty to tell the truth and not lie or deceive people. Community health nurses may have difficulty observing this duty. Information may be withheld from the client, and the client may be deceived because the nurse may think the information will cause the

client anxiety, or the nurse may think the client does not really want to know the truth.

3. Confidentiality: Confidentiality helps protect the functioning of professional-client relationships and helps protect the client's right to privacy. Sometimes the nurse's duty to protect the client's privacy may be overridden when the duty is in conflict with other duties, such as the preservation of life, prevention of harm, protection of the health of others, or the enhancement of the health of the community.
4. Advocacy: The *Code for Nurses* specifies a duty of advocacy whereby the community nurse is only required to protect, speak for, and support the interests of the clients to not be harmed in the provision of health care services.
5. Caring: To provide care to clients is a moral obligation of the nurse. Caring has a relationship to human health and involves a nursing commitment to protect human dignity and the welfare of health clients. Caring is a significant element in health care because it occurs within the context of providing for health needs.
6. Accountability: The *Code for Nurses* defines accountability as being answerable for one's behavior toward another. Accountability seems to define the relationships between client, nurse, other professionals, and society. Accountability in nursing practice dates back to Florence Nightingale, who included "humanistic orientations" in her early training for nurses.

II. Ethical principles in community health

A. Relationship of ethical rules, principles, and theories: Rules imply that certain actions should or should not be performed because they are right or wrong. Principles serve as the foundation of rules, whereas theories are collections of principles and rules.

B. Principle of beneficence

1. Definition: Do good and avoid harm are the basic tenets of the principle of beneficence. Although this principle implies a duty to help or provide benefit to others, it does not include the obligation to jeopardize self-welfare or self-interests.
2. Applications in community health
   a. Balancing harms and benefits: The rule of utility derived from the principle of beneficence includes the moral duty to balance benefits against harms to maximize the outcomes of an action and reduce the risks of potential actions. This rule may be applied in community health when deciding which programs to fund, which screening programs to conduct, and which research projects adequately protect the person's rights.
   b. Cost benefit analysis: Cost benefit analysis is a specific application of the principle of beneficence whereby the harms and benefits of a health care method or program are converted into a monetary unit and weighed against the selection of other methods and programs that provide similar outcomes.
3. Problems and conflicts
   a. Paternalism: Paternalism is a principle that raises a moral question about the limiting of clients' liberties to make decisions about their health care.
   b. Extent of rule of utility: Balancing of benefit over harms in community health leads to two potential problems. First is the potential of overlooking or ignoring individual liberties and values for the common good. The second problem occurs when the rule of utility is applied to long-term health policy decisions.

C. Principle of autonomy

1. Definition: The moral principle of autonomy is an acknowledgment of and respect of the individual's rights to make choices and to act according to individual determinations.
2. Applications in community health
   a. Respect for persons: Community health nurses acknowledge respect for clients by allowing them to have opinions and choices about their health care while protecting them from harm to self and others.
   b. Protection of privacy: Observations of clients, touching, and access to personal health and economic data about clients may be invasion of clients' privacy. Community health nursing services are responsible for seeing that policies appropriately protect clients' privacy and that informed consent is obtained before information is released to any source.
   c. Provision of informed consent: The principle of autonomy requires that clients be given a voluntary choice to consent to health care services. There are three essential elements required for clients to make decisions about consent: adequate information about care; adequate time to comprehend information and to ask questions; and freedom from coercion or undue influence to volunteer the information.

d. Individual freedom of choice: Community health nurses should respect the right of clients and their legal guardians to make decisions about life and health, which may include refusal of treatment.
e. Protecting diminished autonomy: Respect for the principle of autonomy requires that community health nurses recognize clients who lack the capacity to act autonomously and who are entitled to protection within the health care system.

3. Problems and conflicts
   a. Coercive health measures: Coercive health measures are a source of conflict for community health nurses. The protection of the community's health may supersede the individual's right to choice in health matters.
   b. Invasions of privacy: Invasions of clients' privacy may be justified on the basis of harm to third parties. The community health nurse should inform the client whose privacy is invaded that the data will be communicated in a manner that will reduce the potential for future infringement of that client's privacy.

D. Principle of justice
   1. Definition: The principle of justice purports that equals should be treated equally and that unequals should be treated differently according to their differences.
   2. Applications in community health
      a. Entitlement theory: Entitlement theory is a theory of justice that states that everyone is entitled to whatever they naturally get at birth. The government has no responsibility for improving the life status of the less fortunate.
      b. Utilitarian theory: The basic premise of this theory is that expenditures and use of resources should be distributed among the citizenry according to how the greatest net total good can be achieved and so the largest number of people can be served.
      c. Maximin theory: The maximin theory of justice speaks to the least advantaged members of society. Free exercise of liberty is permitted on the part of all citizens, allowing for social and economic inequalities to evolve in a manner that will benefit the least advantaged members of society.
      d. Egalitarian theory: This theory of justice provides for an equal claim to all goods and resources by all citizens.
   3. Problems and conflicts
      a. Distributing basic goods and services: Assigning priorities of health interests for the distribution of goods and services creates conflicts of interest among health care providers, with subsequent influence on the actual delivery of needed services.
      b. Distributing nursing resources: Once priorities for health within a community are designated, community health nurses must decide who will receive their services and how the services can be distributed equally. The moral requirements of justice create numerous conflicts of interest when specific choices must be made.

III. Application of ethics to community health nursing practice
   A. The priority of ethical principles: Ethical principles direct and guide nursing actions with individuals and aggregate groups.
   B. Accountability in community health nursing: Moral accountability in nursing practice implies that nurses are answerable for the promotion, protection, and meeting of health needs of clients while respecting the clients' right to make decisions about their health care. Community health nurses are primarily answerable for the health of aggregates, thereby making their accountability requirements different from those in other spheres of nursing practice.
   C. Future directions: If the principle of beneficence is to be emphasized as a moral requirement in community health nursing, then the nursing process applied to the community must be clearly differentiated from the nursing process applied to other spheres of nursing practice. Also, there is a need to determine how accountability will be measured in community health nursing and how effectively the nursing services are meeting accountability requirements.

IV. Clinical applications for the student: Students are encouraged to read and analyze several case situations commonly encountered in community health nursing practice. The case situations apply the moral concepts of societal obligations and professional responsibilities to clients; also, the duties of veracity, the protection of confidentiality, and advocacy are applied. Additional case situations apply the principles of autonomy, beneficence, and justice.

V. Summary: Community health nursing practice, a synthesis of public health service and nursing, is influenced by both traditional ethics of professional nursing and the aggregate focus of community health.

How community health nursing views the moral requirements of practice will determine the future direction and influence of the discipline in meeting the health needs of communities.

Additional Critical Thinking Activities

1. Review at least six issues of the *American Journal of Nursing* from the current year. Also, review six issues of the same journal from a year prior to 1950. Prepare a class report, comparing and analyzing the differences in the following topics covered in the articles:
   A. Types of ethical dilemmas discussed.
   B. Recommendations for resolution of ethical dilemmas.
   C. Differences between the old and the current journal topics as they relate to types of ethical principles and conflicts.
2. Review a copy of the informed consent form from a local hospital for the three essential components (listed in your textbook) that are required for clients to make decisions about consent. Prepare a report of your analysis. Next, obtain an informed consent form from a local community health agency or primary care center. Compare this form with the one used in the hospital.
3. Conduct research at a local public health agency to determine how certain demographic groups such as the elderly or adolescents are targeted and funded for health care. Analyze how priorities are set and what, if any, decisions could result in ethical conflict. Explain your answer, using a specific theory of distributive justice.
4. Select one of the following situations, which involve potential ethical conflict. Discuss and analyze the situation according to the ethical principles that you have learned in this chapter. How would the utilization of a different priority of ethical principles affect possible outcomes?
   A. A high school student with acquired immunodeficiency syndrome (AIDS) wishes to attend class.
   B. A student has confided in a school worker that her father is sexually abusing her. She does not want her mother, who is a teacher at the school, to know and does not want the nurse or the counselor/principal to discuss this with anyone.
5. Interview three or four practicing community health nurses. Ask each to describe the most difficult ethical conflict they have experienced in community health nursing practice (be sure to obtain all the important facts relating to the conflict, persons involved, etc.). Analyze each conflict and note the following:
   A. Moral judgments made by the nurse and other persons involved in the conflict.
   B. Nonmoral judgments made by the nurse and other persons involved in the conflict.
   C. The issue that makes this conflict a situation of moral (or nonmoral) conflict.
   D. The ethical principles that seem to be in conflict.
   E. Ethical principles, rules, or theories used by the nurse (and others) in resolving the issue.
   F. Alternative approaches to the conflict using a different priority of ethical principles and potential outcomes.

   Evaluate your analyses. Do they contain information that might provide insight and direction for future or similar areas of conflict? Explain.

Critical Analysis Questions

1. In community health nursing, the nurse is *primarily* accountable for which of the following factors?
   1. how the moral requirements of the principle of beneficence are met by nursing services
   2. the provision of health care services to maximize total net health in aggregate groups
   3. how the moral requirements of the principle of autonomy are met by nursing services
   4. demonstration of the increased health of aggregate groups through various research methods and studies while containing costs

   a. 2, 3, 4
   b. 1, 2, 3
   c. 1, 2
   d. 1, 2, 4
   e. all of the above
2. According to the American Nurses' Association in the *Code of Nurses,* "Accountability refers to being answerable to someone for something one has done." Accountability also includes which of the following factors?
   1. providing an explanation to self, the client, the employing agency, and the nursing profession
   2. being held legally responsible for judgments exercised and actions taken in the course of nursing practice
   3. providing an explanation to self, the client, the physician, and the nursing profession
   4. evaluating the effectiveness of one's performance of nursing responsibilities

   a. 2, 3, 4
   b. 2, 4
   c. 1, 2, 4
   d. 1, 2, 3
   e. all of the above
3. It can be argued that community health nurses have a duty to tell the truth and forbear from

lying or deceiving for all of the following reasons. Which of the following reasons indicates a duty in response to the client's right to know or his right to self-determination?

1. The implicit contract relationship between client and nurse engenders a duty to tell the truth.
2. To *not* tell the truth or to deceive clients may, in the long run, undermine relationships and bring about undesirable consequences for future relationships with clients.
3. Telling the truth is part of the respect nurses owe clients as persons.
4. Nurses have a duty to protect and to strengthen other health care relationships in general.

a. 3 only
b. 2, 3
c. 1, 2, 4
d. 2, 4
e. all of the above

4. In health care relationships, the duty to observe the rule of confidentiality is not an absolute duty. This means which of the following statements is true?
   1. The community health nurse may use professional judgment in deciding how to communicate confidential information about clients.
   2. Observing confidentiality is a *prima facie* (meaning that it may be overridden when in conflict with other duties that are morally stronger).
   3. Even if a client tells the nurse in confidence that he wishes to kill another member in the community, the nurse has a duty to protect others from harm by warning the intended victim of the client.
   4. The nurse may occasionally be required to give testimony in a court of law in relation to confidential information about a client.

   a. 1, 4
   b. 2, 3
   c. 2 only
   d. all of the above
5. True or False? Ethical principles are abstract guides that serve as the foundations for such moral rules as "always tell the truth" and "treat equals equally."
6. True or False? In utilitarian theory, the ethical principle of beneficence often carries more weight than the ethical principles of autonomy and justice.
7. True or False? Decision-making in community health settings on the basis of a principle of beneficence raises moral questions concerning the extent of the rule of utility in decisions.
8. True or False? The formal principle of justice claims that equals ought to do good and prevent or avoid doing harm.

Answer Key ▼

1. d
2. c
3. a
4. d
5. True
6. True
7. True
8. False

7 Cultural Diversity and Community Health Nursing Practice

Chapter Summary

Caring for culturally diverse groups has been a focus of community health nursing since its inception. As early as 1893, public health nursing was started by nurses in New York City, who provided home care to immigrants, particularly to recent arrivals. These nurses were not from the same cultural background as the immigrants, and had to deal with the cultural differences between themselves and the persons in their care.

There is great diversity among cultural groups in expectations and experiences. In turn, their perceptions of health and illness also differ. Hence, the workplace offers enormous challenges for community health nurses, who want to understand their clients' perceptions of health and illness as they provide interventions that promote wellness.

In many instances, especially in home care, community health nurses must assist well persons from various cultures over a period of weeks or months to adjust to alterations in their health status, to adapt individual and family behaviors so as to improve health status, and, overall, to develop health-promoting patterns. In addition, there are an insufficient number of ethnic minority nurses to help other nurses understand the experiences of diverse cultural groups.

Annotated Outline

I. Culture, ethnicity, and race: Culture, ethnicity, and race play a strong role in understanding cultural behavior.

   A. Culture: Consists of a set of ideals, values, and assumptions about life that are widely shared among a group of people. It provides the organizational structure for what members of the cultural group determine as acceptable. The organization of each culture distinguishes one culture from another. Organizational elements include language and the arts, child-rearing practices, religious practices, family structure and values, and attitudes. It is important that nurses know these organizational elements in order to provide culturally appropriate care.

   B. Ethnicity: Involves the shared feeling of peoplehood among a group of individuals. It is based on individuals sharing similar cultural patterns (such as values, beliefs, customs, behavior, and traditions) that over time create a common history. There are intraethnic variations, and not all individuals of a particular ethnic group express the same level of ethnicity.

   C. Race: Refers primarily to a social classification that relies on physical markers, such as skin color, to identify group membership. Individuals may be of the same race, but differ in ethnic affiliations.

II. Cultural competent behaviors: Cultural competence is an ongoing life process that results from an interplay of factors that motivate persons to develop knowledge, skill, and ability to care for individuals, families, and communities. Culturally competent nursing care includes four principles. First, care is designed for the specific client. Second, care is based on the uniqueness of the person's culture and includes cultural norms and values. Third, care includes empowerment strategies to facilitate client decision making in health behavior. And fourth, care is provided with sensitivity to the cultural uniqueness of clients.

   A. Cultural competence: In today's climate of increased diversity, nurses are caring for a greater number of culturally diverse clients than ever before. Cultural competence is needed to provide nursing care that meets the needs of these persons. Being culturally competent helps nurses to (1) meet the cultural needs of clients who are often from a different culture than the nurse, (2) decrease the cost of health care and increase opportunities for positive outcomes, and (3) facilitate achievement of specific objectives for persons of different cultures as delineated in Healthy People 2000.

   B. Developing cultural competence: Nurses develop cultural competence in different ways, but mainly through having experiences with individuals of other cultures and being receptive to these experiences. Also critical to the development process is having cultural awareness, cultural knowledge, cultural skill, and engaging in cultural encounters.

C. Dimensions of cultural competence: Nurses integrate their professional care knowledge with the clients' care knowledge and practices to negotiate and promote care that reflects the clients' values. Their decisions and actions are guided by cultural preservation, cultural accommodation, cultural repatterning, and culture brokering. Decisions of cultural preservation support clients in maintaining those aspects of their culture that promote healthy behaviors. Decisions of cultural accommodation include those aspects of the culture that are crucial to providing satisfying care. Decisions of cultural repatterning involve working with clients to develop health-promoting behaviors.

III. Inhibitors to developing cultural competence

A. Stereotyping: Relates to ascribing certain beliefs and behaviors to groups without recognizing individual differences within the groups. Stereotyping blocks the willingness of people to be open and thus to learn about specific individuals or groups.

B. Prejudice and racism: Prejudice is the emotional manifestation of deeply held beliefs about other groups. It usually denotes negative attitudes. Some individuals believe that persons of a particular race, skin color, cultural practice, or social standing are inferior and cannot benefit fully from society's offerings of education, good jobs, and community activities. To justify these beliefs, individuals may then deny persons who are different from themselves the opportunity to benefit from societal offerings. Racism, a form of prejudice, refers to the belief that persons who are born into a particular group are inferior in intelligence, morals, beauty, self-worth, and so forth. Prejudice and racism may be (1) overtly intentional, (2) overtly unintentional, (3) covertly intentional, or (4) covertly unintentional.

C. Ethnocentrism or cultural prejudice: This is the belief that a person's cultural group determines the standards of behavior by which all other groups are to be judged. Persons with ethnocentric beliefs devalue behaviors that differ from their own and judge other behaviors to be inferior.

D. Cultural Imposition: Refers to the process of imposing an individual's values on others. It is the belief in one's own superiority.

E. Cultural Conflict: This may occur when there is a misunderstanding of expectations between clients and nurses, when either group is not aware of or denies cultural differences.

F. Cultural shock: This may be a normal reaction to beliefs and practices of clients' cultures that are disallowed or disapproved of in the nurse's own culture. Being aware of their own cultural beliefs and having knowledge of other cultures may help nurses to be less judgmental and more accepting of differences in other cultures.

IV. Cultural nursing assessment

A. Nurses use a cultural nursing assessment to help them identify and understand clients' perspectives of health and illness. By adopting a relativistic approach, nurses avoid judging or evaluating clients' beliefs and values in terms of the nurses' own culture. A variety of tools are available to assist nurses in conducting cultural assessments. The focus of such tools varies, and selection should be determined by the dimensions of culture to be assessed. During initial contacts with clients, nurses should perform either a brief cultural assessment or begin an in-depth one. To help them in conducting cultural assessments, nurses should be aware of a variety of principles; these should include the following:

1. Be cognizant of the environment.
2. Know about community social organizations such as schools, churches, hospitals, tribalcouncils, restaurants, taverns, and bars.
3. Know the specific areas to be focused on before beginning the cultural assessment.
4. Select a strategy for gathering cultural data. Strategies may include in-depth interviews, informal conversations, observations of everyday activities or specific events of the client, survey research, and a case-method approach to study certain aspects of a client.
5. Identify a confidante who will help "bridge the gap" between cultures.
6. Know the appropriate questions to ask without offending the client.
7. Interview other nurses or health care professionals who have worked with the specific client to get their input.
8. Talk with formal and informal community leaders to gain a comprehensive understanding about significant aspects of community life.
9. Verify and cross-check the information that is collected before acting on it.
10. Avoid pitfalls in making premature generalizations.
11. Be sincere, open, and honest with oneself and the client.

B. Using a translator: When nurses do not speak or understand the client's language, they should make every effort to obtain assistance from a translator. Consider the following when a translator is needed:

1. Use a translator who has knowledge of health-related terminology.

2. Observe the client for non-verbal messages, such as facial expressions.
3. Accuracy in transmission of information may be increased by asking the translator to translate the client's own words and asking the client to repeat the information that was communicated.
4. Use family members as translators cautiously.
5. Some individuals prefer that questions about sexuality or childbirth be posed by a translator of the same gender.
6. Differences in socioeconomic status and educational level between the client and the translator may lead to problems in interpretation of information. Confidentiality may also be threatened if the client and the translator are from the same community.
7. Birth origin and language or dialect spoken should be identified before selecting a translator.
8. Avoid using professional jargon, colloquialisms, abstractions, idiomatic expressions, slang, similes, and metaphors.
9. Clarify roles with the translator, and review the situation and information to be translated prior to and at the end of each health care encounter.

V. Variations among cultural groups: While all cultures are not the same, all cultures have the same basic organizational factors. The organization of these factors within cultures differentiates one group from another.

A. Communication: Verbal and nonverbal communication vary across cultures, and if nurses do not understand the client's cultural rules in communication, the client's acceptance of a treatment regimen may be jeopardized. For example, in the Asian culture, confrontation or disagreement with those in authority are often unacceptable behaviors. Community health nurses should not interpret a smile as acceptance of their intervention strategies.

B. Space: Personal space is the area that persons need between themselves and others in order to feel comfortable. Cultural groups, such as Hispanics, who may touch persons with whom they are speaking, may be more comfortable with less space than Asians, who view touching strangers as inappropriate. Community health nurses should understand spatial requirements and should take cues from clients in order to place themselves in the appropriate spatial zone.

C. Social organization: Families are significant to the organization of cultural groups and have a significant influence on its members. When working with clients, nurses should be cognizant of family involvement in decision making and should advocate that the individual's needs also be considered.

D. Time perception: It is important for community health nurses to recognize that time is perceived differently across cultures. Individuals may be future-, present-, or past-oriented. Nurses should clarify the meaning of time before instituting health-promotion and disease-prevention strategies, to increase their benefits and minimize misunderstanding.

E. Environmental control: Individuals' relationships with the environment are directly related to their perceived control in health promotion and disease prevention. Individuals may believe that they can overcome any illness that they may develop (mastery-over-nature), that they may have very little control over what happens to them in health and illness (subjugation-to-nature), or that illness represents a disharmony with nature and that they must look to nature for solutions to return them to a healthy state (harmony-with-nature).

F. Biological variations: Each culture has its own unique variations in areas of growth and development, skin color, enzymatic differences, and susceptibility to disease. Mongolian spots and lactose intolerance are often found among minority groups, while sickle cell anemia is often associated with African-Americans, thalassemia with Asians, and cleft uvula with Native Americans. Variations in growth and development may be influenced by environmental conditions such as nutrition, climate, and disease.

VI. Dietary practices and cultural orientation: Dietary practices are an integral part of the assessment for families, especially since they play a prominent role in all health problems. Efforts to understand dietary patterns of clients need to go beyond relying on membership in a defined group. Knowing clients' assimilative practices makes it possible to develop treatment regimens that will not conflict with their cultural food practices. Awareness of the religious origin of some dietary practices is necessary to avoid creating additional tensions in the nurse-client relationship as nurses negotiate with clients to meet their health needs.

VII. Socioeconomic factors and culture: Members of minority groups are disproportionately represented on the lower tiers in the socioeconomic ladder. Poor economic achievement is also a common characteristic among populations at risk, such as those in poverty, the homeless, migrant workers, and refugees. Nurses should be able to distinguish between culture and socioeconomic class issues, and not interpret behavior as having a cultural origin when in fact it is attributed to socioeconomic class.

Additional Critical Thinking Activities

1. Invite a folk practitioner to speak to the class about beliefs and practices of his/her cultural group. Have the person discuss ways in which health professionals and folk practitioners can work together to meet year 2000 objectives.
2. Using the outline provided — Variations Among Selected Cultural Groups— have students discuss variations that they observe among other cultural groups in the community.
3. Have each student in the class invite a student who is of a different cultural background to lunch. Have them discuss differences in cultural practices as they relate to health-illness perception.
4. Have members of the class bring a food dish that represents their culture and share it with each other in a Culture Kitchen. Then, have the students discuss:
   A. The origin of the particular dish in their culture.
   B. The significance of the food for the family.
   C. The holidays on which the foods are most frequently used.
   D. The nutritional value of the food.

Critical Analysis Questions

1. Understanding the effects of culture on behavior is important to the community health nurse because culture:
   a. is a blueprint for behavior of minority groups.
   b. is genetically transmitted to all individuals.
   c. is a learned process that is transmitted by the family, ethnic group, and society.
   d. determines the client's capacity to respond to a health problem.
2. The basic perspectives on health include all of the following *except*:
   a. health reflects a balance between the self and nature.
   b. health is a result of "good luck."
   c. health results from harmony between the yin and yang forces.
   d. health is the sum total of all the organs functioning in the body.
3. The folk healer in African-American culture is called a:
   a. yerbero.
   b. voodoo priest.
   c. shaman.
   d. curandero.

An Anglo-American senior nursing student scheduled a 2 pm appointment with a female Hispanic client to make a home visit for a post-partum followup. The client agreed to the appointment date and time. The student stressed to the client the importance of keeping the appointment. Two hours before the scheduled appointment, the student called. The client did not answer the phone. The student consulted her instructor.

4. The instructor agreed that the student should:
   a. call the client every thirty minutes until she reaches her.
   b. reschedule the visit for the next day.
   c. assume that the client is not interested in the visit and report the matter to the administrator.
   d. ask the client to call when she is ready for her to make the visit.
5. One possible explanation for the instructor's and student's response is that they were aware that in the client's culture, time is viewed:
   a. from a past orientation.
   b. from a present orientation.
   c. from a future orientation.
   d. as relative, depending on the situation.
6. The student's behavior is an example of:
   a. cultural acceptance.
   b. cultural frustration.
   c. cultural relativism.
   d. cultural blindness.
7. In post-conference, designed to elicit comments about values and their relationship to health practices, the instructor asked the student to share the experience with her colleagues. Which of the following statements does not reflect a reason for the instructor requesting this exchange?
   a. Knowledge of values allows nurses to care more competently for clients.
   b. Unexamined values get in the way of the nurse-client relationship.
   c. Nurses act on implicit values even when they have not been overtly expressed.
   d. When the nurse and client have different values, it is impossible for them to work together.
8. When serving a culturally diverse population, which of the following essential resources should community health agencies have available?
   a. a translator
   b. a culture care specialist
   c. expert, caring nurses
   d. all of the above
9. Nurse Evans overhears Dr. Peters telling Ms. Lopez that her seven-year-old daughter needs to have her tonsils removed. Ms. Lopez is hesitant and wants to get another opinion. Dr. Peters wants to have the surgery done immediately. As the nurse responsible for the care management, you would:
   a. obtain more information from the client on the nature of her concerns.
   b. ignore the conversation as it was between the client and the doctor.
   c. schedule the client for the surgery.

d. refer the mother to the on-site folk healer.

10. Culturally competent nursing care is characterized by:
    a. care that is consistent with the client's beliefs.
    b. an understanding by the client that their care reflects current Western health care practices.
    c. the substitution of folk medicine for scientific medicine.
    d. a match between the ethnicity of the client and the nurse.
11. One of the reasons why cultural competence is being stressed in baccalaureate programs is that:
    a. technological changes have made nursing impersonal.
    b. self-determination of clients is minimized where cultural differences are considered.
    c. the United States is becoming more heterogeneous.
    d. cultural care is universal care and all people need to be treated the same.
12. Nurses develop cultural competence in many ways, but mainly by:
    a. working with clients who are culturally similar to themselves.
    b. being afraid to make mistakes when confronted with situations that are different.
    c. refusing to allow awareness of cultural differences to have any effect when conducting a cultural assessment.
    d. learning from clients as they express their experiences and problem-solving strategies.

Select the statement below that best defines the concept in 13-17.

a. understanding an individual's culture within the context of your own culture
b. the tendency to judge all individuals as the same
c. insisting that Asian clients make direct eye contact with nurses during a health-teaching program
d. an intense emotional response when working with clients from cultures other than one's own
e. negative responses of clients to unacceptable nursing practices

13. _____ cultural conflict

14. _____ cultural imposition

15. _____ cultural shock

16. _____ ethnocentrism

17. _____ stereotyping

Answer Key

1. c
2. d
3. b
4. a
5. b
6. c
7. a
8. d
9. a
10. a
11. c
12. d
13. e
14. c
15. d
16. a
17. b

8 Environmental Health

Chapter Summary

Maintenance of a safe and healthy environment has been a community health problem since early civilization. In recent years, the degradation of the environment has increased through pollution of waters, air, and the soil in which food is grown, as well as through the cumulative stressors that occur in fast-paced industrialized societies. In the broadest sense, environmental health includes all aspects of the relationship between a host and its health, as well as the effect of hazardous biologic and chemical agents on health. Community health nurses are often called upon to address environmental health problems. The report, *Health People 2000*, specifies priority objectives for the nation in environmental health, including (1) eliminating blood levels of lead above 25 ug/dL in children under age five; (2) increasing protection from air pollution so that at least 85 percent of people live in counties that meet Environmental Protection Agency (EPA) standards; and (3) increasing protection from radon so that at least 40 percent of people live in homes that have been tested by homeowners and have been found to be safe.

Annotated Outline

I. The role of community health nurses: Florence Nightingale, the founder of modern nursing, was particularly interested in environmental health. In her work with the military hospitals during the Crimean War, she recognized that environmental contamination led to health hazards for the ailing soldiers. She immediately began collecting epidemiological data about the effects of sanitation on morbidity and mortality.

   Community health nurses are in ideal roles to evaluate the extent of hazardous substances in the homes and environments of the clients they serve. Many pollutants are more concentrated indoors, which makes the home, school, and worksite important areas to evaluate in terms of pollution from tobacco smoke, wood stoves, gas ranges, building materials (especially asbestos), radon, and a wide range of commonly used household products.

   Hazards in the external environment include pesticides and lawn care products, lead products (often found in paints and in wastes), contaminated water and soil, and hazardous wastes, as well as those hazards that occur in recreational areas such as polluted lakes and streams. Natural disasters and emergency spills also have a devastating effect on environmental health. Biologic agents such as bacteria and viruses can also contaminate food, soil, and water and can infect blood-sucking insects, which then transmit disease to humans.

   Outdoor air pollution results from a mixture of gases and particulates. These (as well as radiation) can cause a range of health hazards.

   Risk assessments are important to enable community health nurses to estimate the probability of health risks in a given population due to environmental factors. Steps in the risk assessment process include (1) exposure assessment, (2) hazard identification, (3) dose-response assessment, and (4) risk characterization. Community health nurses are involved in conducting risk assessments, interpreting the findings, reporting the hazards, and implementing other interventions to protect the health of the people.

II. Environmental health information resources: Community health nurses play a key role in identifying and accessing environmental health information and in conveying that information to members of the community. A wide variety of resources are listed in the chapter, as well as suggestions for using consultants to assist in recognizing and dealing with environmental health hazards.

   A. Key sources for environmental health information are the local health departments and environmental agencies. These resources can help identify exposure pathways, information about dealing with environmental exposure, and trends in environmental health problems in the community.

   B. At the state level, three important environmental health agencies are the state health department, the environmental health agency, and the poison control center. Each of these agencies plays a special role in providing information about hazardous wastes, chemical spills, toxic substances, and other environmental health irritants.

   C. A variety of federal agencies provide resources to support the community health nursing role in environmental health. Specifically, the EPA and the Agency for Toxic Substances and Disease Registry are key sources of information through their many electronic databases and printed materials.

III. Environmental health assessment and analysis at the community and client level: The community health nurse uses many data-gathering tools described in the chapters on epidemiology and communicable disease, as well as in this chapter, to assess the health of the environment. Two approaches are especially useful.
   A. Community-wide health assessments are designed to provide a framework whereby health-related data can be collected from the community. For example, information can be gathered through "windshield surveys," from government agencies, or from interviews with community members. In the assessment, it is crucial to determine the exposure pathway; e.g., the routes the pollution might take from its original site to the community residents.
   B. Client and family assessments are a next step once the community-wide health assessment has been completed. An environmental-exposure history for a client or family includes an exposure survey, an environmental history, and a health history.
   C. For most chemical and physical agents in the environment, the adverse health effects are unsuspected, undetected, or poorly understood. An adverse health effect is a response that either impairs an organ's functioning at the subclinical level, or one that results in illness, injury, or death. The nursing diagnosis for adverse health effects is important.

IV. Nursing diagnosis: Community-based nursing diagnoses identify aggregates and population responses to environmental health risks. It is important for the nurse to look carefully at physiological as well as psychological responses to exposures. Identifying the exposure pathway is crucial.
   A. Planning ways to intervene in environmental health risks should include both removing the contaminant and educating the population at risk.
   B. Intervention strategies require a team approach to develop comprehensive action plans for addressing the environmental health threat or problem. Intervention includes preventive actions, communication, referral, education, treatment, and enforcement of public health guidelines.

V. Health-risk communication
   A. The first step in health- risk communication is defining the need. Exposure situations can be delineated into *less risky* and *more risky* categories.
   B. The goal of health risk communication is to involve concerned citizens in the community assessment and the subsequent care plan.

VI. Future trends in environmental health: New techniques are continually being developed for examining questions related to causation. For example, meta analysis involves the re-examination of results from previous studies and is becoming an increasingly useful tool because it combines several studies to give greater statistical power than would be available in each separate study.

Additional Critical Thinking Activities

1. Ask each student to read a current news magazine or newspaper to identify at least three possible or actual environmental health and safety hazards.
   a. Who is at risk?
   b. What might the exposure pathway be?
   c. What local, state, or federal agency would have information about this potential environmental health threat?
   d. What could/should community health nurses do?
2. At the beginning of your course, begin a file of news articles from either printed materials, television, or radio that describe environmental health hazards. Discuss with your class the impact on the health of the citizens if these hazards actually occur.
3. Assign a panel of students to debate a timely topic related to environmental health such as the following: It is the responsibility of the locality to make certain the environment is safe for the residents (versus the responsibility of the companies in the community or of the residents themselves).
4. Give the whole class this assignment and have them compare results at the end of the week: For a week, keep a diary of ways in which you personally contribute to the contamination of your environment. Identify three ways in which you can change your own behavior to become more protective of the environment.
5. Let each student choose an environmental health issue or concern in your community and, using the many resources described in this chapter, thoroughly review the hazard; the effect on people; the interventions that could/should take place; and the role that community health nurses should play in reducing or eliminating this hazard.

Critical Analysis Questions

1. Name four major environmental health hazards.
2. True or False? People experience higher concentrations of air pollution outside versus inside.
3. List five common sources of indoor air pollution.
4. Identify three ways in which pesticide exposure can occur.
5. True or False? Lead poisoning is no longer a major environmental health problem in the United States.
6. List at least five possible health hazards that a community health nurse might observe while driving through a middle-sized United States city.
7. Briefly discuss the extent of the problem of hazardous wastes.
8. List three common gases that comprise air pollution.
9. Explain the difference between ionizing and non-ionizing radiation.
10. Define exposure pathway.

Answer Key

1. Air pollution, water pollution, hazardous wastes, and toxic substances
2. False
3. Tobacco smoke, wood stoves, gas ranges, building materials, asbestos, radon, household products
4. Dermal contact, inhalation, or ingestion.
5. False
6. Inadequate collection of waste, standing and polluted water, poor air quality, inferior or unsafe housing, poor road conditions, suspected presence of lead-based paint, noise, crowding
7. About 275 million tons of hazardous waste are generated annually in the United States; this is 1,900 pounds/person. More than 64,000 areas are contaminated; of these, about 1300-1400 either are on—or are proposed for—the National Priorities List of worst waste sites in the United States. An estimated 41 million United States residents live within 4 miles of hazardous waste.
8. Carbon monoxide, nitrogen oxides, sulfur oxides, and hydrocarbons
9. Ionizing radiation contains enough energy to release electrons; non-ionizing radiation has insufficient energy to release electrons; e.g., as the protective atmospheric ozone layer is depleted, non-ionizing radiation in the atmosphere increases.
10. An exposure pathway is the process by which an individual is exposed to contaminants that originate from some source of contamination.

9 Policy, Politics and the Law: Influence on the Practice of Community Health Nursing

Chapter Summary

Community health nurses are an integral part of the health care system and are significantly affected by government and the legal system. Many nurses who select community health nursing as an area of practice are intrigued by the interdependence of law, health, nursing practice, and government.

An understanding can be gained from two major bodies of literature: law and political science. Within these fields, one can gain insight into how government, law, philosophy, and political viewpoints have emerged as important factors in our health care system and how these factors have greatly shaped the care that is delivered.

Annotated Outline

I. Governmental role in health care: The central issue addressed in this section is that an understanding of how law and government relate to health care can be gained from two major bodies of literature: law and political science.
   A. Legal basis for government's role in health care: Most legal bases for Congressional action in health care are found in Article I, Section 8, of the United States Constitution.
   B. Trends and shifts in government roles: In reference to trends, many historical events have played a significant part in developing the role of government in health care. Many of the federal functions are being shifted to the states and are becoming their responsibility.
   C. Major government health care functions: The federal government has four major health care functions.
      1. Direct services
      2. Financing
      3. Information
      4. Policy setting

II. Organization of government agencies: This section discusses the structure in which governments function. In addition, it looks at international organizations and their activities in the health care field and at different roles of community health nurses in different governmental agencies.
   A. International organizations: Describes the goal, the location, and the composition of the World Health Organization and its activities in the health care field.
   B. Federal agencies: Discusses the major components of the Department of Health and Human Services and other federal agencies, and the functions of each component in relation to health care.
   C. State and local government departments: At the state level, three executive branch departments are described—health, education, and corrections. The organization of a local health department and the roles on community health are discussed.
   D. Social welfare programs: Summarized are insurance, welfare, and other programs that are health related and administered through DHHS and the state and local governments.
   E. Impact of government health functions and structures on community health nursing: Government funding, in particular, has shaped the functions of community health nurses within all levels of government. The categorization of money by governments to special needs has led to special, more narrowly focused community health nursing roles.

III. Community health nurses' role in politics and the political arena: Gives an overview of the political system and ways in which community health nurses can be involved.

IV. Private section influence on regulation and health policy: Describes the process of regulation writing, ways to influence it, and other means of participating in shaping health policy.
   A. Process of regulation. The regulatory process includes the following:
      1. Study
      2. Initial drafts
      3. Final drafts
      4. Proposed regulations published
      5. Public comment/public hearing
      6. Further study or final regulation published
      7. Changes in practice

V. Laws affecting community health nursing practice: This part of the chapter examines selected legal aspects of community health nursing, including those aspects that are unique to the practice. How laws and regulations have shaped community health nursing are addressed, including examples of different types of laws.

A. Types of law: Laws have had a major impact on community health nursing practice. Some of these laws are the following:
   1. Constitutional law: From this type of law, community health nurses can get answers to questions in selected practice situations; for example, on what basis the state can require quarantine or isolation of individuals (with tuberculosis) in the community.
   2. Legislation and regulation: Much legislation affects community health nursing directly. For instance, in dealing with a person with a communicable disease, the state exercises its power through legislation. Regulations are specific statements of law that relate to individual pieces of legislation.
   3. Judicial and common law: Judicial law is that law based on court or jury decisions. Representatives from both sides of an issue present evidence, written or oral, before a court and/or jury who decides the outcome. One principle of common law is observed when the court uses other types of laws to make its decision, including previous court decisions or cases.
B. General community health nursing practice and law: Two legal aspects apply to most community health nursing practice situations. The first aspect is the tort of professional negligence or malpractice; the second aspect is the scope of practice defined by custom and state practice acts.
   1. Professional negligence: An act or failure to act when a duty was owed to another, that was not reasonable and led to injuries compensable by laws.
   2. Scope of practice: The scope-of-practice issue involves differentiating the practice of physicians, nurses, and other health care providers. Scope of practice is assessed by examining the usual and customary practice of a profession and by taking into account how the legislation defines the practice of a particular profession in a jurisdiction.
C. Special community health nursing practice and law: Four special areas of community health nursing practice and their respective legal aspects are highlighted. Those four areas are school and family health, occupational health, home care and hospice, and correctional health.
D. Legal resources: There are many resources available in public libraries, as well as law libraries, that can help community health nurses find laws that are pertinent to their practice. Possible sources are as follows:
   1. State code
   2. State annotated code
   3. Indexes to codes
   4. Supplements to codes and indexes
   5. Federal Register and State Register
   6. Codes of regulations (federal and state)
   7. Administrative agency rules and decisions
   8. Case law
   9. Opinions of the Attorney General
   10. Legal dictionaries
   11. Legislative histories
   12. Legal periodicals

VI. Clinical applications: This section reviews chapter material and how law affects daily community health nursing practice.

Additional Critical Thinking Activities

1. Talk with a community health nurse who works in a nearby health department. See if the two of you can identify categories of government function other than those identified in this chapter.
2. Interview a member of your state nurses' association. Ask them to discuss with you the enforcement of the ANA Code for Nurses. Be sure you have reviewed a copy of it beforehand.
3. In your career plan, you may have identified a community health nursing role in which you would like to work. Identify that role and prepare a packet of possible current legislation, regulations, and judicial opinions related to it.
4. Locate and tour the nearest law library. In addition to a school library, you might find one at the county courthouse or at an attorney's office. Ask for a listing of the main sources. If it is a courthouse, tour the entire facility, identifying all of its services. See if you can locate cases in which nursing malpractice or negligence was the issue by going to the index of the Reporter System for your jurisdiction.
5. Contact your state nurses' association and find out what proposals, if any, they plan to introduce to the state legislature this year. Develop a fact sheet on the law and indicate what changes need to be made in the act. Participate in the state nurses' association legislative committee and get involved with contacting your legislator about the proposals. Identify the legislator's staff person who follows health and social issues.

Critical Analysis Questions

1. True or False? What government accomplishes in the area of health often depends on the particular executive administration and political party in majority.

2. True or False? The federal government has had little effect on health care delivery in the last 20 years.
3. True or False? The major effect of government on health care has been the provision of money for grants, training, and research.
4. True or False? The legal basis on which the federal government has functions in health care is found in the Fourteenth Amendment to the United States Constitution.
5. True or False? The major function of government in health care is direct delivery of care to many American citizens.
6. True or False? Aid to Families with Dependent Children is just one program classified as a social welfare program.
7. The most notable recent development from HCFA is ________________________________.
8. Many community health nursing roles are found in state and local departments of health, education, corrections, social services, housing, and others. Briefly identify what these roles are.
9. Who writes federal regulations? (Select one)
   a. Courts
   b. Congress
   c. Executive branch
10. Which is written first?
    a. Laws
    b. Regulations
    c. Both a and b—written at the same time.
11. As part of shaping health policy, several methods of lobbying were listed. Identify four of these, and briefly state which can be most effective.
12. If you were a community health nurse employed in an industry, which of the following federal laws would affect you the most?
    a. National Child Abuse Act
    b. Freedom of Information/Privacy Act
    c. OSHA
13. List the key components of professional negligence involving a community health nurse.
14. A nurse practice act can be found in which of the following sources?
    a. Federal procedure
    b. State Code of Laws
    c. Judicial opinions
    d. State regulations
15. True or False? Often one of the best methods of keeping current with the law and community health nursing practice is to read a community newspaper on a regular basis.

Answer Key

1. True
2. False
3. True
4. False
5. False
6. True
7. The prospective payment mechanism known as diagnostic-related groups (DRGs).
8. Community health nurses may be consultants, teachers, practitioners, administrators, clinical nurse specialists, and researchers. Many address the needs of special groups of clients; others address the general needs of whole populations, communities, and families.
9. c
10. a
11. Methods include face-to-face encounter, personal letters, mailgrams, telegrams, telephone calls, testimony, petitions, reports, position papers, fact sheets, letters to the editor, news releases, talk shows, speeches, demonstrations, and litigation. Depending on the issue, each of these can be equally effective.
12. c
13. Duty, breach of duty, proximate cause—causation, damages
14. b
15. True

10 Organizing Frameworks Applied to Community Health Nursing Practice

Chapter Summary

Community health nursing is the specialty area that blends nursing and public health theory into a population-focused practice designed to promote and preserve the health of communities. The practice of community health nursing is guided by theories, models, and concepts. Two models have particular relevance for guiding community health nursing: the Neuman Systems Model and the Omaha System. The Neuman Systems Model has been used effectively and extensively in both community health nursing education and practice. The Omaha System, however, is the only model for practice developed by practicing community health nurses. This chapter introduces the use of conceptual models and theories in community health nursing and provides extensive discussion of how both the Neuman Systems Model and the Omaha System have actually been used.

Annotated Outline

I. Definitions
   A. A model is a way of defining or describing something, assisting with analysis of systems, specifying relationships and processes, and representing situations in symbolic terms that may be manipulated. Models can be physical, symbolic, or mental. A conceptual model is a set of images and thought patterns that are conveyed via language.
   B. A theory is a set of interrelated constructs (concepts) and propositions that presents a systematic view of phenomena.

II. Using conceptual models
   A. Conceptual models with the greatest utility to community health nursing are those that view people as being in continuous interaction with the environment.
   B. All people have developed conceptual models about some aspects of their lives. Everyone has a unique set of concepts guiding how ideas and information are categorized, and how situations are perceived.
   C. In nursing, conceptual models refer to person, environment, health, and nursing.
   D. Some nurses use primarily one conceptual model; others merge more than one model into a synthetic model for guiding practice.
   E. Conceptual models give direction, simplify, and help to organize information in practice. Models assist nursing practitioners to think about clinical situations by using concepts to sort out events and situations.

III. The ANA model of community health nursing practice is a conceptual model that emphasizes health promotion and consumer participation; it considers health as being influenced by many factors, both within people and within the environments in which they live.

IV. The APHA definition of public health nursing emphasizes that nursing is a synthesis of knowledge from both the public health sciences and professional nursing, designed to guide the improvement of the health of the entire community.

V. Systems models have special applicability to community health nursing because of their emphasis on the interaction of parts, the idea that the whole is greater than the sum of the parts, and the concepts of openness, boundary, feedback, entropy, and negentropy. Communities are excellent examples of the concepts of systems theory. According to systems theory, communities are open systems that exchange materials such as energy, goods and services, values, and ideals, with the environment inside and outside the community.

VI. The Neuman Systems Model was designed to help graduate students understand their clients in a holistic perspective. Neuman defines from a systems viewpoint the main concepts of person, environment, health, and nursing.
   A. The Neuman Systems Model sees people as being open systems in dynamic interaction with their environment. The client system is comprised of five interacting variables: physiological, psychological, sociocultural, developmental, and spiritual.
   B. The Neuman Systems Model can be used with individuals, families, groups, and communities.
   C. The major goal of nursing in the Neuman model is to keep the client system stable through accurate assessment of actual and po-

tential stressors, followed by implementation of appropriate stressors. Three intervention modalities are recommended by this model: *primary prevention*, to strengthen the lines of defense by reducing risk factors and preventing stress; *secondary prevention*, to begin following the occurrence of symptoms in order to strengthen the lines of resistance by establishing relevant goals and interventions to reduce the reaction; and *tertiary prevention*, which can be initiated at any point following treatment when some degree of system stability has occurred.

D. The three prevention-as-intervention modes can be used separately or simultaneously to direct nursing actions.

E. To date, the Neuman Systems Model has been adopted by nurses in fourteen countries to guide curriculum development and nursing practice with individuals, families, and communities.

F. The example provided in this chapter of the Neuman Systems Model in education includes a basic core plus the following subsystems: communication and transportation; health and safety; economics; education; law and politics; and religion.

G. The Neuman System has been effectively used in community health nursing practice in Canada to organize the delivery of long-term care services.

VII. The Omaha System has direct applicability to community health nursing practice.

A. Nursing diagnosis is a clinical judgment about individual, family, or community responses to actual and potential health problems/life processes.

B. Nursing intervention describes activity that follows a thought process or written exercise, usually referred to as planning.

C. Evaluation is a process designed to determine value or amount, or to compare accomplishments with some standards.

D. Nursing process is a framework for making decisions like the problem-solving process, scientific method, program-management process, community-assessment process, or quality-assurance process.

E. In the early 1970s, the Visiting Nurse Association of Omaha, Nebraska, began addressing practice, documentation, and data-management concerns by converting their narrative method of documentation to a problem-oriented approach. After several successful projects, they designed schema to rate the outcomes of care. This system allows nurses who practice in diverse community settings to gather comprehensive data in order to manage client data and needs.

F. The Omaha Problem Classification Scheme is a client-focused taxonomy of nursing diagnoses, comprised of simple and concrete terminology, and the language is organized at four discrete levels of abstraction.

G. The levels of the Omaha Problem Classification Scheme are as follows: domains, problems, modifiers, and signs and symptoms. The four domains are environmental, psychosocial, physiological, and health-related behaviors. Forty client problems form the second level of the scheme. The modifiers are family/individual, actual, or potential health promotion. The fourth level involves a cluster of signs and symptoms specific to each problem.

H. The Intervention Scheme is a systematic arrangement of nursing actions or activities designed to help nurses and other health-care professionals document both plans and interventions. The scheme is designed for use in making nursing diagnoses.

I. The Problem Rating Scale for Outcomes is a five point Likerty type scale that provides a systematic, recurring method of measuring client progress throughout the time of service.

Additional Critical Thinking Activities

1. Divide the class into two groups and ask one group to debate that the ANA conceptual model of community health nursing is more applicable than the model developed by the APHA; ask the other group to respond as proponents of the APHA model.
2. Have the students read at least three articles on community health nursing and see if they can identify the conceptual model guiding the nurse-author's practice.
3. Assign several students to interview one staff nurse in public health nursing, one supervisor, and one director of public health nursing (if the community lends itself to this) to determine the basis that guides their practice. Then ask each student to take either a pro or con position to this statement: The practice of community health nursing is truly based on one or more conceptual models.
4. Assign several students to read a research article from a current nursing journal and determine which conceptual framework the author is using to guide his or her study.
5. Present each student with the following problem: You are a community health nurse who receives a referral and makes an initial home visit to a cli-

ent. To apply the Omaha Problem Classification Scheme, what steps would you follow?

A. Consider all subjective and objective data generated by the referral and home visit.
B. Compare those data in relation to the four domains, forty problems, two sets of modifiers, and clusters of signs/symptoms of the Problem Classification Scheme.
C. Differentiate client data between that which suggests specific problems and that which rules out problems.
D. For problems, identify the appropriate modifiers and the signs/symptoms for actual problems.
E. Reconsider steps A through D before finalizing decisions and recording those decisions in the client's record.

6. For this exercise, allow students to work with a partner or in small groups. Each student should select a client that they have visited, or create a fictitious client. Ask each student to share typical referral and first-visit data, including both pertinent and irrelevant client information. Have team members apply the Omaha Problem Classification Scheme to the client data, and complete a problem list that is of reasonable length. Finally, ask them to compare problems, modifiers, and signs/symptoms selections, and discuss their findings. Remind them that two students may disagree and both be correct. Inherent within a correct answer are logical explanations that are supported by actual data, not by assumptions read into the data or events expected to occur in the future.

Critical Analysis Questions

1. An internally consistent group of relational statements that presents a systematic view about the subject being studied and is useful in describing, explaining, or predicting is a definition of:
   a. science.
   b. systems.
   c. theory.
   d. law.
   e. model.
2. An analogy or example that is used to help visualize and understand something through expression of structure is a definition of:
   a. science.
   b. systems.
   c. theory.
   d. law.
   e. model.
3. Properties of systems include all of the following except:
   a. wholeness
   b. openness
   c. orderliness
   d. randomness
4. According to Neuman's model, nursing intervention is implemented through:
   a. promoting adaptation.
   b. primary, secondary, and tertiary prevention.
   c. facilitating effective behavior.
   d. repatterning of behavior.
5. True or False? Nursing diagnosis and client problem can be described as synonymous.
6. Describe the relationship of nursing diagnosis to other concepts such as nursing process, quality assurance, medical diagnosis, and general problem-solving.
7. Who is usually credited with originating interest in the nursing process and establishing the scientific basis of nursing?
8. Which of the following community health developments provided the greatest linkage to nursing diagnosis?
   a. commitment to preventive and therapeutic services
   b. population-based philosophy
   c. public health principles
   d. practice based on nursing model
9. A significant milestone occurred in 1980 when a definition of nursing included diagnosis. The definition was developed by a member of the ____________. (fill in blank)
   a. National League for Nursing
   b. American Nurses' Association
   c. Visiting Nurse Association of Omaha
   d. North American Nursing Diagnosis Association
10. Development of the Omaha Problem Classification Scheme involved:
    a. empirical data from diverse clients.
    b. nurses from various agencies and locations.
    c. establishment of reliability and validity.
    d. research.
    e. all of the above.
11. List the four levels of the Omaha Problem classification Scheme.
12. The Omaha Problem Classification Scheme consists of __________ nursing diagnoses/client problems.
13. True or False? Nursing diagnosis offers important benefits involving nursing practice, documentation, and data management.
14. True or False? Nursing diagnosis is useful to novice nurses, but not to experienced nurses.

Answer Key

1. c
2. e
3. d
4. b
5. True
6. Nursing diagnosis is closely linked to those concepts and is an important component or subset of all the other more general concepts.
7. Florence Nightingale
8. d
9. b
10. e
11. Domains, problems, modifiers, and signs/symptoms
12. Forty
13. True
14. False

11 Epidemiological Applications in Community Health Nursing

Chapter Summary

Epidemiology, the "mother science" of public health, is a multidisciplinary enterprise, encompassing clinical medicine and laboratory sciences, quantitative methods, such as biostatistics, and public health policy and goals. While clinical medicine focuses on the diagnosis and treatment of disease in *individuals*, epidemiology studies *populations* in order to understand causes of disease and to develop and evaluate effective interventions to prevent disease and maintain health. Community health nursing bridges these disciplines in its focus on individual clients and services, and in its appropriation of epidemiologic methods and findings in community health nursing practice.

Annotated Outline

I. Definition and history: Epidemiology is the study of the distribution and determinants of health-related events in human populations, and the application of this knowledge to improving the health of communities. Descriptive epidemiology studies the distribution of disease and other health-related states and events in terms of personal characteristics, geographic distribution (place), and temporal patterns (time). Analytic epidemiology is directed toward understanding the origins and causal factors of these events. The origins and development of epidemiology are discussed, with particular reference to the broadening scope of epidemiologic research and development of methods.

II. Basic concepts in epidemiology: To facilitate the study of complex health events, epidemiologists rely on two sets of concepts, among many others:

   A. The epidemiologic triangle—agent-host-environment: This concept indicates the relations among causal agents, susceptible persons, and environmental factors. The web of causality, a related concept, more adequately illustrates the complex interrelationships of numerous factors interacting to increase (or decrease) the risk of disease.

   B. Stages of health and prevention: The disease process is understood to be a continuum from prepathogenesis (susceptibility) through asymptomatic stages, to clinical manifestations and eventual resolution. Levels of prevention are related to these stages of health and disease. Primary prevention involves interventions to reduce the incidence of disease by promoting health and preventing disease processes from developing. Secondary prevention includes programs designed to detect disease in the early stages, before signs and symptoms are clinically evident, to allow early diagnosis and treatment. Tertiary prevention provides interventions directed toward persons with clinically apparent disease, with the aim of curing, ameliorating the course of disease, reducing disability, or rehabilitating.

III. Basic methods in epidemiology

   A. Sources of data: Three categories of common sources of data for epidemiologic studies are discussed:

      1. Routinely collected data such as census data, vital records, and surveillance data.
      2. Data collected for other purposes such as medical and insurance records.
      3. Original data collected for specific epidemiologic studies.

   B. Measures of morbidity and mortality

      1. Rates in epidemiology: The use of rates as the basic measure in epidemiologic studies is explained. A rate is a measure of the frequency of a health event in a defined population during a specified period of time. Most rates have three common factors: a numerator consisting of the number of persons who experienced the event of interest (e.g., deaths, cases of disease), a denominator representing the population at risk of the event, and the time period during which the events were enumerated.
      2. The concept of risk: Risk is the probability that an event will occur within a specified time period. It is distinguished from a population at risk, those persons for whom there is some finite probability of the event.
      3. Mortality rates: The most common mortality rates are defined and illustrated, and the limitations of mortality rates as indicators of morbidity are discussed. Both overall and

group-specific mortality rates are described. Cause-specific rates are presented and distinguished from the proportionate mortality ratio and case fatality rate. The infant mortality rate and related neonatal and postneonatal rates are also described.

4. Rate adjustment: The concept of age adjustment is introduced and explained in general terms as a statistical adjustment using a standard population in order to make fair comparisons in rates. Both direct and indirect adjustment are discussed.
5. Measures of morbidity: Incidence and prevalence rates are the most commonly used measures of levels of disease in a population.
   a. Prevalence rate. The prevalence rate measures existing disease in a population at a particular time; e.g., the number of existing cases divided by the current population.
   b. Incidence rate. The incidence rate reflects the number of *new* cases developing in a population at risk during a specified time. It estimates the risk of developing the disease in the observed population within a specified time.
   c. Incidence and prevalence compared. The relation of prevalence to both incidence and duration is explained. The critical distinction in interpretation and application is emphasized.
   d. Attack rate. The attack rate is a form of incidence rate commonly employed in investigations of infectious agents.
6. An example of an investigation of congestive heart failure in a community setting is presented to illustrate the use and interpretation of these measures of morbidity and mortality.

C. Comparison groups: The use of comparison groups and the ability to compare rates in comparable groups who differ on factors of interest is emphasized as central to epidemiologic research.

IV. Descriptive epidemiology

A. Descriptive versus analytic epidemiology: Descriptive epidemiology describes the distribution of health outcomes according to person, place, and time—- the who, where, and when of disease patterns. Analytic epidemiology searches for the determinants of the patterns observed— the how and why. Experimental studies include interventions to test preventive or treatment measures, techniques, materials, policies, or drugs.

B. Descriptive epidemiology

1. Person: Some examples of variation in morbidity and mortality by personal characteristics are presented. Personal characteristics of interest in epidemiology include gender, age, race, education, occupation, income (and related socio-economic status), and marital status.
2. Place: Factors influencing geographic variations in the distribution of disease are discussed. These include differences in the chemical, physical, or biological environment.
3. Time: Several temporal patterns of disease variation are discussed, including secular (long- term) trends, point epidemic, cyclical (including seasonal) patterns, and event-related clusters.

V. Analytic epidemiology: Analytic epidemiology seeks to discover the factors that influence observed patterns of health and disease, and to increase or decrease the risk of adverse outcomes.

A. Ecological studies: The ecological study is presented as a bridge between descriptive epidemiology and analytic epidemiology. In ecological studies, only aggregate data such as population rates are used. Advantages and disadvantages are discussed, with particular focus on the "ecological fallacy" and the uncertainty concerning temporal sequence.

B. Cross-sectional studies: In cross-sectional designs, subjects are simultaneously classified on exposure and outcome status. The prevalence ratio is presented as a measure of association. Selective survival bias is explained.

C. Case-control studies: Subject selection based on outcome status is described. Given the way subjects are selected for a case-control study, neither incidence nor prevalence can be calculated directly. The odds ratio as a measure of association is defined and illustrated. Advantages (cost and time savings) and disadvantages (susceptibility to bias) of the case-control method are presented.

D. Cohort studies: In cohort studies, subjects are classified on factors of interest and are followed over a period of time to observe some health outcome. Cohort study designs allow for calculation of incidence rates and, therefore, estimates of risk of disease. Cohort studies may be prospective or retrospective.

1. Prospective cohort studies: Subject selection and follow-up are described. The relative risk as the preferred measure of association is defined and illustrated. Measures of impact (excess risk and population-attributable risk) are also defined and interpreted, with examples. The advantages of the cohort design for studies of disease etiology

are discussed, along with disadvantages, particularly sample size, cost, and long periods of follow-up.

2. Retrospective cohort studies: The use of existing historical records for this design is explained. Advantages and disadvantages are discussed.

VI. Experimental studies: In contrast to observational studies, in experimental or intervention studies the investigator initiates some treatment or intervention which may influence the risk or course of disease. Two types of experimental studies, clinical trials and community trials, are described.

A. Clinical trials: In clinical trials, the research issue is generally the efficacy of a medical treatment for disease. Common characteristics of clinical trials are described, including randomization and "blinding" of treatment assignments.

B. Community trials: In community trials, the issue is often health promotion and disease prevention, rather than treatment of existing disease. The intervention is undertaken on a large scale—with the unit of treatment allocation being a community, region, or group, rather than individuals—and often involves educational, programmatic, or policy interventions.

VII. Screening: Screening is defined, and characteristics of successful screening programs are presented. Concepts of reliability and validity as measures of a screening test's performance are introduced.

A. Reliability: Reliability is presented as the precision or reproducibility of a measure. Major sources of errors affecting the reliability of tests are described.

B. Validity: Validity in a screening test is measured in terms of the probability of correctly classifying an individual with regard to the disease or outcome of interest, usually measured by sensitivity and specificity. An example illustrates the calculation of sensitivity, specificity, and positive predictive value.

VIII. Causality

A. Statistical associations: The concept of statistical association is introduced and related to the discussion of null values for measures of association described earlier.

B. Bias: The concept of bias is defined as a systematic error in the estimate of an association. The three major categories of bias are described:

1. Selection bias is bias resulting from the way subjects enter a study.

2. Information bias is bias due to misclassification of subjects in the study.

3. Confounding bias is bias resulting from the relation of the outcome and study factor with some third factor not accounted for.

C. Criteria for causality: Because statistical associations may be due to random error or bias, other criteria for causality are used to determine when associations are likely to be causal. No single epidemiologic study can satisfy all criteria. Epidemiologists rely on the accumulation of evidence, as well as on the strength of individual studies, to provide a basis for effective public health interventions and policies. Seven criteria on which there is general agreement are presented.

IX. Applications of epidemiology in community health nursing: Community health nurses work in diverse settings and agencies, with a range of responsibilities. The practice of community health nursing is enhanced by the understanding and application of epidemiologic concepts and methods. Epidemiologic measures are used to assess the health needs of a population. Planning and implementation of health care services, interventions, and policies depend upon understanding factors which influence health and disease, and upon the ability to evaluate interventions, programs, and policy.

X. Clinical application: A hypothetical situation is presented to illustrate the use of the epidemiologic approach in a situation wherein nurses both provide direct services and are involved in planning at the community level.

XI. Summary: This chapter presents epidemiology as a multidisciplinary enterprise whose concepts and methods are a critical foundation for the practice of community health nursing. Epidemiology provides basic tools for the study of health and disease in communities served, in order to shape policies and programs. The knowledge gained from epidemiologic studies enables community health practitioners to target programs and allocate resources more effectively and to develop effective intervention strategies. Using the skills gained from the study of epidemiology allows the community health practitioner to be more effective in evaluating research literature for its applicability in a given situation and in critically assessing the significance of health-related statistics, as well as in understanding and evaluating specific clinical situations.

Additional Critical Thinking Activities

1. Ask students to look at a recent issue of the Monthly Vital Statistics Report with Final Mortality Statistics from the National Center for Health Statistics or the most recent issue of *Health: United States*. Ask them to find a table which shows the number of deaths and the rate for leading causes of death by age group. Finally, they should solve the following, using that table:
   A. Calculate the proportionate mortality ratio for malignant neoplasms in the 5- to 14-year-old age group (number of deaths due to that cause divided by the total number of deaths in that age group). Do the same for the 45- to 64-year-olds. Compare the two numbers.
   B. Now compare the rates given for deaths from malignant neoplasms in the two age groups. How does this comparison differ from the comparison in Question **a** above?

   After studying the difference in cause-specific rates and proportionate mortality ratios, the student should see that the PMR is not an indication of the risk of death, and comparisons of PMRs across populations do not indicate the relative risk of death for a given cause in one group compared to another.
2. Hormone replacement therapy (HRT) for women undergoing menopause, either natural or surgical, is the subject of a number of studies and debate. On one hand, it relieves many of the unpleasant symptoms of menopause and reduces the risk of CHD and osteoporosis in post-menopausal women, both major sources of morbidity and mortality. On the other hand, it may increase the risk of endometrial cancer or breast cancer in some women. Have students study the recent literature on the risks and benefits of HRT and debate or write their responses to the following: How does the epidemiologic evidence contribute to a woman's decision to use or not to use HRT? What is the role of the nurse in interpreting the evidence and assisting in the decision-making process?

   These considerations should take into account not only the epidemiologic weight of the evidence, but also the necessity of weighing the risks and benefits differently for women in different risk groups. That is, the population at risk is peri-menopausal women, but the levels of risk for different outcomes will vary considerably within that population, and these differing risk profiles should be considered. Further, the values and preferences of the woman should play a central role in her decision to use or forego HRT. Clarification of the nurse's professional role, which includes expert knowledge and epidemiologic skills, is important in facilitating informed decision making while protecting the autonomy of the subject.
3. Observational studies, especially prospective cohort studies, sometimes raise ethical issues concerning the right of subjects to know potential risks of exposures under study. For example, the adverse effects of cigarette smoking on pregnancy outcomes are well established, though there are still questions to be answered. Using this example, ask students to break into groups to discuss the following: The research brief by Lieberman et al. (1994) studied the role of timing of fetal exposure to maternal smoking on fetal growth retardation. How would you design a study to determine the joint effects of timing of maternal smoking during pregnancy and maternal age on birth weight? What steps would you take in the study design to protect subjects and to ensure both the validity of the study and the provision of interventions that will contribute to a healthy pregnancy outcome?

   Here questions of research and professional ethics are considered along with issues of scientific validity. Clearly the study design will have to incorporate means of monitoring or collecting information on smoking status at various stages of pregnancy, while also offering information on the effects of smoking and smoking cessation programs.
4. Divide students into teams of two or three for the following assignment: Study news reports for your community, looking for issues or events that have an impact on the health of the community.

   Who is at risk? Are some persons or groups affected more than others?

   What are the most likely adverse outcomes?

   What solutions are being offered? Are they likely to be effective from a community health nursing perspective?

   What primary, secondary, and tertiary prevention programs would you propose?

   How do your nursing education and your understanding of epidemiology equip you to address this problem?
5. If time permits, encourage student groups to participate in the following: Form a journal club. Meet once a month to discuss an article of importance to community health nursing. Set up a rotating schedule to have one person pick the article and lead the discussion each month. Use both your understanding of nursing principles and of epidemiology to critically evaluate the article and decide what its implications are for your own practice.

Critical Analysis Questions

1. Mausner and Kramer (1985) report that at the initial examination for the Framingham Study (a long-term cohort study of heart disease), the prevalence of coronary heart disease (CHD) was about the same in men as in women aged 30 to 44 (about 5 per 1000 in each group). Do these equal rates mean that men and women in this age group have equal risk of developing CHD?
2. The Center for Epidemiologic Studies Depression Scale (CES-D) is a screening questionnaire designed to detect depressive symptoms. Suppose it were used in a school situation to screen for depression in adolescents. Of the 1680 students who answered the questions, 126 were determined on the basis of psychiatric interviews to suffer from major depression. Of these 126 true cases, 107 had been positive on the CES-D. Of the 1554 students who were not diagnosed with major depression, 373 had been positive on the CES-D. Given these results, calculate the following:
   a. the actual prevalence of major depression in this population
   b. the sensitivity, specificity and positive predictive value of the CES-D as a screen for major depression in this population
3. In a study to determine the validity of a screening test, the following statement was made: "The test has a sensitivity of 95% and a specificity of 90%." Indicate whether each of the following is true or false:
   a. 10% of the people with the disease were missed by the test.
   b. 90% of the people who do not have the disease were negative on the screening test.
   c. 5% of the people with the disease were negative on the screening test.
   d. 95% of the people who did not have the disease were positive on the screening test.
4. An obstetrician noticed an increase in early fetal losses (EFL) in his practice the year following the availability to the public of at-home pregnancy tests. What is the most likely explanation for this observation? What might explain this observation *in the absence* of a true increase in EFL?
5. Mark each of the following as primary, secondary, or tertiary prevention.
   a. screening for glaucoma
   b. environmental control measures
   c. rehabilitation in stroke victims
   d. a health fair exhibit distributing information about radon exposure in the home
   e. a health fair offering blood pressure checks
   f. immunization of children against measles
   g. educating young women about birth control and prenatal care
   h. a midnight basketball program for at-risk youth
   i. use of neonatal intensive care units

Answer Key

1. No. The rates are prevalence rates—existing disease was diagnosed at the initial exam. As such, they do not provide an estimate of risk of disease and are, instead, affected both by incidence and duration—e.g., by the course of disease and determinants of survival. Men tend to experience acute events with higher fatality, while women in this age group tend to develop chronic heart conditions. The longer duration for CHD in women compared to men contributes to the nearly equal prevalence, in spite of the higher incidence (and therefore higher risk) in men.
2. a. The prevalence of major depression is 7.5%.
   b. The sensitivity of the test is107/126 = 0.85 or 85%.
      The specificity of the test is 1181/1554 = 0.76 or 76%.
      The positive predictive value is 107/480 = 0.22 or 22%.
      While major depression is not a rare event in an adolescent population, the specificity of this test is so low that the number of false positives is large,and the resulting positive predictive value of the test is very low. Only about one in five of the students with a positive test actually has a diagnosis of depression. This means great care has to be taken in the interpretation of these test results with the children and their parents.
3. a. False. The percentage of persons with the disease missed by the test is 1-Se, or 5%.
   b. True.
   c. True. See **a** above.
   d. False. The false positive rate is 1-Sp or 10%.
4. The easy availability of home pregnancy tests may have increased the ascertainment of early pregnancy losses. That is, in the past, many women might have experienced a loss before they knew they were pregnant and, therefore, would not have reported it. Now, because their use of the test kit has increased their awareness of pregnancies, they are also more aware of a loss and might report the loss to their doctor.
5. a. Secondary
   b. Primary
   c. Tertiary
   d. Primary
   e. Secondary
   f. Primary
   g. Primary

h. Primary (preventing problems from developing and developing healthy behaviors) or secondary (intervening where problems may be latent)
i. Tertiary

12 Research Applications in Community Health Nursing

Chapter Summary

Research in community health nursing has developed over the years. Because practicing community health nurses work at the grassroots level with community members in improving their health care, they are in key positions to identify practice problems in need of research. The role of the community health nurse includes identifying topics for research and, sometimes, conducting the research. Community health nurses work both independently and collaboratively with other researchers for the development of research-based knowledge for practice.

Annotated Outline

I. Relationship of community health nursing to primary health care: Links between community health nursing and primary health care are described as community-based practice, involvement of the community in health care decisions, focus on disease prevention and health promotion, and use of a multisectoral approach in planning and implementing appropriate solutions to health problems.

II. The research process
   A. Assessment: Includes initiating the idea for a researchable topic, initial review of the related literature, identifying the purpose of the research, and delineating the population for study.
   B. Planning: Includes stating the specific research problem, continuing review of the literature, delineating the conceptual framework, selecting the research approach and design, selecting the appropriate data-gathering method, developing the data-analysis plan, gaining human subjects' approval, and conducting pilot studies and revisions in design.
   C. Implementation: Includes inviting the participants to take part in the research, implementing the data-gathering plan, and implementing the data-analysis plan.
   D. Evaluation: Includes analyzing findings, interpreting the results, and drawing conclusions.
   E. Action: Includes communicating research findings via publications and presentations, applying results in practice, taking action for social and policy change, and planning additional research.

III. Practice-generated questions for research: Significant research questions are generated from community health nursing practice and focus on concepts of primary health care.
   A. Accessible health care: Research questions relate to accessibility, distribution, and utilization of services by those in need.
   B. Community involvement: Research questions relate to the level and mechanism of community involvement in health decision-making.
   C. Disease prevention and health promotion: Research is needed on questions relative to preventable diseases, healthful lifestyle changes, and conditions that increase morbidity and mortality in the community.
   D. Appropriate technology: This concept raises research questions about technology that is relevant to people's defined health care needs. Issues raised relate to cost, affordability, and effectiveness.
   E. Multisectoral approach: Relevant research questions relate to what mechanisms exist that promote and/or hinder intersectoral collaboration and ways to remove barriers.
   F. Examples: Examples of research studies related to the key concepts of primary health care and health promotion are presented.

IV. Roles and issues in nursing
   A. Relationships: The relationships of the practicing community health nurse, the administrator of an agency, and the researcher are discussed. Research for community health nursing is described as a joint endeavor or partnership. The importance of a partnership of the researcher with the community is also discussed. Problems in conducting research in the community relate to sharing activities, establishing priorities in research and health care activities, gaining access to records and files, maintaining confidentiality, and reporting results.
   B. Communication: Good two-way communication must occur between the researcher and the people in the field involved in the research. Issues addressed include receptivity to research

methods and findings, dissemination of information, bridging the gap between practitioner and researcher, and presentation of research findings.

C. Ethics: Ethical issues must be carefully addressed when designing and conducting research. Ethical issues may arise throughout the research process.

D. Position of researcher in employment settings: The issue of who employs the researcher, with resultant potential uncertainties about the authority structure, is often a major source of role strain. The researcher should have a clear understanding with employers and administrators about the organization and expectations for their work.

E. Funding of research: Alternative funding mechanisms are suggested for research projects in competitive economic times.

V. Participation in research: Suggestions are made as to how the practicing baccalaureate community health nurse can become involved in the research process.

VI. Clinical application: Selected examples of research studies and implications for community health nursing practice are presented.

Additional Critical Thinking Activities

1. Identify a problem or issue concerning health in your neighborhood, your dormitory, or your apartment complex. Specify and illustrate the steps you would go through, including problem identification and research question formulation, if you were going to conduct a research study concerning this problem or issue. Prepare a brief outline of these steps.
2. Read a research article from a recent nursing journal in community health, and answer the following questions:
   A. What research methodology was utilized?
   B. Identify any potential ethical problems with the study.
   C. Identify the funding source, if specified.
   D. Identify practice implications of the findings for community health nursing.
3. Find an article in the research literature that was authored and/or co-authored by a practicing community health nurse. Determine the nurse's function or role in the research process.

Critical Analysis Questions

1. What are the priority areas for research with consideration of the WHO and UNICEF (1978) definition of primary health care?
2. What are the major concepts of importance to consider in the Ottawa Charter for Health Promotion (1986) when planning and conducting research?
3. What are the stages of the research process?
4. What are some of the roles and issues in research?
5. Describe at least ten ways a practicing community health nurse can become involved in research.

Answer Key

1. Equitable distribution, community involvement, focus on prevention, appropriate technology, multisectoral approach, and conceptual or theoretical base for practice
2. Building healthy public policy, creating supportive environments, strengthening community action, developing personal skills, and reorienting health services
3. The research process is a problem-solving process and includes assessment, planning, implementation, evaluation, and action.
4. Partner relationships between professionals and the community, community health nurse, and researcher; communication related to ethical concerns; funding sources; and job clarification with employer
5. Identifying clinical problems in need of research, taking anecdotal notes to help identify key variables, reading research, discussing observations with nursing colleagues, collaborating with researchers in joint research endeavors, accessing populations for study, assisting in securing institutional approval for research, collecting data, serving as a research participant, assisting in interpreting and explaining study findings, using relevant study results in practice, identifying relevant groups for reporting findings of research

13 Educational Theories, Models, and Principles Applied to Community Health Nursing

Chapter Summary

Health education is a vital part of community health nursing. The promotion, maintenance, and restoration of health requires that community health clients receive a practical understanding of health-related information. Because community health nurses see clients with varying needs and abilities in a variety of settings, they are in key positions to deliver health education.

In an era of growing health costs and increasing collaboration between health service providers and consumers, clients are increasingly encouraged to share responsibility for their own health maintenance. Community health nurse educators empower consumers by educating them about ways to more effectively manage their own health processes. As lifespan increases, people are more likely to experience the chronic illnesses related to aging that require complex changes in diet, exercise, lifestyle, and medical treatments. Health education becomes crucial to health care in light of such social changes.

The ability to apply learning theories in a variety of educational settings is essential to guide the thinking, decision-making, and practice of community health nurses. To promote the health of clients, it is necessary to teach practical health concepts and self-care skills in understandable ways. This chapter provides a necessary theoretical foundation, along with practical strategies to enable community health nurses to successfully educate clients.

Annotated Outline

I. General educational theories: Educational theories help to provide community health nurses with a variety of ways in which to approach client education. They also offer pragmatic insights into the ways in which people learn.
   A. Behavioral: The goal of behavioral theorists is behavioral change. The educator attempts to modify a selected behavior through the consistent use of a reinforcer, a punishment, or the withdrawal of a reinforcer.
   B. Social: Social learning theorists build on the principles of behavioral theorists; however, they believe that behavior is a function of an individual's expectations about the value of an outcome. The educator attempts to change behaviors by enabling clients to change expectations about the value of a certain outcome and/or the ability to achieve the desired outcome.
   C. Cognitive: Cognitive theorists believe that by changing thought patterns and providing information, learners' behavior will change. The educator seeks to provide information in a variety of ways that will change clients' thought patterns and that will ultimately be followed by changes in behavior.
   D. Humanist: Humanistic theorists emphasize the importance of feelings, emotions, and personal relationships in determining behavior. The educator strives to avoid being overly controlling and restrictive with learners, but rather seeks to help them grow and develop according to their natural inclinations.
   E. Developmental: Developmental theorists believe that learning occurs in concert with developmental stages. Each stage is a major transformation from the previous one, and learning occurs quite differently in each developmental period. The educator recognizes that readiness to learn is dependent on the individual's developmental stage.
   F. Critical: Critical theorists approach learning as an ongoing dialogue. The educator attempts to change beliefs through the process of discourse, which ultimately changes thinking and behavior.
   G. Community health nurses' application of general educational theories: Community health nurse educators should understand general educational theories and should be able to choose and then apply the most appropriate theory in a wide variety of health education situations. Often it is necessary to combine any number of these perspectives as aids in the education process.

II. Health-education models: Conceptual models are used to organize global ideas and to simplify complete systems into succinct formats. They provide meaningful tools to guide the thinking, observations, and practice of educators.

A. PRECEDE-PROCEED: This model focuses primarily on planning and evaluating health education programs in communities. PRECEDE-PROCEED is an acronym for Predisposing, Reinforcing, and Enabling Causes in Educational Diagnosis and Evaluation - Policy, Regulatory, and Organizational Constructs in Educational and Environmental Development.

B. Health Belief: The Health Belief Model was developed to provide a framework for understanding why some people take specific actions to avoid illness while others fail to protect themselves. The model was designed to predict which people would and which people would not use preventive measures, and to suggest interventions that might reduce client reluctance to access health care.

C. Health Promotion: The Health Promotion Model was developed as a complement to other health-protecting models such as the Health Belief Model. The Health Promotion Model is designed to determine the likelihood that healthy lifestyle patterns or health-promoting behaviors will occur.

D. Community Health Nurses' Application of Health Education Models: Many other health education models also exist. Community health nurses must select the most appropriate model upon which to base or frame educational interventions.

III. Educational principles: A variety of educational principles may be used to guide community health nurses to effectively provide health education to their clients.

A. Nature of learning: The nature of learning is organized into three domains: (1) cognitive, (2) affective, and (3) psychomotor.

B. Principles associated with the events of instruction: The nine basic steps in the sequence of instruction are the following: (1) gaining attention, (2) informing the learner of the objectives of instruction, (3) stimulating recall of prior learning, (4) presenting the stimulus, (5) providing learning guidance, (6) eliciting performance, (7) providing feedback, (8) assessing performance, and (9) enhancing retention and transfer of knowledge.

C. Principles that guide the educator: Six basic principles that guide the effective educator are these: (1) sending a clear message, (2) selecting the learning format, (3) setting the learning environment, (4) organizing learning experiences, (5) encouraging participatory learning, and (6) utilizing evaluation and feedback.

D. Community health nurses' application of educational principles: Principles of education create a framework for providing effective health education, which may be used to guide community health nurses.

IV. The educational process: A solid knowledge of the educational process is essential for the community health nurse.

A. Identify educational needs: Community health nurses must understand the health education needs of their clients. Nurses may determine educational needs by performing a systematic and thorough assessment of clients' needs. Once needs have been identified, they must be prioritized so that the most critical educational needs may be met first.

B. Establish educational goals and objectives: Goals and objectives that will guide the educational program must be identified. Goals are broad, long-term expected outcomes and should directly address the client's overall learning needs. Objectives are specific, short-term criteria which need to be met as steps toward achieving the long-term goal. Objectives must be stated clearly, and the expected outcomes must be defined in measurable terms.

C. Select appropriate educational methods: Methods should be chosen which facilitate the efficient and successful accomplishment of program goals and objectives. The methods should also be appropriately matched to the client's strengths and needs. The educator should choose the simplest, clearest, and most succinct manner of presentation.

D. Implement the educational plan: Implementation consists of the management of the educational process. The educator must be flexible and able to modify educational methods and strategies to meet unexpected challenges that may confront both the educator and the learner.

E. Educational evaluation: Educational evaluation involves three areas: (1) educator evaluation, (2) process evaluation, and (3) product evaluation.

V. Evaluation of the educational product: The educational product is the outcome of the education process. As applied to community health nursing, the educational product is a measurable change in the health or behavior of the client.

A. Evaluation of health and behavioral changes: The community health nurse educator seeks to measure health and behavioral changes that result from health education. There are a variety of approaches, methods, and tools that can be used to assist in evaluating the educational product, including questionnaires, surveys, skills demonstrations, testing, subjective client feedback, and direct observation of improvements in client mastery of materials.

B. Short-term evaluation: It is important to evaluate short-term health and behavioral effects of health education programs and to determine whether these are really caused by the educational program.

C. Long-term evaluation: The ultimate goal of health education is to help clients make lasting behavioral changes that will improve their overall health status. Long-term evaluation may be geared toward following and assessing the status of an individual client, family, or community over time.

VI. Clinical application: The key points of this chapter are brought together in a clinical example of applied health education.

Additional Critical Thinking Activities

1. Review the general theories of learning summarized in the chapter and decide which one would most effectively fit the learning needs of an individual who has been recently diagnosed with lung cancer; a family caring for an individual with Alzheimer's disease; and a community in which adolescent cigarette smoking is on the rise.
2. Based on one of the three health education models outlined in this chapter, plan a health education program for a group of pregnant teenagers.
3. Recall an educational interaction with a client that did not seem to go well. Identify what might have been the problem, based on educational principles. Develop a plan for ways in which the interaction could have been improved, based on educational principles.
4. Recall a learning experience in which one of the following was problematic: message, format, environment, experience, participation, or evaluation. Then, develop a plan for how the problem could have been overcome and turned from a negative or neutral learning situation into a positive one.
5. Review the phases of the educational process and apply this process to an individual with hypertension; a family with a child with attention deficit disorder; and a community in which tuberculosis is on the rise.
6. Develop a short-term and long-term evaluation of the educational product of a program designed to teach elementary school students health-promoting behaviors such as eating a well-balanced diet and exercising at least three times a week.

Critical Analysis Questions

1. True or False? Health education is a vital part of community health nursing.
2. True or False? If health education is successful, the patient should not have to change any behaviors.
3. List four of the six types of general educational theories mentioned in this chapter that may guide community health nurses as they develop educational programs.
4. True or False? Typically, only one general educational theory should be necessary to apply in any given situation.
5. Identify two of the three health education models outlined in this chapter, and differentiate between the major purpose of each model.
6. All of the following are types of domains that comprise the nature of learning except:
   a. spiritual.
   b. cognitive.
   c. affective.
   d. psychomotor.
7. List six of the nine basic steps outlined in this chapter that comprise the events of instruction.
8. List four of the six basic principles described in this chapter that guide the effective educator.
9. Outline the five steps of the educational process.
10. All of the following are components of educational evaluation except:
    a. educator evaluation.
    b. process evaluation.
    c. product evaluation.
    d. needs evaluation.
11. True or False? The goal of the education product is a measurable change in the health status or behavior of a client.
12. Define and differentiate between short-term and long-term evaluation.

Answer Key

1. True
2. False
3. 1. Behavioral, 2. Social Learning, 3. Cognitive, 4. Humanist, 5. Developmental, and 6. Critical.
4. False
5. 1. PRECEDE-PROCEED: focuses primarily on planning and evaluating health education programs

   2. Health Belief: designed to predict which people would and which people would not use preventative measures, and to suggest interventions that might reduce client reluctance to access health care

   3. Health Promotion: developed as a complement to other health-protecting models; designed to determine the likelihood that healthy lifestyle patterns or health-promoting behaviors will occur
6. a

7. 1. gaining attention, 2. informing the learner of the objectives of instruction, 3. stimulating recall of prior learning, 4. presenting the stimulus, 5. providing learning guidance, 6. eliciting performance, 7. providing feedback, 8. assessing performance, and 9. enhancing retention and transfer of knowledge
8. 1. sending a clear message, 2. selecting the learning format, 3. setting the learning environment, 4. organizing learning experiences, 5. encouraging participatory learning, and 6. utilizing evaluation and feedback
9. 1. identify educational needs, 2. establish educational goals and objectives, 3. select appropriate educational methods, 4. implement the educational plan, and 5. utilize educational evaluation
10. d
11. True
12. 1. Short-term evaluation: It is important to evaluate short-term health and behavioral effects of health education programs and to determine if they are really caused by the educational program.
    2. Long-term evaluation: The ultimate goal of health education is to help clients make lasting behavioral changes that will improve their overall health status. Long-term evaluation may be geared toward following and assessing the status of an individual client, family, or community over time.

14 Community Health Promotion: A Multi-Level Framework for Practice

Chapter Summary

Community health nursing is based on a synthesis of public health and nursing knowledge. Three concepts provide the major cornerstones for a multi-level framework for community health nursing practice: health, health promotion, and community. This chapter is focused on the historical roots and definitions of the three concepts and on a discussion of the community frameworks used by community health nurses to guide their practice, their education, and their research.

Lifestyle is one of the most critical modifiable factors influencing the health of Americans today. Many Americans exercise regularly, maintain their weight at recommended levels, and deliberately attempt to manage their stress. Some drive at reduced speeds, drink fewer alcoholic beverages than in the past, and smoke less or not at all. Others jog or walk on country lanes and in city parks, participate in structured physical fitness programs, and engage in a variety of relaxation techniques at home and at work. But lifestyle changes are not enough. Changes must also occur in the environment and in health care. Many nurses are interested in the promotion of the health of populations through healthy lifestyles and healthy families, aggregates, and communities.

Annotated Outline

I. Health and health promotion: The concept of health shapes the process of community health nursing from assessment of the health-related needs of individuals, families, aggregates, and communities, to evaluation of behavioral outcomes.

   A. Historical perspectives: The belief in people helping themselves can be traced to the Old Testament; the holistic view of health is found in classical Greek writings and throughout history.

   B. Definitions of health: The idea of health was consistently described as a comparative concept, allowing for "more" or "less" or gradations, along a health-illness continuum. Four models of health, ordered from narrow and concrete to broad and abstract are as follows: (1) clinical-health, the absence of disease; (2) role-performance-health, the ability to satisfactorily perform one's social roles; (3) adaptive-health, flexible adaptation to the environment; and (4) eudaemonistic-health, self-actualization and the attainment of one's greatest human potential.

   C. Definitions of health promotion: Health promotion is an accepted aim of community health nursing practice, although few authors distinguish between health promotion, disease prevention, and health maintenance. Health promotion is directed toward achieving an optimum level of health and well-being. Disease prevention is directed toward reducing the threat of illness, disease, or complications. Health maintenance is directed toward keeping a current state of health and well-being. These definitions require that one assess not only health behaviors, but also the basis upon which one makes a choice to perform a given behavior.

   D. Definitions of self-care: The term "self-care" has been very influential in nursing's approach to health promotion. Self-care was used to describe activities that individuals initiate and perform on their own behalf to maintain life, health, and well-being. Self-care activities may be carried out by an individual, a community, or a society, and are based on scientific, economic, religious, philosophical, and cultural influences.

   E. Disease prevention, risk appraisal and risk reduction: Risk appraisal and reduction are ways professionals can assist individuals and groups in developing a part of their self-care plan. The goal of risk appraisal and reduction is aimed at primary prevention or early detection of disease, and many tools and techniques are available for determining level or risk.

      1. Health-hazard appraisal: The objectives of the health-hazard appraisal are as follows: to assess the total risks to a client's health; to initiate life-style changes in the client to avoid disease precursors or to minimize their pathogenic influence; and to institute medical treatment and life-style changes as early in the course of disease as possible.

2. Clinical preventive services guidelines: The *Guide to Clinical Preventive Services* was based on review of the scientific evidence on 169 clinical preventive services for 60 target conditions. The *Guide* includes information about the appropriate content of periodic health examinations. Clinical preventive services refer to disease prevention and health promotion services delivered to individuals in health care settings—immunizations, screening, counseling, and chemoprophylactic regimens. Many of these preventive measures are routine nursing interventions.
3. Wellness inventories: Wellness inventories are different from most health-risk appraisal instruments and guidelines for preventive services, because they tend to define health risks more broadly, and because they emphasize the empowerment of individuals to achieve health. Wellness appraisals lead to disease prevention, but do so by advocating health enhancement or promotion. Typical wellness instruments include inventories related to self-responsibility, nutritional awareness, physical fitness, stress management, and environmental sensitivity.
4. Advantages and disadvantages: Risk appraisals are useful in supporting individual's self-care behaviors and in measuring the effectiveness of planned interventions for risk reduction. The limitations include questionable validity and reliability of the instruments, the inconsistency with which different appraisal instruments measure and analyze health characteristics, and an overemphasis on life-style factors and lack of attention to other important risks, such as environmental hazards and inadequate health care.

II. Community

A. Historical perspectives: The emphasis on community versus the individual as the focus of practice is not new, but is receiving greater attention since the mid-1970s. For example, declining mortality and morbidity rates were attributed to better standards of living and better nutrition. In 1990, the importance of the environment and the community in maintaining an individual's health were made very clear in the *National Health Promotion and Disease Prevention Objectives, Healthy People 2000.* It has been argued that the contribution of community health nursing to problems of the environment lies in our ability to integrate personal choices and environmental forces that affect health.

B. Models and frameworks: In community health nursing practice, nurses soon become aware that the community is more than the sum of the individuals, families, and aggregates within it, and that for any real change to occur, the larger community must be considered. Existing community models are often based on an assumption that a healthy community is facilitated by assessing the various components of the community system. Interventions are planned at the system level by participating with relevant components or subsystems. Although these models provide guidance for assessing community and aggregate systems, less guidance is provided for community health promotion interventions.

C. Community studies: Two of the most influential community-wide studies of health risks are the Framingham Heart Study and the Human Population Laboratory's longitudinal survey in Alameda County, California. Both of these studies supported the hypothesis that selected risk factors are directly related to morbidity and mortality. Findings from large community surveys prompted a number of multi-level intervention programs based on a public health model. These programs have provided a scientific knowledge base for the implementation of risk-appraisal and risk-reduction programs. However, information on the relative effectiveness of specific individual and community level interventions in reducing risk still remains limited.

D. Community health nursing applications: The aim of community health nursing is to facilitate community residents' ability to increase their awareness of their own health situations, and to become empowered to determine what they want for themselves, their families, and their community. Nursing concerns seen from a community health nursing perspective require a framework that can take into account aspects of health promotion, disease and illness prevention, and illness care of individuals, families, aggregates, and the total community. Community health nursing activity must take into consideration the people, the community, and the pattern of the interrelationships among them.

III. Shifting emphasis from illness to wellness: In community health nursing practice, it is clear that many factors have an impact on the health of individuals, families, and communities. The biomedical model of health cannot explain why some individuals exposed to recognized illness-producing stressors do not become ill, whereas other individuals who appear to be in the most health-conducive circumstances do become ill.

Both the disease paradigm and the health paradigm are useful for advancing the specific aims and processes of community health nursing. The disease approach directs CHN practice toward disease prevention, risk-reduction, prompt treatment, and rehabilitation. The health approach directs CHN practice toward promotion of greater levels of positive health.

IV. A model of community health promotion: Laffrey and Kulbok's model of community health promotion is based on the health paradigm and the disease paradigm. The health paradigm is focused on promoting health as a dynamic, creative, and positive quality of life. The disease paradigm is focused on reducing known risks and threats to health and on preventing disease. Clinical strategies may be similar within the two paradigms; however, the ultimate goal of each paradigm contains fundamental differences. These differences are evident when viewing the specific purpose of the nursing care: to promote well-being or to prevent disease. The model includes two major dimensions: client system and focus of care. Client system refers to the level of client; e.g., individual, family, aggregate, or community, toward which community health nursing is targeted. The focus of care within the model is illness care, illness prevention, or health promotion. Community health nursing care, within this model, must extend beyond resolving a specific illness, to preventing the illness and promoting optimal health for the individual, the family, the aggregate, and the total community. All levels are important to the health of the community and its populations.

Additional Critical Thinking Activities

1. Read newspapers and view national news shows for three days to determine media exposure of individual, family, aggregate, and community health risk reduction measures. Specify which of the determinants (lifestyle, biology, environment, health care) is the focus of the identified risk reduction measures. Analyze the potential of the measures for influencing the health of individuals, families, high-risk aggregates within the community, and the total community. Include examples in your written report.
2. Complete the lifestyle assessment questionaire and health risk appraisal form included in Appendix G. Compare and contrast the health risk and wellness perspectives. Consider whether these lifestyle assessment forms will stimulate you to initiate a health behavior change program. Why or why not?
3. Identify at least three organizations in your community that sponsor health promotion and disease prevention programs. For each organization, provide information on the type of program, the type of interventions, eligibility for service, and costs of services. Determine whether the program activities are self-care in focus. If possible, interview the director of one of the programs to determine the effectiveness of these activities in your community. Write a report on your findings.
4. Discuss with a classmate the relative advantages and disadvantages of risk reduction programs at the individual and community levels. Compare and contrast them in terms of effectiveness, cost, ethical concerns, and types of consumer and professional involvement.
5. Discuss with a classmate the relative advantages and disadvantages of health promotion programs at the individual and community levels. Compare and contrast them in terms of effectiveness, cost, ethical concerns, and types of consumer and professional involvement.
6. Select a health situation, such as teen pregnancy in a high school in your community. Using the multi-level framework, describe illness care, illness/disease prevention, and health promotion care at each of the four client levels (individual, family, aggregate, and community).

Critical Analysis Questions

1. Which of the following factors was most influential in deemphasizing the holistic view of health and self-care?
   a. religious beliefs
   b. professional attitude
   c. scientific and biologic view of disease
   d. economic constraints
   e. political ideologies
2. Which of the following factors has consistently been most important in the cyclical popularization of self-care?
   a. religious beliefs
   b. professional attitude
   c. scientific and biologic view of disease
   d. economic constraints
   e. political ideologies
3. In 1975, Milton Terris expanded the WHO definition of health. Select the response(s) that correctly represents changes made by Terris. (Select one or more.)
   a. deletion of the word "complete"
   b. addition of the words "social well-being"
   c. addition of the words "ability to function"
   d. addition of the words "flexible adaptation"
4. Which of the following exemplifies secondary prevention?
   a. provision of adequate housing
   b. nutrition education
   c. genetic counseling

d. screening

5. Which of the following terms is the correct descriptor of "behavior directed toward keeping a current state of health and well-being"?
   a. health promotion behavior
   b. illness/disease prevention behavior
   c. health maintenance behavior
6. Which of the following health-risk appraisal approaches is most appropriate for use in planning health care for age-specific populations in a community?
   a. health hazard appraisals
   b. clinical guidelines and recommendations for preventive services
   c. wellness appraisals or inventories
7. Which of the four determinants of health and/or disease is not generally covered in risk appraisal instruments?
   a. human biology
   b. environment
   c. lifestyle
   d. health care
8. The Stanford three-community study established the efficacy of which models of intervention? (Select one or more.)
   a. small group discussion
   b. face-to-face instruction
   c. mass media
   d. health hazard appraisal
9. Which of the following statements is not consistent with Milio's set of propositions for improving health behavior?
   a. Health education has a maximal impact on behavior patterns and options for investing personal resources.
   b. Organizational decisions determine the range of personal resources available.
   c. Social change is reflective of change in population behavior.
   d. Health status of populations is a function of lack or excess of health resources.
10. Which of the following concepts formed the basis for the community and professional partnership reported by Flick and others?
    a. multidimensional health
    b. reciprocity and trust
    c. social justice
    d. educational empowerment
    e. all of the above
11. Create a plan to address the problem of adolescent substance use among students in an urban public high school. Use the model of community health promotion, and propose illness/disease prevention activities for each level of client system.

Answer Key

1. c
2. e
3. a and c
4. d
5. c
6. b
7. d
8. b and c
9. a
10. e
11. The plan should describe appropriate disease prevention activities; e.g., risk appraisal or reduction for individual, family, aggregate, and community client systems.

15 Community as Client: Using the Nursing Process to Promote Health

Chapter Summary

Nurses, especially community health nurses, have traditionally considered the community as one of their clients. Some nurses have viewed the community as their principal client. Irrespective of the relative emphasis given to the community, the concept of "community as client" has not been adequately defined. Nursing diagnoses related to the community level, for example, are just being developed. Nursing practice directed to the community client has been neglected. The effects of that practice have yet to be fully documented. Empirical data, either corroborating or refuting the importance of nursing practice "with" the client, will be helpful. Students' and staff nurses' case examples are important. Program evaluation efforts and the dissemination of those findings to nurses in practice and in the area of health policy are also needed.

The purpose of this chapter is to provide both conceptual clarity and guidelines for nursing practice with the community client.

Annotated Outline

I. Community defined: *Community* can be simply defined as people in relationship with others or can include a bounded geographical setting and/or common values or interests; it can also include emotional as well as geographical and functional relationships.
   A. Community analyzed: Most definitions of community include the following: networks of interpersonal relationships that provide friendship and support to members, residence in a common locality, and emotional solidarity.
   B. Community specified: In this chapter, the definition of community includes people, place, and function dimensions.

II. Community as client: The community as client has been described as the setting, unit, and target of service.
   A. The community client: The community is considered the client or target of service when nursing practice, regardless of setting or unit of service, is community oriented. Healthful change is sought for the community's benefit.
   B. Relevance of the community client to nursing practice: The direct care of clients can occur within the context of a community orientation when changes in clients' health will affect the health of the community. The improved health of the collective is the nursing goal.

III. Defining goals and means of community-oriented practice.
   A. Community health: The goal of community-oriented practice. Common characteristics include status, structure, and process.
      1. The status dimension: Includes physical, emotional, and social parameters, such as measures of morbidity and mortality, life expectancy/indexes and risk factor profiles (physical parameters), consumer satisfaction and mental health indexes (emotional parameters), crime rates and function levels (social parameters).
      2. The structural dimension: Includes community health services and resources and attributes of the community structure itself, commonly identified as social indicators or correlates of health.
      3. The process dimension: Community health as the process of effective community functioning or problem solving is the least well-established definition; it can include the notion of community competence. According to Cottrell, there are eight essential conditions of community competence.
      4. Community health, a synthesis: The definition offered in this chapter integrates the status, structural, and process dimensions.
   B. Partnership: The means of community-oriented practice. Most changes aimed at improving community health involve partnerships between health care providers and community residents. This chapter proposes that community resident participation should be active rather than passive, and also that nurses should be actively involved in change for improved community health.
      1. Partnership defined: Partnership is the informed, flexible, and negotiated distribution (and redistribution) of power among all par-

ticipants in the process of change for improved community health.

2. Partnership justified: Partnership is important because health is not given, but is generated. Optimally, health is created from the interaction among providers, recipients, and their environments. Providers have preferred compliance to collaboration and have kept consumers of health care in a subservient position.
3. Conclusion: The goal of community health nursing is to form a partnership with consumers to work towards improved health.

IV. Assessing community health: Requires that relevant existing data be gathered, additional data be generated, and the data base be interpreted.

A. Data collection: The goal is to acquire usable information about the community and its health. A variety of data are gathered, including vital statistics and demographic data. Additional data may need to be generated, such as those pertaining to community beliefs; values; goals; perceived needs; power, leadership, and influence structures; and problem solving processes. Data collection should provide information about community health problems and community health strengths.

B. Data assessment: Data are analyzed, themes are noted, and community health problems, strengths, and needs for action are identified. Lay participation is important to this process. Five key methods of data assessment include informant interviewing, participant observation, secondary analyses of existing data, surveys, and windshield surveys.

C. Assessment guides: The assessment guide presented with this chapter includes three dimensions of the definition of community as defined by the author—place or space, people, and function—and the three dimensions of community health—status, structure, and process. Each of these dimensions is represented by a variety of indicators.

D. Assessment issues: Gaining entry is a major hurdle to assessment. Once entry is attained, role negotiation must begin. Confidentiality, differing perceptions of community health problems, and the lack of reliable statistical data about small communities are also issues.

V. Community health nursing diagnosis: Diagnosis consists of three parts.

A. "Risk of" identifies the specific problem faced by the community.

B. "Among" specifies the community the nurse will be working with in relation to the identified problem.

C. "Related to" identifies factors contributing to the problem.

VI. Planning for community health: This phase includes analyzing and assigning priorities to the community health problems previously identified by the nursing diagnosis, establishing goals and objectives, and identifying interventions to accomplish the objectives.

A. Problem analysis and prioritization: Problem analysis seeks to clarify the nature of the problem and should be undertaken for each identified problem; this requires the assistance of a group rather than the work of an individual. Problems must be ranked, and this process also involves the community members, experts, administrators, and other resource controllers.

B. Establishing goals and objectives: The goal is generally a global statement of the desired outcome, and objectives are more specific.

C. Identifying intervention activities: Intervention activities are the means by which objectives are realized. They reflect strategies that spell out what must be done to achieve the objectives, the ways in which change is effected, and how the problem cycle can be interrupted.

VII. Implementing intervention for community health: During this phase, the plan for improved community health is transformed into reality.

A. Factors influencing implementation: A variety of factors influence the implementation stage, including the nurse's preferred mode of action, the nature of the problem, community readiness to solve the problem, and the characteristics of the social change process. Nurses can act as content experts, fact gatherers, analysts, program implementors, enabler-catalysts, teachers of problem-solving skills, and activist-advocates.

B. Nurse's preferred role: The nurse can act as a content expert, helping communities select and attain task-related goals; as a process expert by increasing the community's ability to solve the problem; or as fact gatherer, analyst, program implementor, enabler-catalyst, teacher of problem-solving skills, and activist-advocate.

C. Implementation mechanisms: Implementation mechanisms represent the vehicles or modes by which innovations are transferred from the planners to the units of service. Influential community leaders or lay advisors, small informal groups, bureaucracies, mass media, and public policy are used as aids to the nurse-intervener and to his or her community partner(s). The nurse must assess how change is viewed by the community, decide who will support the change, and determine what level and type of resistance can be expected.

VIII. Evaluating intervention for community health: Evaluation is the appraisal of the effects of some organized activity or program. It begins in the planning phase of community action. Evaluation by objective and the more formalized program evaluation are mentioned.

Additional Critical Thinking Activities

1. A 6-month-old infant is brought to the county's public health department because of fever and diarrhea. During an interview with the 16-year-old mother, the nurse discovers that the infant has not had his "baby shots" or routine well-baby check-ups. The mother says, "Folks don't bring their babies to the doctor unless they're sick." Identify and justify the unit of service and target of service in this situation.
2. Go to the library. Identify, review, and critique one article in the nursing literature in which the relevance of the nursing process to community-oriented nursing practice is discussed or exemplified.
3. You have been asked to collect data about a community's health facilities, vital statistics, and values regarding health. Which method of data collection would you select for each type of data and why?
4. Interviews with community residents consistently reveal that they believe their water supplies are contaminated. The health department's sanitarian tells you the latest tests reveal the water is safe. Is contaminated water a community health problem? Why or why not?
5. Health and welfare professionals working in the community where several of your patients live have decided to institute an after-school recreation program for teenagers. The county government is reluctant to appropriate funds, although school officials are eager to donate school sports facilities, and teenagers and their parents agree about the importance of an after-school program. Your objective: To develop a community-wide recreation program for teenagers by June 1994. Select the two best intervention activities for this objective, and state the reasons for your choice.
6. See Activity 1. Sketch a community-oriented nursing care plan appropriate to this situation. Identify a goal, three objectives, and two activities for each objective.
7. Develop a community-oriented nursing care plan to aid in alleviating the isolation of the elderly in an urban high-rise building. About one third of the elderly wish to decrease the isolation; others wish to be "left alone." Although limited resources are available, several health workers and the high-rise manager are ready to meet to discuss the possibilities. Identify a goal, three objectives, and two activities for each objective.

Critical Analysis Questions

1. In treating a worker injured at a construction site, the nurse interviews the worker, the foreman, and several of the co-workers. Does this exemplify community-oriented nursing practice? Why or why not?
2. In a routine day, the community health nurse conducts a scoliosis screening clinic at a junior high school, makes a home visit to the parents of a child with a high absenteeism rate, bandages a child injured on the playground, and plans a first-aid course to teachers. Which of these activities exemplify community-oriented nursing practice? Why?
3. Which of the following examples best illustrates partnership for health?
   a. telling interagency council members that teenage pregnancy is the major health problem in their service area
   b. helping a rural community council to survey area water supplies
   c. developing a volunteer program for local health and welfare agencies
   d. assisting a high school counselor and school nurse to determine the students' health education needs
4. Which two of the following best illustrate the definition of community presented in the chapter?
   a. residents of a small Appalachian hollow
   b. members of the American Public Health Association
   c. an urban neighborhood of East Asian migrants
   d. senior nursing students enrolled in a community health course
5. Define "target of service" and "unit of service" in Question 2, and give an example of each.
6. State two of the reasons for using the nursing process in community-oriented practice.
7. Give an example of how each element of the nursing process — assessment, planning, intervention, and evaluation — is used in a community-oriented nursing practice.
8. Identify the most appropriate method(s) of data collection for a particular type of data:

   Type of data
   1. Environmental hazards
   2. Health manpower
   3. Norms about preventive care
   4. Crime patterns
   5. Incidence of reportable infectious disease

   Data collection method
   a. participant observation
   b. informant interviewing
   c. reviewing existing records of meetings
   d. analyzing existing demographic and vital statistics
   e. survey

9. Suppose you needed to document such correlates of inadequate transportation as unemployment and an unreliable system of public transportation. Which methods of data collection would you use?
10. You are concerned about the high school drop-out problem, but the residents assure you, "That's the way it is here." Would you interpret this as a problem? Why or why not?
11. The elderly residents of a working-class neighborhood are anxious about teenage vandalism, yet the crime rates among teenagers are actually very low. Would you interpret this as a problem? Why or why not?
12. Briefly describe how interacting groups, lay advisors, the mass media, and public policy can be used as mechanisms for implementing community-oriented nursing intervention.
13. Briefly list two benefits of needs assessment.
14. The principal of the local elementary school (Monroe School) has noticed that many entering kindergartners lack the required immunizations, and he complains to you in October that the problem is worse this year than last. Develop an objective you would work toward immediately, as well as one activity you would reject. Defend your choices.
15. For three years, you have heard residents of an isolated, rural area complain about the lack of medical services in their community. You also know that many of your clients fail to keep medical appointments in the nearest town. What goal would be appropriate and why?

Answer Key

1. Yes, if the target of service is the entire workforce and not just the injured individual. The goal, for example, might be to establish and maintain employee awareness and adherence to safety regulations.
2. The scoliosis screening clinic, the home visit to the parents of a child with a high absenteeism rate, and the planning of a first-aide course for teachers all exemplify community-oriented nursing practice. In each case, the target of service is a population group with known health risks. Bandaging the injured child without addressing the larger problem of accidents to children is focusing nursing care on the individual and not on the community.
3. b
4. a and c
5. Target of service: The population group for whom healthful change is sought; e.g., elementary school children. Unit of service: The entity to whom nursing care is delivered; e.g., individual, family aggregate, organization, or community. The entity from whom healthful change is sought; e.g., parents and teachers of injured elementary school children.
6. Systematizes thinking. Facilitates the application of existing nursing knowledge. Emphasizes the commonalities within nursing, irrespective of the setting, target, and unit of service.
7. Assessment: Collecting data about community health problems and capabilities through methods such as windshield surveys, information interviewing, participant observation, and secondary analyses of existing data. Planning: Analyzing and assigning priorities to community health problems, establishing goals and objectives, identifying intervention activities to accomplish the objectives. Intervention: Developing strategies in partnership with relevant others in the community. Evaluation: Determining whether the objectives were met and how effective and efficient the intervener's activities were.
8. (1) b, d (2) b, f (3) a, b (4) e (5) e
9. Unemployment: Analyze existing demographic data; interview heads of key businesses and industries. Unreliable public transportation: participant observation on buses, subways, etc.; interview selected informants such as bus and taxi company representatives and area rescue squad members.
10. A nurse might consider this a problem because the basic skills acquired in high school are important for employment, managing a home, etc. If the community does not view this as a problem, the nurse would be advised, however, not to begin community-oriented intervention on this point. It is more important to begin with a mutually agreed-on problem.
11. It is a problem if the elderly people perceive it as such. As the vandalism is perceived to be problematical, the nurse might accept the elderlys' definition and work with them to clarify the actual problem. The problem could be that teenagers are loitering on the street corners because job and recreational opportunities are limited.
12. Interacting groups link individuals to society. Lay advisors are influential in the approval and dissemination of change. They are especially useful with late adopters and those resisting change. The mass media is efficient in dealing with money, and is especially effective with early adopters. Public policy can constrain individual choice for the common good and can mandate certain healthful behaviors.
13. Needs assessment may raise consciousness of providers; can serve to link residents and health providers; and leads to more accurate assessment.
14. Objective: Determine the percentage of children lacking required preschool immunization at Monroe School in each of the past five years. This is

essential to confirm the principal's impression. Activities: (1) Compile the data from school records. (2) Contact PTA for assistance in compiling data. The second activity should be selected, as it involves significant others in a process that would increase their awareness of any problem.

15. The problem is, as yet, unspecified. The goal is to specify the problem; e.g., inaccessible health services. From that, you can infer lack of reliable and inexpensive transportation, long waits in physician offices, and/or inadequate self-care skills.

16 Community Health Nursing in Rural Environments

Chapter Summary

Universal access to health care has become a national priority. Recruiting and retaining qualified health professionals in underserved communities, particularly in the inner city and rural areas of the United States, is difficult. Not much has been written about the special challenges, problems, and opportunities of community health nursing practice in rural settings. This chapter discusses the issues surrounding health care delivery in rural environments and presents the following: the definitions and perceptions of the term "rural," the lifestyle and health status of rural populations, an explanation of barriers to obtaining a continuum of health care services, a description of nursing practice issues, and strategies to deliver more effective community-based services to clients who live in more isolated environments with sparse resources.

Annotated Outline

I. Historical overview: Formal rural community health nursing originated with the Red Cross Rural Nursing Service. Before that agency came into existence, care of the sick in a small community was provided by informal social support systems. Historically, this task was assigned to healing women who lived within the geographical area, if self-care and family-care did not prove effective in bringing about healing. The health needs of rural Americans have been numerous—not necessarily unique, but nevertheless different from those of urban populations. Consistent problems of maldistribution of health professionals, poverty, limited access to services, ignorance, and social neglect have plagued many rural communities for generations. Concern for rural health is often a passing fad that is preempted by other areas of greater need. Hopefully, this will not be the case with health care reform in its efforts to assure universal access to care for rural as well as urban residents.

II. Definitions and terms

- A. Rurality—a subjective concept: Everyone has an idea of what constitutes "rural" versus "urban." Rural can be defined in terms of the geographic location and population density, or it may be specific and use distance (e.g., 20 miles) or time (e.g., 30 minutes) needed to commute to an urban center.
- B. Rural versus urban—a continuum: Frequently-used definitions to describe rural-urban are provided by several federal agencies. Their definitions, often dichotomous in nature, fail to take into account the relative nature of ruralness. Rural-urban residency is a continuum ranging from living on a remote farm, to a village or small town, to a larger town or city, to a large metropolitan area with a "core inner city." About 25% of all United States residents live in rural settings. For this chapter, rural refers to areas having fewer than 99 persons per square mile, and communities having a population of 20,000 or less.

III. Current perspectives

- A. Population characteristics: In rural areas there are a number of under-represented groups (minorities; subgroups) who reside across the fifty states. There is a higher proportion of caucasians in rural areas (about 82%) than in core metropolitan areas (about 62%). There are regional variations, and some rural counties have significant numbers of minorities. Of the total rural population, nearly four million are African-American, almost two million are Native American, thirty-four million are Asian-Pacific Islanders, and seventy-five million are of other races. Little is documented on the needs and health status of those populations.
- B. Health status of rural populations
  1. Perceived health status: Even though rural communities constitute about one-fourth of the total population, we do not fully understand the health problems or the health behaviors of those residents. The health status measures that are addressed herein are the following: perceived health status, diagnosed chronic conditions, physical limitations, frequency of seeking medical treatment, usual source of care, maternal-infant health, children's health, mental health, minorities health, and environmental and occupational health risks.

2. Chronic illness: Rural populations have a poorer perception of their overall health and functional status than their urban counterparts do. Those over the age of 18 assess their health status less favorably than urban residents do. Studies show that rural adults are less likely to engage in preventive behavior, which increases their exposure to risk. They are less likely to wear seat belts, have regular blood pressure checks, have pap smears, and have complete self-breast examinations. Failure to participate in these lifestyle behaviors affects the overall health status of rural residents, as well as their level of function, physical limitations, degree of mobility, and level of self-care activities.
3. Physical limitations: Limitations in mobility and self-care are strong indicators of an individual's overall health status. Rural adults under age 65 are more likely than urban adults to assess their health status as fair to poor, and a greater percentage have been diagnosed with a chronic health condition. Community health nurses in rural practice settings play an important role in providing a continuum of care to clients living in these underserved areas. For instance, they teach rural clients how to prevent accidents, how to engage in more healthful lifestyle behaviors, and how to reduce the risk of chronic health problems. Once a client is diagnosed with a long term problem, community health nurses can help clients in rural environments manage chronic conditions to maintain an optimal level of health and function.
4. Utilization patterns of health care: Despite their overall poorer health status and higher incidence of chronic health conditions, rural adults seek medical care less often than urban adults. In part, this discrepancy can be attributed to scarce resources and lack of providers in rural areas.
5. Sources of care, and time/distance to services: The ability to identify a "usual" source of care has been viewed as a favorable indicator of access to health care and to a person's overall health status. Having the same provider of care can enhance continuity of care, as well as a client's perceived perception of the quality of that care. Rural adults (85%) are more likely than urban (78%) to identify a particular medical provider as their usual source of care. General practitioners are usually seen by rural adults, while urban adults are more likely to seek care from a specialist. Rural persons who seek ambulatory care are more likely to travel more than 30 minutes to reach their usual source of care. Rural residents' ability to identify a usual site of care or a particular provider often stems from a community or county having only one, perhaps two, health care providers.
6. Maternal-infant health: Conflicting reports exist in the literature regarding pregnancy outcomes in rural areas. Overall, rural populations have higher infant and maternal morbidity rates, especially in counties designated as HPSA. In these counties one also finds fewer specialists such as pediatricians, obstetricians, and gynecologists to provide care to at-risk populations.
7. Children's health: Reports on the health status of rural children show regional variations and conflicting data. School nurses are an important factor in the overall health status of children in the United States. The availability of school nurses in rural communities also varies from region to region. In rural areas of the United States, school nurses are usually scarce.
8. Mental health: The facts about the mental health status of rural populations are ambiguous and conflicting. Stress, stress-related conditions, and mental illness are prevalent among populations when severe economic difficulties persist. The depressed agriculture, lumber, and mining industries have resulted in numerous job losses in rural communities; hence, the term "farm stress." Economic recession is also a contributing factor to a family not having insurance or being under-insured, a situation with a higher incidence in rural communities.
9. Minorities' health: There are a significant number of at-risk minority groups in rural America who have some rather unique concerns; in particular, children, the elderly, American Indians, Native Alaskans, Native Hawaiians, migrant workers, African-Americans, and the homeless.
10. Environmental and occupational health risks: A community's primary industry is an influencing factor in the local lifestyle, the health status of its residents, and in the number and types of health care services it may need. Three high-risk industries identified by OSHA that are found in predominantly rural environments are lumbering/forestry, mining, and agriculture. Associated health risks of those industries are machinery and vehicular accidents, trauma, and select types of cancer and respiratory disease stemming from repeated

exposure to toxins, pesticides and herbicides.

C. Rural health care delivery issues and barriers to care: Even though each rural community is unique, the experience of living in a small town has several common characteristics. Barriers to health care may be associated with these characteristics; e.g., whether or not services and professionals are available, affordable, accessible, or acceptable to rural consumers. To design community-based programs, health officials must design strategies and implement interventions that mesh with a client's belief system. This means that a family and a community must be actively involved in planning and delivering their own care. There is minimal empirical data about rural family systems in terms of their health beliefs, values, perceptions of illness, health care seeking behaviors, and their ideas of what constitutes appropriate care.

IV. Assessing, planning, implementing, and evaluating nursing care

A. Rural nursing theory, research and practice: There is a growing body of literature on nursing practice in small towns and rural environments, and several themes emerge. Researchers from the University of Montana contend that existing theories do not fully explain rural nursing practice and they have examined the four concepts pertinent to a nursing theory (health; person; environment; nursing/caring).

B. Community health nursing in rural environments: The work-related stressors of community health nursing have received some attention in the literature. Rural nurses report stressors associated with geographic distance, isolation, sparse resources, and other rural environmental factors.

C. Future research needs: There only are a few empirical studies on rural nursing practice, and since much of it consists of anecdotal reports by nurses, the research needs are endless. Specific areas that are of particular importance to community health nursing practice in rural environments include the following: factors related to satisfaction and dissatisfaction with rural practice; stressors/rewards of rural practice; and empirical data on the community nursing needs of rural under-represented groups, minorities, and other at-risk populations that vary by region and state.

D. Preparing nurses for rural practice settings: Nurses in rural practice must have broad knowledge about nursing theory. Health promotion, primary prevention, rehabilitation, obstetrics, medical-surgical, pediatrics, competency in planning and implementing community assessments, and an awareness and understanding of the particular health concerns in a specific state are important in this practice environment. A community's demographic profile and its principal industry can present a snapshot of some of its social, political, and health risks. From this kind of information, a community health nurse can anticipate the particular skills that will be needed to care for clients in a catchment area.

V. Future Perspectives: Residents of rural communities and their elected representatives, as well as the administrators of public and private health care agencies, should be aware of the problems inherent in providing a continuum of care to underserved populations. Media accounts focus almost exclusively on rural hospitals and the lack of primary care providers, but tend to neglect the public and community health perspective. Case management and community oriented primary care have proven to be effective models in helping to address some of those deficits.

A. Scarce resources and a comprehensive health care continuum: A fragmented health care system perpetuates problems in providing a comprehensive continuum of care to populations living in areas having scarce resources (money, personnel, equipment, ancillary services). In rural communities, the most critically needed services usually are preventive services, such as health screening clinics, nutrition counseling, and wellness education. Community health nursing needs vary by community. There is great need for school nurses, family planning services, prenatal care, care for individuals with AIDS and their families, emergency care services, services for children with special needs (including those who are physically and mentally challenged), mental health services, and community-based programs for the elderly.

B. Appropriate year 2000 objectives: Since the demographic profile varies from community to community, each state has variations in the health status of its populations. *Healthy People 2000* and *Healthy Communities: 2000* have important implications for community health nurses in that a significant number of at-risk populations cited in that policy-guiding document reside in rural areas across the 50 states. Priority objectives vary, depending on population mix, health risks, and health status of residents in the state, and the documents can assist officials to tailor the objectives to their community's needs.

VI. Building professional-community-client partnerships: The Federal Office of Rural Health Policy emphasizes that community-based programming, which actively involves the state and local element, is an essential element for any kind of reform to be successful, especially in rural areas. Professional-client/community partnerships are critical elements for reform to be meaningful at the local level.

A. Case management: Case management is an effective strategy for arranging a continuum of care for rural clients, with the case manager tailoring and blending formal and informal resources. Collaborative efforts between a client and case manager allow clients to participate in their plan of care in an acceptable and appropriate way, especially if resources are scarce.

B. Community Oriented Primary Care: Community Oriented Primary Care (COPC) is an effective model for delivering available, accessible, and acceptable services to vulnerable populations living in underserved areas. It emphasizes flexibility, grass-root involvement, and professional-community partnerships. This model blends primary care, public health, and prevention services, which are offered in a familiar and accessible setting. The COPC model is interdisciplinary in nature, uses a problem-oriented approach, and mandates community involvement in all phases of the process.

Additional Critical Thinking Activities

1. In class, or in conference with several of your peers, discuss the definitions and compare them to your own.
   A. How are they similar or different?
   B. How is rural defined in your geographic area?
   C. Identify vulnerable or at-risk populations that live in rural areas of your state. What is known about those communities? What are their particular health care needs? If possible, contact a community health or school nurse who works with that population to learn more about their health care needs.
   D. What are the particular health care delivery problems and/or barriers that rural populations in your state must confront?
   E. Is there a rural health care agency in your state? If so, where is it located, and who is responsible for this agency?
   F. Review nursing research studies that target rural populations. How is rural defined? Describe methodological issues pertinent to this study as they relate to the definition. Are the findings true for other rural populations?
   G. List and discuss research priority areas for community nurses in rural practice settings in your area.
   H. What are the characteristics of rural health care delivery in your region? How can community health nursing mesh with existing resources in that system?
   I. Which informal systems (e.g., extended family, neighbors, churches, barter/exchange/voucher systems, self-help, mutual aid groups) may substitute for unavailable or inaccessible services in rural areas?
   J. What characteristics of rural communities and the rural lifestyle facilitate or impede rural community nursing practice in your state?
   K. Do models exist that facilitate the development of home and community-based nursing services in rural areas of your state?
   L. What are the best strategies to educate and support informal support systems to augment and enhance limited community nursing resources in your area (e.g., extended family, neighbors, or members of church and civic groups)?
2. Interview one or more nurses who work in a rural environment; if possible, one who works in a community health setting.
   A. What do they find to be most rewarding and challenging about rural practice?
   B. What nursing skills do they believe are essential for a nurse to practice in a rural health setting?
   C. How would they describe their work-related stressors?
   D. Have they implemented any creative strategies to deliver care to their rural clients?

Critical Analysis Questions

1. Define the following terms:
   a. Frontier
   b. Rural
   c. Farm Residency and Non-farm Residency
   d. Urban
   c. Suburban
   f. Metropolitan Statistical Area (MSA)
   g. Non-Metropolitan Statistical Area (non-MSA)
   h. Core Metropolitan
   i. Other Metropolitan
2. Which of the following approaches is an effective way to deliver a continuum of care to clients living in areas with scarce resources?
   a. managed care
   b. case management
   c. hospice services
   d. primary care
3. True or False? Rural can be equated with farm residency.

4. True or False? In some ways, the access to health care concerns experienced in rural areas are similar to those confronted by underserved residents living in the inner city.
5. True or False? Overall, the health of rural residents is better than their urban counterparts'.
6. Generally speaking, of the following health problems, which are more prevalent in rural populations? (Select one or more.)
   a. Chronic illness
   b. Occupational-related injuries
   c. Infectious childhood diseases
   d. HIV-infection
   e. Machinery accidents
   f. Substance abuse

Answer Key

1. a. Frontier: An area with fewer than six persons per square mile.
   b. Rural: Can be defined as either a community with less than 2,500 residents; or one with less than 99 persons per square mile; or a community with less than 20,000 residents.
   c. Farm Residency: Residence outside the city limits; involvement in agriculture industry.
   Non-farm Residency: Residence within the city limits.
   d. Urban: Can be defined as a community with more than 2,500 residents; or as one with more than 99 persons per square mile.
   e. Suburban: Areas outlying highly populated cities.
   f. Metropolitan Statistical Area: County with a central city of at least 50,000 residents.
   g. Non-Metropolitan Statistical Area: Counties that do not meet MSA criteria above.
   h. Core Metropolitan: Densely populated counties with more than 1 million people.
   i. Other Metropolitan: Fringe counties surrounding the core metropolitan area.
2. b
3. False
4. False
5. False
6. a, b, e

17 Health Promotion Through Healthy Cities

Chapter Summary

The Healthy Cities movement is mobilizing local governments, professionals, citizens, and private and voluntary organizations to put health promotion on the political agendas of cities. Guiding this movement are the World Health Organization (WHO) principles of primary health care and health promotion. These principles may be implemented by community health nurses using the nine-step CITYNET-Healthy Cities process as a guide.

Annotated Outline

I. The history of the Healthy Cities movement began in the middle 1980s in Canada and Europe (WHO Regional Office for Europe). It is now an international movement involving thousands of cities.

II. Models of community practice
   - A. Locality development is a process-oriented model that emphasizes consensus, cooperation, a need to build group identity, and a sense of community.
   - B. Social planning uses rational-empirical problem solving, usually by outside professional experts.
   - C. Social action is focused on increasing the problem solving ability of the community, along with concrete actions to correct the imbalance of power and privilege of an oppressed or disadvantaged group.
   - D. Arnstein's ladder of participation suggests partnership, delegated power, and citizen control as the higher levels of participation.

III. Examples of Healthy Cities in Europe and North America suggest that different models of community practice are being implemented in the Healthy Cities movement.

IV. An understanding of the facilitators and barriers of the Healthy Cities movement can assist in sustaining the Healthy Cities process. The Healthy Cities movement supports the promotion of healthy public policy at the local level through multisectoral action and community participation.

V. Implications for community health nursing include facilitating the Healthy Cities process using the nine-step CITYNET-Healthy Cities process. Examples of community health nursing roles in implementing the steps are presented.

VI. Outcomes of Healthy Cities are related to the principles of health promotion and provide evidence of the successes of the multisectoral community partnership formed.

Additional Critical Thinking Activities

1. Consider either the city where you go to school or your hometown in terms of its similarity to a Healthy City. Identify at least three characteristics of the city you choose to study that are consistent with the precepts of a Healthy City.
   - A. What partnerships exist among public, private, and not-for-profit groups in this city?
   - B. What barriers/obstacles do you observe that exist in your city to keep it from becoming a Healthy City?
   - C. What strengths exist in your city to promote the Healthy City concepts?
2. Evaluate the existence (or absence) of at least three of the Healthy City guiding principles for health for all in the city that you evaluate. They are equity, health promotion, community participation, multisectoral cooperation, appropriate technology, primary health care, and international cooperation.
3. Interview at least ten people to determine the type, amount, and site of the health promotion that they personally practice. Determine to what extent the city supports, encourages, or poses obstacles to their chosen form of health promotion.
4. Consider the city in which you live (or if you live in a rural area, choose a city with which you are familiar) and identify four specific ways in which community health nurses can initiate Healthy City activities if they do not currently exist.

Critical Analysis Questions

1. List the principles that guide the Healthy Cities process.
2. Trace the Healthy Cities movement.

3. Describe the steps in the CITYNET-Healthy Cities process.
4. Identify examples of the roles of community health nurses in Healthy Cities using the CITYNET-Healthy Cities process.
5. Identify examples of outcomes of the Healthy Cities process.

Answer Key

1. The principles that guide the Healthy Cities process are the principles of Health For All and five elements that make up the strategic framework in the *Ottawa Charter for Health Promotion.* The principles of Health for All include equity, health promotion, community participation, multisectoral cooperation, appropriate technology, primary health care, and international cooperation. The five elements in the *Ottawa Charter for Health Promotion* are building healthy public policy, creating supportive environments, strengthening community action, developing personal skills, and reorienting health services.
2. The Healthy Cities movement began in Canada in 1984. In 1986, the World Health Organization Regional Office for Europe initiated the WHO Healthy Cities Project. The movement spread in Europe and currently includes 35 participating cities, 23 national networks, and over 650 cities and towns. Healthy Cities also are found in Africa, Southeast Asia, and the Western Pacific regions, to name a few. Multi-City Action Plans (MCAP) developed to provide European Healthy Cities with the means for international cooperation in health planning and the sharing of professional experts. CITYNET-Healthy Cities was developed in Indiana as a nine-step process to facilitate a city becoming a Healthy City.
3. The first step of the CITYNET-Healthy Cities process involves building partnership to orient community leaders to the Healthy Cities process. The second step involves establishing city leaders' commitment to the Healthy Cities process. The third step involves developing a Healthy City Committee that includes multisectoral representation of the community and local resident participation. The fourth step focuses on development of leaders in communities that understand a city's potential for health promotion. The fifth step involves community assessment to identify health concerns of the community. The sixth step involves community-wide planning, which refers to identifying community priorities for health and strategic planning for local health action. The seventh step is community action for health, which includes redirecting community health services toward local health priorities and plans. The eighth step is providing data-based information to policy makers. This refers to providing policy makers with necessary data to show progress on community health action. The final step is monitoring and evaluating progress. This refers to continual collection of data, reevaluation, and redirection of health programs and policies.
4. One example of the community health nurse's role in Healthy Cities is conducting a community assessment. The nurse can use her skills to conduct surveys such as windshield and needs assessment surveys to identify community strengths and problems. Another example is providing policy makers with data-based information, such as testimony at town hall meetings on community health needs, or progress on specific health action.
5. One example of an outcome in the Healthy Cities process is found in New Castle Healthy City. The New Castle Healthy City Committee was able to promote healthy public policy by providing testimony to the city council which resulted in drafting, supporting, and passing an ordinance banning cigarette smoking in city buildings. An example of an outcome for improving personal skills is a family fitness walk, as held by Seymour Healthy City.

18 The Nursing Center: A Model for Community Health Nursing Practice

Chapter Summary

Nursing centers are well positioned to increase access to quality health care at reasonable cost. This chapter focuses on the nursing center model within the context of community health nursing and the *Healthy People 2000* goals.

Annotated Outline

I. Definition and theme
   A. Nursing center: Nurse-conducted clinic; nurse-anchored system; care that is managed by nurses.
   B. Theme: Nurses are in charge of providing care to clients in a community setting.

II. Historical perspective: The roots of nursing centers are found in the work of Lillian Wald, Margaret Sanger, and Mary Breckinridge. Visiting nursing gave way to public health nursing. Also relevant was the development of the nurse practitioner role, followed by nurses establishing independent practices. These historical influences led to the development of nursing centers. Schools of nursing began establishing nursing centers during the 1970s to provide educational experiences for students, practice opportunities for faculty, health services to the community, and sites for nursing research.

III. Contemporary conceptual model of a nursing center: The nursing center is an organization where the client has direct access to nursing services; nurses diagnose and treat, and promote health and optimal functioning; services are client-centered and reimbursed; accountability and responsibility for client care remain with the nurse; and overall accountability for the center remains with the nurse executive. The contemporary nursing center is represented by a model with four concentric circles. The outer circle is the larger community. The community determines the purposes of the nursing center; these purposes are the next inner circle. The purposes determine the roles of nurses in the center, which is the next inner circle. These roles frequently include advanced practice nurse, community health nurse, nurse executive, and clinic nurse. These roles determine the services, which is the next circle. At the very center of the model is the client.

IV. Populations served: Nursing centers serve general communities, the elderly, the poor, rural residents, culturally diverse individuals and families, the homeless, university students and families, women, HIV positive individuals, migrants, the mentally ill, the developmentally disabled or handicapped, victims of abuse, and prisoners.

V. Services provided by nursing centers: Primary prevention services provided by nursing centers include exercise classes, nutrition classes, parenting classes, prenatal care, family planning, and immunizations. Examples of secondary prevention services in centers are weight control programs, smoking cessation programs, screening for chronic diseases, developmental screening, and primary care. Tertiary prevention services include outpatient transfusion services, enterstomal therapy services, home health services, and HIV services.

VI. Nursing centers' contributions to the Healthy People 2000 goals and objectives: Populations served and services provided by nursing centers are related to these national goals and objectives.
   A. Goal I — Increase the span of healthy life for Americans: Nursing centers contribute to this goal by providing health education, aerobic exercise activities, screening tests, smoking cessation programs, and chronic disease monitoring.
   B. Goal II — Reduce health disparities among Americans: Nursing centers continue to serve an unusually high proportion of disadvantaged groups. Important services to these groups are primary care, prenatal care, and immunizations.
   C. Goal III — Achieve access to preventive services for all Americans: Nursing centers offer health promotion services such as nutrition education, and preventive services such as prenatal care. Nursing centers have increased access by focusing on reducing barriers to care.

VII. Nursing centers and the year 2000 objectives: The national health promotion and disease prevention objectives are organized in four priority areas. In the area of health promotion, nursing centers address seven of the eight priorities. Concerning health protection, nursing centers address one (oral health) of five priorities. In the area of preventive services, centers provide services in all eight priority areas. To address surveillance and data systems, nursing centers are selecting management information systems which enable them to collect data on clients served, services provided, and the efficiency, effectiveness, and cost of services.

VIII. Developing a nursing center: Nurses must have knowledge and skills in five areas to develop nursing centers: (1) integrating the center into the community; (2) determining services; (3) obtaining funding; (4) marketing; and (5) handling legal and regulatory issues. A sound business plan is needed to ensure that all aspects of beginning a center have been considered.

A. Integrating the center into the community: The steps or activities outlined in Healthy Communities 2000: Model Standards can be used in developing a plan for the center. Involving the community and developing collaborative relationships with existing community agencies and providers are critical in the planning process.

B. Determining services: The community needs assessment identifies gaps in health services that are needed and wanted by the community. Hours of service and recipients of service must be decided, along with the specific services to be offered.

C. Obtaining funding: Sources of start-up funding include personal funds, borrowed funds, or grants from federal, state, or local government agencies and foundations. There are at least five different ways to finance a center over time: grants, fees for services, contracts, third-party reimbursements, and charities. It is most advantageous to use a combination of these methods.

D. Marketing: Everything done to promote the center is marketing. A planned marketing process generates clients; provides trend analysis for growth decisions; assesses the competition; and assists in setting fees. Strategies frequently used by nursing centers include brochures, television and radio spots, newspaper public interest pieces, and word of mouth.

E. Handling legal and regulatory issues: Nurses face three major legal and regulatory restrictions as they develop nursing centers.

1. Scope of practice: State nurse practice acts that restrict the practice of advanced practice nurses (APNs) limit the services provided in nursing centers.
2. Prescriptive authority: State laws that limit the authority of APNs to prescribe are problematic for nursing centers providing primary care.
3. Eligibility for reimbursement: Nursing centers must be eligible to receive direct reimbursement for nursing services. The ability to be reimbursed by third party insurers depends largely on state statute. Federal reimbursement policy has been more favorable than that of the states.

IX. Research: While research exists on nursing centers, additional studies are needed on quality of care, efficiency, cost effectiveness, and outcomes.

Additional Critical Thinking Activities

1. Review your state's nurse practice act. What is the regulatory environment the practice act provides for advanced practice nurses?
2. What are the laws in your state on prescriptive authority and third party reimbursement? Determine your recommendations for changes in these laws to be more supportive of the practice of advanced practice nurses.
3. Visit a nursing center in your region or state. Estimate the probability of the center remaining open in the next decade. Use supporting evidence to justify your position.

Critical Analysis Questions

1. In a nursing center:
   a. the client has direct access to nursing services.
   b. nurses diagnose and treat.
   c. nurses promote health and optimal functioning.
   d. services are reimbursed.
   e. all of the above
2. Nursing centers are responsive to the needs of the community when:
   a. the staff determines the needs of the community.
   b. the nurse executive determines the services needed by the community.
   c. the community is involved in assessing its needs.
3. Advanced practice nurses are:
   a. nurse practitioners.
   b. clinical nurse specialists.
   c. nurse midwives.
   d. all of the above.
4. The following nursing role is not found in a nursing center:
   a. staff nurse
   b. clinic nurse
   c. advanced practice nurse
   d. nurse executive
5. Nursing centers care for an unusually high proportion of:
   a. the middle class.

b. racial minorities.
c. American workers.
d. all of the above.

6. Services provided by nursing centers:
   a. are mostly primary preventive services.
   b. are primary and secondary preventive services.
   c. address primary, secondary, and tertiary levels of prevention.
7. Primary care is:
   a. not provided by nursing centers.
   b. provided by some nursing centers.
   c. provided by many nursing centers.
8. Nursing center services address the following year 2000 goals:
   a. reduce the number of hospitalizations for Americans
   b. reduce health disparities among Americans
   c. reduce the rate of chronic diseases for Americans
   d. all of the above
9. A nursing center can be financed by:
   a. grants.
   b. fee for service.
   c. contracts.
   d. all of the above.
10. Nurses face major legal and regulatory restrictions in developing a nursing center that can include:
    a. obtaining a business license.
    b. the state nurse practice act.
    c. state clinic certification.
    d. all of the above.

Answer Key

1. e
2. c
3. d
4. a
5. b
6. c
7. c
8. b
9. d
10. b

19 Case Management

Chapter Summary

As the emphasis on prevention, health promotion, health protection, and risk reduction becomes more pronounced in the health care delivery system, the community health nurse will play a predominate role in supporting continuity of care along the health care continuum. Two essential nursing functions are necessary to provide uninterrupted access to community resources: advocacy; and case/care management with individuals, families, groups, and communities. Regardless of the target group for community health nursing services, a systematic process for each is congruent with the five steps of the nursing process.

Self-care responsibility for consumers of health care is a value upheld in current health policy and is pointedly articulated in the Health Objectives for the Year 2000. Health care consumers are capable of informed decision making based on education and the integration of personal health values in their life style. For clients who are not realizing their capacity for self-determinism, the nurse can empower clients through nursing action that seeks to engage and support decision making.

Annotated Outline

I. Case/care management: A health care delivery process that seeks to plan, organize, coordinate, and monitor services and resources to respond to an individual's health care needs.
   A. Managed care is an organized program to control access and utilization of health services. An example of a managed care organization is a health maintenance organization like Kaiser Permanente or Group Health Association. Managed care organizations will consume a larger portion of the health care options in the future. Managed health care is a delivery system, while case/care management is a process existing in those systems. Case management can also exist outside of managed care organizations.
   B. Community health nurses are uniquely positioned to provide case management within their scope of practice due to their experience with multiple disciplines and providers, linkages with community structures, and knowledge of client health status in the community.
   C. Activities of case management include case finding, screening and intake, assessment, identification of the problems, problem prioritizing and planning, advocation of client's interests, arrangement for service delivery, monitoring of clients during service, reassessment, evaluation, documentation, and designing and monitoring caremaps/critical paths/multidisciplinary action plans.
   D. Case management activities may or may not include physical/psychological care with the client.
   E. Providers of case management include public nonproviders, private nonproviders, acute provider systems, and long-term provider systems.
   F. The regulation of case managers through credentialing is being explored by federal and state entities.
   G. Legal and ethical issues for case management include kickbacks from recipients of referrals, informed consent and decision making, self-determinism, competition for scarce resources, liability, and accountability of case managers.
   H. Case management is a nursing action inherent in community health nursing practice to promote continuity of care.

II. Advocacy: Nursing actions that inform, support, and affirm clients in their goal of self-determination. It is one function of nursing that supports the goal of continuity of care.
   A. To fulfill the role of advocacy, nursing actions are predicated on the clients' current and future capacity for self-determination.
   B. The clients' health-illness trajectory and the community resource capacity will influence the scope of actions the nurse uses to implement the advocacy role.
   C. Conflict potential is present in advocacy. Sources of conflict include role expectations, scope of practice, provider and community values, client values, interdisciplinary practice patterns, conflict of loyalties, functions, and scarce resources.

D. The information exchange process used with clients promotes amplification, clarification, and verification of the client goals and actions. Clients who decline to be informed and participative need to understand the consequences of their decision.

E. Affirmation activity with clients recognizes the dynamic nature of changing resources and client needs as it encourages reevaluation and rededication to self-determination after initial choices are made.

F. Strengthening one's capacity for problem solving is an important responsibility for professional and client growth. It can be enhanced by implementing techniques to illuminate values and generate alternatives. Brainstorming and problem-purpose-expansion are two methods to enhance problem-solving skills.

G. Ethical issues in advocacy include barriers to self-determinism in the midst of scarce resources, accountability to employer and client, and informed consent.

III. Conflict management skills: Essential to effective case management to promote continuity of care. Activities to manage conflict range from simple to complex, depending on the conflict perspective—facts, methods, objectives, and values.

A. Each individual exhibits a behavioral orientation of assertiveness and cooperation when engaging in conflict management—competing, collaborating, accommodating, avoiding, or compromising. Orientations can change, depending on the situation and progress in the conflict process.

B. Conflicts can follow stages that are cyclical—antecedent conditions, trigger events, escalation, de-escalation, and aftermath.

C. Negotiation is a strategic process used to move conflicting parties toward an outcome. The outcome may be distributive (enlarging one's gain at another's expense) or integrative (mutual advantages overriding individual gains). Negotiation stages include prenegotiation, negotiation, and aftermath.

1. Prenegotiation: Activities to get parties' agreement to enter negotiation.
2. Negotiation: Period when parties establish issues and agenda, advance demands and uncover interests, discover new options, and work out an agreement.
3. Aftermath: Period after agreement when parties experience the consequence of their decision.

D. The community health nurse must have knowledge of resources available to provide care postdischarge, and must coordinate the resources to be delivered. Inherent in the success of this process are the skills of teamwork and collaboration.

IV. Achieving collaboration: A developmental process that encompasses seven steps: awareness, tentative exploration and mutual acknowledgment, trust building, collegiality, consensus, commitment, and collaboration.

V. Continuity of care: A desirable goal in the delivery of health care as a client utilizes multiple providers and services. It includes linkages with providers and services which contribute to a client's health status through an identifiable process.

A. The goal of continuity of care can be facilitated through nursing actions in advocacy and case/care management. Advocacy and continuity of care are both standards in the American Nurses Association of Standards for Community Health and Home Health Nursing Practice.

B. Case management is based on the following client data: (1) sociodemographic/financial, (2) health status, (3) functional status, (4) environmental barriers, (5) nursing and other health care requirements, (6) family and community support, (7) patient/family/significant others, (8) formal and informal goals, resources, and options, and (9) benefit coverage.

C. When nurses make referrals, they are directing clients for information, treatment, assistance, support, or help with decisions. Referrals should be written and augmented with the opportunity for verbal discussion.

D. Coordination includes planning, linking clients with services, and communicating among clients and providers. Activities may include completing paperwork, supervising staff, exchanging information, arranging services, and collaboratively planning care.

Additional Critical Thinking Activities

1. From your readings, define the following terms:
   A. Continuity of care.
   B. Advocacy.
   C. Autonomy.
   D. Case/care management.
   E. Managed care.
   F. Conflict management.
   G. Collaboration.
   H. Self-determinism.
   I. CareMAPS/critical paths.
2. In class or in a conference with your peers, discuss the definitions and compare them to your own.
   A. How are they similar or different?
   B. Give reasons why they differ.
   C. What actions have you observed in nursing staff to support these activities?

3. Interview a nurse and a social worker. Ask the following of each one:
   A. How do they see their roles in client advocacy and case management?
   B. What activities are performed as an advocate and/or a case manager?
   C. What conflicts do they confront as an advocate and/or case manager?

   Compare and discuss their responses.
4. Attend a community action meeting that focuses on the health care needs of a community.
   A. Identify the consumer advocates.
   B. Who appears to be in conflict?
   C. What techniques are used to manage the conflict?
5. Spend two days with a nurse case manager.
   A. Identify his/her activities.
   B. Measure the amount of time he/she spends on each of the following: referrals, coordinations, screening, monitoring, and documenting.
   C. Discuss his/her opinion of the necessity of credentialing for those performing in the role of case manager.
   D. Ask that person to share perceptions of legal and ethical issues in that role.

Critical Analysis Questions

1. Define the following terms:
   a. Continuity of care
   b. Advocacy
   c. Autonomy
   d. Case/care management
   e. Managed care
   f. Conflict management
   g. Collaboration
   h. Self-determinism
   i. CareMAPS/critical paths
2. Identify and explain the seven stages necessary to achieve collaboration.
3. Identify three activities used by the nurse to fulfill the advocacy function.
4. Identify the activities used in case/care management.
5. Name three ethical and legal issues common to performing advocacy and case management activities.

Answer Key

1. See answers in text chapter and glossary.
2. Awareness, tentative exploration and mutual acknowledgment, trust building, collegiality, consensus, and commitment.
3. Amplification, clarification, and verification.
4. Case finding; screening; intake assessment; identification of problems; advocation of client interests; arrangement for service delivery; monitoring; reassessment; and evaluation and documentation.
5. Among those that could be included are informed consent, conflict of allegiance between employer, payor, and client, competition for scarce resources, abandonment, negligence, fraud, abuse, and referral kickbacks.

20 Disaster Management

Chapter Summary

Disasters, man-made and natural, are inevitable in this country and around the world. However, there are ways that people and their communities can prevent or manage disasters to decrease the likelihood of morbidity and mortality. This chapter will describe such management techniques throughout the preparedness, response, and recovery phases of disaster. The community health nurse's role throughout these phases will be highlighted.

Annotated Outline

I. Definitions
   A. A disaster is any man-made or natural event that causes destruction and devastation that cannot be alleviated without assistance.
   B. Preparedness is personal, professional, or community knowledge and plans used to prevent or alleviate a disaster.
   C. A natural disaster is an event controlled by nature, such as floods, tornadoes, and drought.
   D. A man-made disaster is an event caused by humans which could be prevented, such as war, vehicular accidents, explosions.
   E. Response is national, regional, local, or individual action taken to prevent or offer assistance in a disaster.
   F. Triage is the process of separating casualties and allocating treatment based on the victim's potential for survival.
   G. Recovery is the stage of a disaster when all involved agencies and individuals pull together to restore the economic and civic life of a community.
   H. A level I disaster requires activation by the local Emergency Medical System in cooperation with local community organizations, such as the American Red Cross and Salvation Army.
   I. A level II disaster requires more of a regional response requiring several casualty protocols.
   J. A level III disaster is one in which a federal emergency has been declared due to widespread destruction.
   K. The federal response plan becomes enacted when it is obvious that a significant disaster or emergency will overwhelm the capability of state and local governments to carry out the extensive emergency operations necessary to save lives and protect property.
   L. Disaster medical assistance teams (DMATS) are specially trained civilian physicians, nurses, and other health care personnel that can be sent to a disaster site within hours of activation.
   M. Emergency support functions are designated tasks that primary agencies within the government are mandated to carry out in the event the federal response plan becomes enacted.
   N. A delayed stress reaction is stress that occurs once the disaster is over.

II. Disasters
   A. Defining disasters: Disasters, whether man-made or natural, are causing increased deaths, destruction, and financial outlay. Overcrowded cities and urbanization have caused stressors that promote civil unrest and ensuing riots. In addition, the overcrowding of cities has forced populations to build their communities in areas that are more vulnerable to disasters, such as coastal and flood plains. Finally, modern warfare has markedly increased the risk of injury and death from disaster.
   B. International decade for natural disaster reduction was a declaration made by the United Nations (for the 1990s) to educate the world regarding disaster reduction, and to end the fatalistic approach that so often accompanies disasters.

III. Preparedness: The first component of the disaster management cycle is preparedness. Successful disaster preparedness depends on the existence of a realistic and well-rehearsed plan.
   A. Personal preparedness entails a plan for keeping oneself ready for disaster, both mentally and physically. Individuals who are not prepared personally will have less to give to family, community, job, and other disaster victims. Personal preparation allow nurses to attend to patient needs sooner than one might anticipate.

Checklists are available to help nurses and their families prepare for disaster before it strikes.

B. Professional preparedness requires nurses to become aware of and to understand the disaster plans at their workplace and how the plan fits in with the community's disaster plan. The more adequately prepared nurses are, the more they will be able to function in a leadership capacity and assist others towards a smoother recovery phase. Disaster training is offered by organizations such as the American Red Cross to help nurses and other professionals provide assistance within their own communities, as well as to other stricken communities and countries that would benefit from their expertise.

C. Community preparedness requires that the community health nurse become familiar with the community disaster plan of the community in which they live. Community health nurses should remain vigilant as to their role in the community and should educate community leaders as to what they have to offer in terms of helping the community prepare for, respond to, and recover from a disaster. Having a realistic, easy-to-understand disaster plan, enacting community-wide mock disaster drills, and having an adequate community disaster warning system are three important ways a community can adequately prepare for disaster.

D. The role of the community health nurse in disaster preparedness is multi-faceted. The nurse, once adequately trained, can initiate or update disaster plans within the place of employment or community, and can ensure that adequate disaster drills are carried out. This role entails a knowledge of available community resources and an understanding of how the community will work together once disaster strikes. The community health nurse is also in a unique position to provide an updated record of vulnerable populations within the community and to educate these populations regarding what impact the disaster might have on them. This role is in addition to educating the general population, including family and colleagues, and the nurse's ongoing role of assessing and reporting environmental hazards.

E. Mass casualty drills or mock disasters are carried out to promote confidence, develop skills, coordinate activities, and coordinate participants. It is critical that those persons who will be involved in the actual disaster be involved in the drill. Mock disaster drills should never create a misplaced sense of security.

F. Agencies involved in disaster preparedness include the American Red Cross, the Salvation Army, many church denominations, and other voluntary organizations. Business and labor organizations should develop and integrate their disaster plans with the overall community disaster plan. Local government coordinates the development of the community plan and conducts evaluation exercises.

IV. Response: The second component of the disaster management cycle is response. Preparing adequately, expecting the unexpected, and remaining flexible are all important in successfully getting through this phase.

A. The level of a disaster determines the extent of agency involvement. A level I disaster is a local disaster requiring activation by the local Emergency Medical System in cooperation with local community organizations. A level II disaster requires more of a regional response and several casualty protocols. A level III disaster is one in which a federal emergency has been declared due to widespread destruction and the inability of local resources to fully respond.

B. The federal response plan becomes activated when it becomes evident that the disaster will overwhelm the capability of state and local governments to carry out the extensive emergency operations necessary to save lives and protect property. The plan sets in motion national interagency coordination with the affected state to deliver twelve emergency support functions such as mass sheltering, mass feeding, and the establishment of surveillance systems. Disaster medial assistance teams (DMATS), which consist of specially trained civilian physicians, nurses, and other health professionals, are available to assist with triage and continuing medical care within hours of activation.

C. Disasters affect communities in many ways depending on the type, cause, and location of the disaster, its magnitude and extent of damage, the duration, and the amount of warning that was provided. Individuals within the community also react differently to disasters depending on their age, cultural background, health status, social support structure, and their general adaptability to crisis. Common initial reactions to disaster include an extreme sense of urgency, an obsession with personal losses, fear, panic, disbelief, reluctance to abandon property, disorientation, difficulty in making decisions, and more. Delayed reactions include insomnia, headaches, guilt, jealousy and resentment, apathy, depression, and domestic violence. The longer it takes for structural repairs and other clean-up, the longer the psychological effects can last.

D. The role of the community health nurse in disaster response depends a great deal on the nurse's past experience, her role in institution and community preparedness, her specialized training, and her special interest. Although community health nurses are most valued for their expertise in community assessment, case-finding and referring, prevention, health education, surveillance, and working with aggregates, the key to a successful response is flexibility and doing whatever it takes to preserve life and to prevent further injury.

E. Shelter management is an ideal assignment for many community health nurses due to their comfort with delivering aggregate health promotion, disease prevention, and emotional support. Although there may be physical health needs to attend to, especially among the elderly and chronically ill, many of the predominant problems in shelters revolve around stress, and even boredom. Community health nurses should use common sense approaches to caring for disaster victims, such as listening, helping in decision making, supporting, and assigning tasks to those who are able to assist. Other activities that the nurse will be involved in include assessment and referral, assurance of medical needs, first aid, meal serving, record keeping, ensuring emergency communications and transportation, and providing a safe environment.

F. International relief efforts occur on a daily basis around the world. Many times other countries request assistance from America, and sometimes American disaster and relief workers are not welcomed, but instead go at the request of the United Nations. Community health nurses can become involved in such efforts after an intense period of training and experience.

G. Psychological stress of disaster workers depends on the nature of the disaster, their role in the disaster, individual stamina, and other environmental factors. Added stress is created when the nurse is from the same community in which the disaster has struck, particularly if the nurse is a victim as well. Stress reactions include anger, powerlessness, feelings of guilt, irritability, and fatigue. Delayed stress reactions, or those that occur once the disaster is over, include exhaustion and an inability to adjust to the slower pace of work or home. Specific strategies for dealing with stress should be adhered to, to prevent prolonging the recovery period. Some of these strategies include getting enough sleep, providing mutual support, and using humor to break the tension and to provide relief.

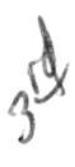

V. Recovery: The third component of the disaster management cycle is recovery. This stage occurs as all involved agencies pull together to restore the economic and civic life of the community.

A. The role of the community health nurse in disaster recovery is multi-faceted. Flexibility remains an important component of assisting others towards recovery. Teaching health promotion and disease prevention are key activities as physical and psychological problems from clean-up efforts are incurred, along with the threat of communicable disease. Case-finding and referral for chronic mental distress and environmental health hazards is important.

Additional Critical Thinking Activities

1. Identify the roles of the community health nurse in the preparedness, response, and recovery stages of a disaster.
2. What roles in a disaster is the community health nurse best suited for, and why?

Critical Analysis Questions

1. The number of man-made disasters and ensuing deaths has risen sharply because of:
   a. urbanization and over-crowding of cities.
   b. people living in areas that are more vulnerable to disasters.
   c. modern warfare techniques.
   d. b and c only.
   e. all of the above.
2. The following should be done to further prevent man-made disasters:
   a. more stringent screening for substance abuse for those involved in mass transportation
   b. increased installation of smoke and carbon-monoxide alarms in homes and businesses
   c. increasingly stringent engineering codes for buildings and bridges
   d. all of the above
3. Which of the following can be classified as a natural disaster?
   a. fire
   b. pollution
   c. drought
   d. a and c only
4. List at least five items that should be stored as disaster emergency items.
5. The most important consideration for a community in preparing for disaster is:
   a. a strong and well-prepared fire and rescue unit.
   b. an adequate warning system to guide citizens to safety.
   c. a concise, realistic, and well-rehearsed disaster plan.

d. open communication and the ability to work together at times of crisis.

6. Community health nurses help prevent man-made disasters by:
   a. assessing for and reporting environmental health hazards.
   b. ensuring up-do-date immunization schedules.
   c. teaching proper hygiene.
   d. a and b only.
   e. all of the above.
7. True or False? A level I disaster does not require the services of community organizations.
8. A mass shooting in a local community building is what level of disaster?
   a. level I
   b. level II
   c. level III
9. All of the following are common reactions to disasters except:
   a. need to help others.
   b. panic and urgency.
   c. chest pain.
   d. disorientation.
10. The most important attribute of a community health nurse assisting in a disaster is:
    a. first aid and CPR certification.
    b. flexibility.
    c. previous hands-on experience with the community's mock disaster drill.
    d. previous critical care experience.
11. Which of the following are types of information included in an initial post-disaster community assessment?
    a. geographic extent of disaster's impact
    b. availability of shelters
    c. clothing needs
    d. a and b only
    e. all of the above
12. All of the following are common examples of delayed stress responses in disaster workers except:
    a. disappointment.
    b. frustration.
    c. guilt over not having done more.
    d. domestic violence.
    e. anger.
13. One of the most important roles for the community health nurse post-disaster is:
    a. case-finding and referral.
    b. health education.
    c. keeping immunization records up to date.
    d. all of the above.

Answer Key

1. e
2. d
3. c
4. Three-day supply of water, and food that won't spoil.
   One change of clothing and footwear per person, and one blanket or sleeping bag per person.
   First aid kit, including prescription medications.
   Emergency tools, including a battery-powered radio, flashlight, and plenty of extra batteries.
   Candles and matches.
   Extra set of car keys, credit card, cash or travelers checks.
   Sanitation supplies, including toilet paper, feminine hygiene products, soap, and plastic garbage bags.
   Special items for infant, elderly, or disabled family members.
   Extra set of glasses.
5. c
6. e
7. False
8. b
9. c
10. b
11. d
12. d
13. d

21 Program Management

Chapter Summary

Assessing, planning, implementation, and evaluation are essential elements of program management for the health care system and nursing.

History indicates that with seemingly unlimited resources, health care services and nursing services developed in a primarily unplanned manner in reaction to perceived crises or needs. Nurses continue to be told that they "react instead of act," implying that perceived crises or needs continue to be the basis for nursing care delivery, instead of planning to act based on assessed needs for nursing care delivery.

This chapter focuses attention on how nurses can act instead of react by planning programs that can be evaluated for their effectiveness and efficacy in meeting their social purpose.

Annotated Outline

I. Definitions and goals
   A. Program—an organized response designed to meet the assessed needs of individuals, families, groups, or communities by reducing or eliminating one or more health problems.
   B. Planning—selecting and carrying out a series of actions designed to achieve stated goals.
   C. Formative evaluation—instituted for the purpose of assessing the degree to which objectives are met or planned activities are conducted.
   D. Summative evaluation—instituted to assess program outcomes or as a follow-up of the results of program activities.

   The term *program* refers to an organized response to a problem, and *evaluation* refers to a process to determine whether the program is achieving its purpose.

II. Historical overview of health care planning and evaluation: Historically, society has financed program planning and evaluation primarily through government. As the health care delivery system has grown in the past years, emphasis in health planning and exploration has increased. Factors fostering increased emphasis are advancements in health care technology, consumer education and increased health care technology, consumer education and increased health care expectations, third party payers, unionization of health workers, urbanization, increased health risks, work force shortages, and increasing health care costs.

III. Benefits of program planning: Systematic planning for meeting client needs benefits clients, nurses, and the employing agencies. Planning usually reflects a desire on the part of the planners to reduce the gap between the program goals and the realities of program implementation and to diminish the unanticipated occurrences that may result during program implementation.

IV. Planning process: The elements of planning include problems diagnosis, identification of problem solutions, analysis and comparison of alternative methods, and selection of the best plan and planning methods. Nutt describes a five-stage process that includes problem formulation, conceptualization, detailing, evaluation, and implementation.
   A. Assessment of need: The initial and most critical step in planning for a health program is the assessment of client need. The following are five basic steps in the needs assessment process: identify the client population and the needs to be met, specify the size and distribution of the client group, set boundaries for the client group, clarify the perspectives of the program clients, and identify the program resources.
   B. Needs assessment tools: The major tools used are census data, key informants, community forums, surveys of existing community agencies, surveys of residents of the community, and statistical indicators.

V. Program evaluation
   A. Benefits of program evaluation: The major benefit of program evaluation is that it determines whether the program is fulfilling its purpose. Evaluation data may be used to justify expanding the program, or they may be used to justify reducing the program size or even closing it.
   B. Planning and the evaluative process: Planning for the evaluative process is an integral part of program planning and should not be considered as something begun after the program has

been in operation for several months. Six steps are used for planning program evaluation:

1. Identify the relevant people for evaluation.
2. Arrange preliminary meetings to discuss the questions of whether the group wants an evaluation.
3. Make a decision about whether the evaluation should be carried out.
4. Examine relevant literature.
5. Plan the evaluative methodology.
6. Write a proposal outlining the program and the evaluative functions and process.

C. Evaluation aspects: Four aspects of evaluation may be employed, depending on the reasons program evaluation is being planned.

1. Evaluation of relevance—need for the program.
2. Progress—the tracking of program activities to meet objectives.
3. Efficiency—the relationship between program outcomes and resources expended.
4. Effectiveness and impact—the ability to meet program objectives and the results of program efforts, as evidenced by the long-term changes in the client population.

D. The evaluative process, which should be operational at the onset of the program, includes goal setting, determining goal measurement, measuring goal attainment, identifying goal-attaining activities, instituting the activities, measuring the goal effect, and making a judgment about achievement of program goals.

E. Formulation of objectives for evaluation: Program objectives should include the specific behavior, the conditions under which the behavior is shown, and the minimum standard of performance.

It is customary for objectives to be stated in levels. Program activities are planned to ensure attainment of all levels of objectives.

F. Sources of program evaluation: Major sources of information for program evaluation are program participants, program records, and community indexes.

VI. Advanced planning methods and evaluation models: Procedural methods are used by the community health nurse clinical specialist when planning and evaluating programs. Five planning methods are discussed.

A. Planning Programming and Budget System (PPBS): This is an outcome-oriented system used to determine the most efficient method of resource allocation. Steps involved in PPBS include (1) setting program goals, (2) defining measurable program objectives, (3) choosing the method for accomplishing the objectives, and (4) developing a program budget with justification for minimizing costs while maximizing program benefits.

B. Program Planning Method (PPM): This is a five-stage process designed to involve clients more directly in the planning process. This process involves clients, procedures, and administrators in identifying the problem, client identification of solutions, problem presentation to administrators by clients and providers, identifying alternatives, and selecting the best plan to resolve the problem.

C. Program Evaluation Review Techniques (PERT): This method is used for large-scale projects that require planning, scheduling, and controlling a large number of activities. This method focuses attention on the key parts of a program, on potential problems with movement toward the goal, on progress evaluation, and on a prompt reporting method to facilitate decision making.

D. Critical Path Method (CPM): This method is somewhat similar to PERT in that it focuses attention on program activities, sequencing of activities, and the estimated time it will take to complete the project from beginning to end. This method is becoming popular in health care delivery as a quality process monitor.

E. The Multi-Attribute Technique (MAUT): This is a planning method based on decision theory, which can be used to make a decision about an individual client or about a national health care program. This method outlines ten steps which include a quantifiable measure to be used in prioritizing and in reaching a decision.

F. Donabedian's Structure-Process-Outcome model, the Tracer method, and case registers are suggested methods for use in program evaluation.

VII. Cost studies applied in health care delivery: Excessive and inefficient use of goods and services in health care delivery is viewed by many as the major cause of rising costs in health care delivery. Four types of cost studies are used to evaluate the safety, efficiency, and efficacy of medical procedures. Few data are available about the costs of nursing.

A. Cost accounting: Cost accounting studies are performed to find the actual budgetary cost of a program, procedure, or technique.

B. Cost benefit: Cost benefit studies are a way of assessing the desirability of a program, procedure, or technique by placing a specific quantifiable value on all costs and all benefits of the variables to be evaluated.

C. Cost efficiency: Cost efficiency analysis involves the analysis of actual costs to perform a number of services at different volumes if the same standards are applied.

D. Cost effectiveness: Cost effectiveness analysis is a measure of the quality of a program, procedure, or technique as it relates to costs.

Additional Critical Thinking Activities

1. You have been asked by a voluntary health agency to evaluate how well it is meeting its target population's needs. Delineate the steps you would take to determine this. Include determination of client needs, appropriate tools, application of model or technique that would be appropriate, data-gathering measures, sources, and analysis of benefits of the program. Write a summary of the report that you would present to the voluntary agency.
2. Select two articles from community health nursing journals that describe the steps of planning and evaluation. Specify, if possible, what kind of model in either planning or evaluation the author is utilizing.
3. Based on your reading in this chapter, discuss the impact that planning and evaluation can have on direct client services.

Critical Analysis Questions

1. True or False? Planning is a conscious design by nurse and client of a desired client future state.
2. True or False? The most critical step in planning for a health program is comparing alternative methods for arriving at problem resolution.
3. True or False? Systematic planning for meeting client needs is only of benefit to the agency sponsoring the program.
4. True or False? Planning for program evaluation begins after the completion of the program.
5. True or False? Program evaluation determines whether client needs are being met and whether the program is fulfilling its purpose.
6. True or False? Outcome evaluation in community health nursing measures the changes in client health status as a result of nursing interventions.
7. True or False? The reactions, judgments, and feelings of program participants are *not* essential to effective program evaluation.
8. True or False? A decline in morbidity or mortality may be an effective measure of a successful program.

Answer Key

1. True
2. False
3. False
4. False
5. True
6. True
7. False
8. True

22 Quality Management

Chapter Summary

As the health care delivery system changes in response to rising costs and decreasing access to care, quality of care continues to be a central issue. Society is demanding greater accountability and increased effectiveness from the system. Both consumers and providers have a vested interest in the quality of health care. Consumers want the best possible health care for their money while providers, though ethically bound to "first do no harm," will gain more in a managed care environment when people remain healthy. Total Quality Management/Continuous Quality Improvement (TQM/CQI) combined with traditional quality assurance/improvement (QA/QI) are tools used in industry to assure the public that it is getting the best value for their health care dollar.

The major thrust of QA/QI programs resulted because of the vast changes that have occurred in the health care system over time, including increasing third party insurance coverage; increasing involvement of federal government in the health care system; increasing demand for service; changing consumer expectations for cost, accessibility, and equality; increasing technological advances; changing population demography; rising costs; increasing numbers of health professionals providing care; and the increasingly monopolistic character of the system. TQM/CQI is relatively new to the health care arena but encompasses traditional QA/QI methods to improve overall system quality. TQM/CQI is a process-driven, customer-oriented philosophy of management. While QA/QI focuses on problem detection, TQM/CQI focuses on the problem prevention with the goal of continuous improvement.

Data are collected and records are maintained on all clients and operational processes of the health care system to provide complete information about the extent and quality of care given within the system. Accurate data are an integral part of a total quality management program.

Annotated Outline

I. Definitions and goals: *Quality* can be defined as a continuous striving for excellence and a conformity to specifications or guidelines. *Total Quality Management/Continuous Quality Improvement* is a process-driven, customer-oriented philosophy of management that embodies teamwork, employee empowerment, individual responsibility, and continuous improvement of system processes which lead to improved outcomes. *Quality assurance/improvement* is defined as the promise or guarantee that certain standards of excellence are being met in the delivery of care.

The goals of quality programs are to ensure client satisfaction, to deliver quality client care, and to demonstrate the health providers' efforts to fulfill their societal responsibility.

II. Historical development of quality improvement in nursing and health care: Quality assurance in the United States dates back to 1892, when licensure of nurses was first introduced. Current developments in quality assurance include the ANA quality assurance model, the ANA study of nurse credentials, and the NLN study of accreditation. Two efforts specifically directed toward strengthening community health nursing practice have been the development of frameworks for community health nursing practice by ANA and APHA and the national consensus conference on public health nursing practice and education.

III. Approaches for quality improvement: Two major categories of approaches exist in quality assurance—the general and the specific. The general approach examines the person's or agency's ability to meet established criteria or standards at a given time.

The general quality control process that indicates the attainment of minimum standards by the person or agency is called *credentialing*, a mechanism for monitoring the quality of structure.

Specific approaches to quality improvement use techniques to evaluate health care delivery processes and identified instances of provider/client interaction. The overall goal of specific quality improvement approaches is to monitor the care delivery processes and outcomes of client care.

A. General approaches

1. Licensure: Legal or mandatory contract between a profession and the state in which the profession is granted control over entry into or exit from the profession and control over the quality of professional practice.

2. Accreditation: Voluntary approach to quality control used for institutions as licensure, primarily used for individuals. Accreditation of institutions assumes that certain standards of physical and organizational structure assure quality health care or quality education at a given time.
3. Certification: Usually a voluntary process within professions that looks at a person's educational achievements, experience, and professional achievements through the process of examination to determine an individual's qualification as a specialist.
4. Other: Three other general approaches to quality assurance/improvement exist and are defined in the ANA study of credentialing in nursing.
   a. Charter: Mechanism by which a state government grants corporate status to institutions, with or without rights to award degrees.
   b. Recognition: Defined as a process whereby one agency accepts the credentialing status of and the credentials conferred by another.
   c. Academic degrees: Titles awarded to individuals who are recognized by degree-granting institutions as having completed a predetermined plan in a branch of learning.

B. Specific approaches
1. Total Quality Management/Continuous Quality Improvement: A process-driven, customer-oriented philosophy of management that embodies leadership, teamwork, employee empowerment, individual responsibility, and continuous improvement to processes which lead to improved client outcomes. The goal of TQM/CQI is to maximize customer satisfaction by delivery of quality care.
2. Peer review committee: Most common specific approach to quality assurance in the United States. These committees were designed to monitor client-specific aspects of care appropriate to levels of care. The audit has been the major tool used by peer review committees.
3. Utilization review: Differs from peer review in that utilization review is directed toward assuring that care was actually needed and the cost was appropriate for the level of care provided. There are basically three types of utilization review: prospective, concurrent, and retrospective.
4. Risk management: Often a part of a quality assurance program. It is designed to reduce grievance and liability of the agency.
5. Professional Standards Review Organizations (PSROs): Established in 1972 as an amendment to the Social Security Act. They were to be publicly mandated utilization and peer review programs. The law provided that medical, hospital, and nursing home care provided under Medicare, Medicaid, and Title V Maternal and Child Health Programs would be reviewed for appropriateness and necessity and would be reimbursed accordingly. As a result of the 1982 Tax Reconciliation Act, PSROs were replaced by Professional Review Organizations (PROs).
6. Evaluative studies: Studies of quality health care that have grown, which have been widely used to evaluate health care. Examples are Donabedian's Evaluative Model, the Sentinel Model, and the Tracer Model.
7. Client satisfaction assessment: Another specific approach to measuring quality of care. The client satisfaction survey can be used to measure structure, process, and outcomes of care given.
8. Malpractice litigation: Nursing is not immune from malpractice litigation.

IV. Model quality assurance program: This program ensures that the results of an organized activity are consistent with the expectations of that activity. ANA has identified seven basic components of a quality assurance program: identifying values, identifying standards and criteria, selecting measures to assess attainment of standards and criteria, making interpretations about the strengths and weaknesses of care given, identifying alternative courses of action, choosing courses of action, and taking action. These are best described using Donabedian's framework for evaluating health care programs.

V. Health provider education: Education is inherent in any quality assurance program. Behaviorally anchored and objectives-oriented ratings are more useful in pinpointing behaviors specific to groups and individuals, respectively, and provide better data for staff development and better data for developing job descriptions.

VI. Records
A. Purposes of records: Records are necessary to the communication structure of the health care organization. Accurate and complete records are required by law and must be kept by all agencies.
B. Community health agency records: Within the community health agency, many types of records are kept and used to predict population trends in a community, to identify health needs and problems, to analyze health trends, to plan programs, to evaluate programs, to prepare and

justify budgets, and to make administrative decisions. Kinds of community health agency records are reports of vital statistics, records of occupational and environmental health and injury and abuse, clinical records, financial records, and service records.

Additional Critical Thinking Activities

1. Compare and contrast the traditional performance standard QA model with the TQM/CQI model.
2. Go to the library and choose a few volumes of the major nursing journals from the 1950s and 1960s.
   A. Scan the journal articles and note the number related to quality assurance/improvement.
   B. Choose several volumes of the same journals in the 1970s and 1980s and 1990s, and note the number of articles related to quality assurance/improvement and total quality management/continuous improvement.
   C. State the differences in the focus of quality assurance/improvement articles of the early decades versus the later decades. Then state the differences in the QA/QI articles versus the TQM/CQI articles.
   D. Analyze the differences in number and focus between the decades.
   E. State your reasons for thinking a difference exists.
3. After gathering data from your reading, do the following:
   A. Develop a total quality program.
   B. Identify the approaches and techniques you would use in this program. Give your reasons.
   C. Include in your plan the mechanisms for evaluating your total quality program.
4. Do the following on your next clinical day:
   A. Ask your instructor or the staff nurse to whom you are assigned to share with you the type of quality program used by your clinical agency. Ask what type of data are collected on work processes and what other records are kept at the community health agency. In addition, ask about the organizational structure of the agency.
   B. Request permission to see examples of work process data and of each kind of record kept at the agency (e.g., clinical, service, financial).
   C. Explore the reasons each record is kept. You may be able to find this information in the agency's policy manual.

Critical Analysis Questions

1. True or False? Total Quality Management/Continuous Quality Improvement exists best in a flat organizational structure.
2. True or False? QA/QI seeks to eliminate errors in process before negative outcomes can occur rather than waiting until after the fact to correct individual performance.
3. True or False? Provider accountability is an implicit goal of quality assurance.
4. True or False? Licensure is the oldest quality assurance approach in nursing in the United States.
5. ____________________ is the general quality control process indicating the attainment of minimum standards by a person or agency.
6. List the four components of quality care.
7. List the general approaches to quality assurance/improvement.
8. List the specific approaches to quality assurance/improvement.
9. Identify the components of a quality productivity model.
10. What purpose do records serve?

Answer Key

1. True
2. False
3. True
4. True
5. Credentialing
6. Professional performance, efficient use of resources, minimal risk to the client of illness or injury associated with care, patient satisfaction.
7. Licensure, accreditation, certification, charter, recognition, education degrees.
8. Total Quality Management/Continuous Quality Improvement, staff review committees, Professional Review Organizations, utilization review, evaluative studies, client satisfaction, malpractice litigation.
9. Quality Control: Measurable process stated in written terms (policy and procedure). Quality Assurance: Standard by which the measurable process is validated (audit). Quality continuation: Constant self-measurement by known standards. Quality improvement: culmination on control, assurance, and continuation.
10. Provide information about client, indicate extent and quality of services, resolve legal issues, provide data for education and research.

23 Group Approaches in Community Health

Chapter Summary

Working with groups is an important skill for community health nurses. In daily practice, nurses routinely plan and implement health-focused action with clients, other nurses, and other health care workers. In some educational programs, nursing students participate in groups and are encouraged to observe their own responses to group membership and group leadership. Such study and experience enrich the students' knowledge of group concepts and aids their application of these concepts to groups of clients, work groups, and community groups.

Basic group concepts presented in this chapter may be used in nursing practice to promote individual health through group work, to identify community groups and their contribution to community life, and to assist groups in working toward community health goals.

Annotated Outline

I. Group concepts: Group concepts are used in nursing practice to promote individual health through groups work, to identify community groups and their contribution to community life, and to assist groups in working toward community health goals.
   A. Group definition: Collection of interacting individuals who have a common purpose. Groups form for several reasons and may occur spontaneously or in response to an identified need.
   B. Group purpose: Dependent on the identified needs, desires, and goals of the actual or prospective members. The purpose may be obvious or subtle.
   C. Cohesion: Refers to the measure of attraction between members. Attraction is increased when members feel accepted by others, see like qualities in each other, perceive that others appreciate them, and believe that a core of similar attitudes and values holds the group together. Both task and maintenance functions influence group cohesion. The attraction members have to the group depends on the nature of the group, including the program, size, type of sponsoring organization, and status of the group in the community.
   D. Norms: Refer to standards that guide, control, and regulate individuals and communities. The group norms represent the standards for group members' behaviors, attitudes, and even perceptions. All groups have norms and mechanisms whereby conformity is accomplished. Groups have both task and maintenance norms.
   E. Leadership: Members' behaviors, including all actions that determine and influence group movement. Examples of leading behaviors include suggestion, probing, questioning, supporting, confronting, advising, clarifying, summarizing, and evaluating. Sources of leader influence are knowledge, ability, access to needed resources, personal attractiveness, status or position in the community or organization, and ability to control sanctions for others. Leadership is often described as patriarchal, paternal, or democratic; each style affects member interaction, satisfaction, and productivity.
   F. Group structure: Describes the particular arrangement of group parts that help to describe the group as a whole. Two structure frameworks are communication and role. A communication structure identifies the parts according to message pathways and member participation in sending and receiving messages. Role structure describes the expected behaviors of members relative to each other as the group interacts over time. Conflicts in groups may develop from competition for roles or from member disagreement about the ascribed roles.

II. Promoting an individual's health through group work: Health behavior is influenced greatly by the groups to which people belong and in which they value membership. People usually consider the responses of others when making decisions regarding personal welfare.
   A. Choosing groups for health change: Either established groups or selected membership groups may be used by community health nurses.
      1. Established groups: Some groups, such as families, exist and work together to meet group needs.

2. Selected membership groups: Some groups form in response to particular community needs to address specific problems or opportunities. Other groups occur spontaneously because of mutual attraction between individuals and as a result of an obvious and keenly felt need. Still other groups form for purposes such as health promotion.

B. Beginning interactions: Once a group forms, work begins on the stated purpose, with early meetings used to clarify individual and group goals. The nurse as leader assists group members in beginning interaction by providing support, inviting participation, giving information, clarifying issues, and suggesting structure.

C. Conflict: When groups work, they experience conflict. Open discussion and work toward problem solving can promote individual and group growth. Nurses can help reduce conflict by demonstrating respect for each person and for that person's point of view.

D. Problem solving for healthful change: Problem-solving and decision-making skills, as well as strategies for implementing change, aid group work. Basic teaching is often used; groups need to be involved in planning the change approach they will use.

E. Evaluation of group progress: The plan for evaluation begins in the earliest phase of a group, and indicators of achievement are written in a group record. Celebration, including special group rewards, is built into the evaluation system.

III. Community groups and their contributions to community life: Groups within a community determine the level of competence exhibited by the community.

A. Identifying community groups: Both formal and informal groups exist in a community. Groups form subsystems of the total community, which is a system. Formal groups can be determined by data in public documents, like comprehensive community plans, as well as from the local media. Informal groups are usually identified through an interview with a key spokesman. Groups are ranked in the community on the basis of characteristics such as social prestige or power.

B. Interlinking subsystems: Subsystems such as family, economy, government, religion, education, and health and welfare are linked vertically to the larger society and horizontally to each other through various communication and cooperative exchanges.

IV. Working with groups toward community health goals: The groups appropriate for meeting community health goals include established, community-sanctioned groups and groups for which nurses select members representing diverse community sectors.

V. Clinical application: Numerous examples of community health nurses' application of group work are presented throughout the chapter. An additional example illustrates the application of groups concepts for multiple groups in one community concerned with numerous chronically ill individuals. Students are challenged to test knowledge of groups concepts through clinical application.

Additional Critical Thinking Activities

1. From any group that you know well, list one specific standard or rule that operates to influence members in the following ways:
   A. To keep all members focused on the group goal.
   B. To affirm and support members.
   C. To influence members to interpret life circumstances in a particular group-accepted way.
2. Read articles from the bibliography at the end of Chapter 23 which focus on (A) promotion of individual health and (B) conflict management.
3. A. List actions that nurses may take to assist groups in various aspects of their work, such as member selection, purpose clarification, arrangements for comfort in participation, and group problem solving.
   B. Observe a nurse working with a health promotion group. Does he or she function in the way you anticipated? What nursing behavior facilitated the group process?
4. Collect local newspapers for five to seven days and note all mentioned groups, clubs, and organizations. Write the name of each group and organization within separate blocks on a piece of paper. Draw lines between these blocks to represent all communication documented within the collected newspapers. With colored lines, draw in other links that you think would exist, such as kinship ties across groups or collaboration for community projects. List the sources from the community that could accurately validate the beginning community group analysis.
5. Describe the role of a community health nurse working with established groups seeking to meet community health goals.
6. Evaluate group effectiveness for either a group you have observed or a group in which you are a member.
7. Identify and describe local political influence groups that speak out for or against health care reform. How do their group purposes relate to the arguments they make?

Critical Analysis Questions

1. Name the two essential components of any group.
2. Define the term *group.*
3. What relationship exists between group cohesion and group effectiveness?
4. Name three qualities that increase group member attraction.
5. List three groups existing in the local community (city, county, region) that address individual health needs of people.
6. What skills and resources are used by community health nurses to facilitate individual health promotion groups?
7. List five kinds of links that connect groups within the community.
8. List two hindering factors in establishing a nursing role in groups working toward community health goals.
9. Differentiate between task and maintenance norms.
10. Describe the value groups hold in encouraging people to promote their own health.
11. What is the ideal size of a small group whose purpose is focused on individual health change?
12. List four interlinking subsystems within a community that influence health.
13. Describe the similarities of working with individuals toward meeting personal versus community health goals.

Answer Key

1. Purpose or goal and member interaction.
2. A collection of interacting individuals who have a common purpose.
3. High group cohesiveness has a positive effect on overall group effectiveness.
4. When members feel accepted by others, see like qualities in one another, perceive that others like them, and believe they share similar attitudes and values.
5. Alcoholics Anonymous, Parents Without Partners, and whatever groups exist locally for the purpose of individual health promotion.
6. Knowledge of group concepts that guide facilitative interventions, knowledge of group health or illness, individual response to crises, health resources, etc.
7. Kinship, resource sharing, common response to community threat, religious and ethnic interests, commonly perceived needs.
8. Any factors that would hinder nursing involvement in community groups constitute correct answers, such as a nurse's internal factors of resistance, family or small group pressures against nursing involvement, community norms, or established ways for allocating responsibility that work against input from professions.
9. Task norms are the compelling force that returns members to the work pressures to ensure affirming actions for members and are helpful in maintaining comfort. These norms address comfort of members and attempt to reduce social and psychological tension.
10. People as social beings belong to a variety of groups; these group affiliations are important to members, and factors such as the values and opinions of members influence the thoughts, feelings, and actions of one another. If the group values health promotion, individual members are likely to subscribe to those values.
11. Ideal size is 8 to 12 participants.
12. Family, the general economy, government, education, religion, health and welfare system (e.g., resources, constraints).
13. The same interventions hold true for both groups (cohesion, group clarity, attraction to the group, commitment and participation, focus on the goal, recognition, encouragement, and evaluation).

24 Family Theories and Development

Chapter Summary

This chapter examines issues relevant to family theory and development. One theoretical framework used to study families is that of family life cycle. This approach emphasizes how families change over time and focuses on interactions and relationships among family members. Other concepts related to the developmental framework are discussed, such as family structures, roles, and functions.

Annotated Outline

I. Defining the family: Emerging definitions of the family are explored. These definitions represent the view of the family as a household unit that is representative of various family structures.

II. Conceptual frameworks: Five frameworks used by community health nurses in their work with families are discussed.

  A. Role theory: This approach assists the community health nurse in understanding the variety of roles played by family members. It offers insights into family behavior.

  B. Systems framework: This approach describes families as units comprised of members whose interactional patterns are viewed as a whole with boundaries permeated by the external environment.

  C. Structural-functional framework: In this framework, the family is viewed as a social system with members that have specific roles and functions.

  D. Interaction framework: This approach focuses on the family as a unit of interacting personalities and examines the symbolic communication processes by which the family members relate to one another.

  E. Family developmental theory: Developmental theory focuses on common, general features of family life and provides a longitudinal view of the family life cycle.

III. Family structures: The family has been experiencing considerable changes affecting the family's structure, functions, and interactions within the family itself and in the community.

  A. Traditional families and other families: Working with and serving the needs of families with varying family structures and functions has numerous implications for health professionals and health and illness care agencies.

IV. Trends in the family life cycle: If the present demographic trends and other trends continue, it can be expected that there will be a decline in the proportion of adults and children experiencing the typical family life cycle.

V. Family demography: Numerous trends are occurring in marriage and the family that have implications for community health nurses working with families. Demographic trends are affecting the family's structure and development.

VI. Family roles and functions: Knowledge about family roles and functions is essential to adequately assess the family and to effectively plan, intervene, and evaluate health care provided to the family.

  A. Family roles: Different types of family roles include child socialization role, child care role, provider role, housekeeper role, kinship role, adult sexual role, therapeutic role, recreational role, and sibling role.

  B. Family functions: All families have certain functions that must be performed for the purpose of meeting the family unit's needs, individual family member's needs, society's expectations, and maintenance of the integrity of the family unit.

    1. Family health functions: It is a basic family function to protect the health of its members and to provide supportive, nurturing care during periods of illness. The community health nurse supports the family in its efforts to perform health-related functions and tasks.

VII. Family developmental theory

  A. Family developmental framework: The family developmental framework identifies points in a family's development where changes (that is, critical transitions) occur in family members' status and roles.

  B. Family developmental tasks: The achievement of family developmental tasks at each family stage is interrelated with the accomplishment of developmental tasks by individual family members.

VIII. Family developmental theory and nontraditional family structures: The life course of many families is not following the typical life cycle of the nuclear family, as demonstrated by variations in childbearing patterns and by the frequency with which disruption occurs before widowhood.

IX. Vulnerable family: When using the family cycle as a framework for assessing the developmental events in the family, the community health nurse should always remember that the enactment of family roles and the appropriateness of the accompanying developmental tasks are defined by the family's culture and by society's expectations and the family's vulnerability. The developmental approach can be used successfully in practice with a variety of family structures, but the community health nurse must recognize that in every family there are individual and family developmental tasks to be accomplished that are peculiar to that particular family. The vulnerable family frequently experiences a shortened family life cycle, resulting in inadequate time to achieve the developmental tasks of each family life stage, blurring the boundaries of the family life stages and resulting in difficulty with subsequent stages, because the previous developmental tasks have not been resolved. The community health nurse can assume that the vulnerable family has developed a variant family structure for the purpose of surviving.

Additional Critical Thinking Activities

1. Marriage is technically a legal relationship based on a mutual contractual agreement. However, marriage and family members rarely "spell out" their expectations and commitments. If you were to marry (or if you are married) and intended to specify your demands as well as your obligations to your spouse and your children (assuming you have or plan to have children), what would they be? Be specific. What degree of personal autonomy would or do you expect? How would or are decisions made? Career expectations met? Household tasks shared? Individual developmental tasks accomplished? Childbearing responsibilities shared, and so on? Can you identify any differences in your intended family structure from your actual family structure, roles, functions, and interactions as they relate to family developmental tasks? Write an analysis of your findings.
2. If you live in a small town or in suburbia, consider the families on your block. If you live on a farm, consider the families who live near you. If you live in an urban apartment or housing complex, review the residents you know. How many of the households represent the traditional nuclear family? How many represent an experimental or nontraditional family form? What variant family forms are there—for parents, widow or widowers living alone, elderly couples, or single persons sharing a home? Analyze the implications of your findings and your knowledge about family forms for community health nursing.
3. Select a family-focused television program and analyze the family's behavior in relation to the family systems framework, interactional framework, structural-functional framework, and developmental framework.

Critical Analysis Questions

1. True or False? The majority of the emerging conceptualizations of the family tend to define the family as a unit consisting of mother, father, and young children.
2. Identify five types of traditional families.
3. List two types of group marriage families and two types of experimental marriage families.
4. List at least eight trends in marriage and the family that have implications for community health nurses working with families.
5. Describe each of the eight family adult roles.
6. Discuss the functions performed within the sibling interactional system.
7. Cite examples of the family's physical, affectional, and social functions.
8. List Duvall's six family functions.
9. Discuss how the family influences family members' development of health habits.
10. What are the family's health functions and tasks?
11. Define the systems, interactional approaches, structural-functional approaches, and developmental approaches for the study of families.
12. Discuss the interrelationship between family developmental tasks and the developmental tasks of individual family members.
13. Select one of the following family types and discuss the application of the developmental framework to assessment, planning, and intervention with the selected family: single-parent family, remarried family, or vulnerable family.

Answer Key

1. False
2. Nuclear family—single adult living alone. Nuclear dyad—middle aged or elderly couple. Single-parent family—kin network. Three generation family. Second career family.
3. Group marriage families: Common residence or compound of households. Sexual swapping

within group. Mix of formerly married couples and singles. Multilateral marriage. Experimental marriage families: Nonrelated adults sharing a common household. Heterosexual cohabitation. Homosexual unions. Affiliated family involving unrelated members of different generations.

4. Postponement of marriage. Large divorce rate. Increase in single-parent families. Changing fertility patterns. Births to unmarried women. Increase in number of elderly. Delayed parenting. Remarriage. Increased singlehood.
5. Behaviors associated with the following roles should be described (see section on adult roles):
   Child socialization
   Child care
   Provider
   Housekeeper
   Kinship
   Sexual
   Therapeutic
   Recreational
6. Discussion should focus on (see section on sibling role):
   Identification
   Differentiation
   Mutual regulation
   Direct services
   Negotiate with parents
   Pioneering
7. Physical functions: Provision of food, clothing, shelter, and health and illness care; protection against danger.
   Affectional functions: Meeting emotional needs.
   Social functions: Provide for a social togetherness, fostering self-esteem, supporting creativity, and initiative.
8. Generating intrafamilial and intergenerational affection.
   Providing personal security and acceptance.
   Providing family members with a sense of satisfaction and purpose.
   Assuring continuity of companionship.
   Providing social placement and socialization.
   Inculcating controls and a sense of what is right.
9. The discussion should include reference to the family members' biophysical and psychosocial development, socialization, transmission of health-related cultural traits, demonstration of health-illness behaviors, and the development of values, beliefs, and attitudes about health and illness.
10. Answer should include reference to providing a health-supporting home environment, provision of resources for meeting holistic needs, health education, health promotion, recognition of health disruptions, seeking health and illness care, and home health-illness care.
11. Systems—views family as a living social system composed of two or more individuals linked together by mutual interaction and interdependence for the purpose of carrying out family functions and attaining goals.
   Interactional—views the family as a unit of interacting personalities and examines the symbolic communication processes by which family members relate to one another.
   Structural-functional—views the family as a social system with members who have specific roles and functions.
   Developmental—views family development as following orderly, sequential changes in the family's growth, development, and dissolution throughout the family's life span.
12. Discussion should include reference to family developmental task's focus on assisting individual members to accomplish their tasks and on individual family members accomplishing many individual developmental tasks to be able to adequately fulfill their family roles.
13. See the respective chapter section regarding the family type selected.

25 Family Health Risks

Chapter Summary

The importance of the family in promoting the health of individuals and communities is well established. Health objectives for the nation emphasize both health promotion and risk reduction. The notion is that reducing the risks to segments of the population is a direct way of improving the health of the general population. Specific risks have been identified, and related objectives to be achieved have been outlined. In order to effectively and appropriately intervene with families to reduce their health risk and thereby promote their health, it is necessary to understand family structure and functioning, family theory, nursing theory, and models of health risk.

In this chapter, health risks in the six categories for families (genetic, age, biologic characteristics, personal health habits, lifestyle, and environment) are identified and analyzed, and approaches to reducing these risks are discussed. Suggestions for structuring community health nursing interventions with families to decrease health risks and to promote their health and well-being are presented.

Annotated Outline

I. Early approaches to family health risks: Early consideration of the family in health and illness focused on three major areas: 1) the impact of illness on families; 2) the role of the family in the etiology of disease; and 3) the role of the family in utilization of services.

   A. Health of families: The family plays an important role in health and illness as a primary unit of health care, and the interrelationship among health, health behavior, and family is highly dynamic. The energized family is characterized by promotion of freedom and change, varied and active contact with other groups and organizations, flexible role relationships, egalitarian power structure, and a high degree of autonomy in family members.

   B. Health of the nation: Paralleling the focus in family studies on health, increased attention was being given to ways to improve the health of the nation. Health objectives for the nation were established and then evaluated and restated for the Year 2000 (Healthy People, 1991).

   C. The notion of "risk": A risk factor predisposes or increases the likelihood of ill health. The reduction of health risks is a major approach to improving the health of the nation.

II. Concepts in family health risk: An examination of several related concepts (family health, family health risk, risk appraisal, risk reduction, life events, lifestyle, and family crisis) is necessary to understand family health risk.

   A. Family health: Family theorists refer to healthy families, but generally do not define family health; definitions of healthy families can be derived within any one of a number of frameworks. Another dimension of family health can be identified by using JL Smith's (1983) four models of health: Clinical model, role-performance model, adaptive model, and eudaimonistic model.

   B. Health risk: While risk factors can singly influence outcomes, the cumulated risks are synergistic; their combined effect is more than the sum of the individual effects.

   C. Health risk appraisal: Health risk appraisal refers to the process of assessing the presence of specific factors within each of the categories that have been identified as being associated with an increased likelihood of an illness, such as cancer, or an unhealthy event, such as an automobile accident.

   D. Health risk reduction: Health risk reduction is based on the assumption that decreasing the number or magnitude or risk will result in a lower probability of the undesired event, for example, substance abuse in adolescents.

   E. Life events: Life events can increase the risk for illness and disability and can be categorized as either normative or non-normative.

   F. Family crisis: A crisis exists when the family is not able to cope with the event and becomes disorganized/dysfunctional.

III. Major family health risks: Risks to families' health arise in several major areas: biological risk, social risk, economic risk, lifestyle risk, and life events leading to crisis.

A. Biological risks: A number of illnesses have a familial component that can be accounted for either from a genetic basis or from established lifestyle patterns.
B. Social risk: The importance of social risks to families' health is gaining increased recognition. Living in high crime neighborhoods, living in communities without adequate recreational or health resources, living in communities that have major chemical, noise, or other contaminants, or living in other high stress environments increases a family's health risk.
C. Economic risk: It is well established that the poor are at greater risk for health problems.
D. Lifestyle risk: Personal health habits continue to contribute to the major causes of morbidity and mortality in this country.
E. Life events: Transitions (movement from one stage or condition to another) are times of potential risk for families.

IV. Community health nursing approaches to health risk reduction: Family health risk appraisal, home visits, contracting, and empowerment are clinical nursing approaches for reducing family health risk.
  A. Family health risk appraisal: Assessment of family health risk requires multiple approaches to address the many components of risk, including biologic health risk, social risk, economic risk, lifestyle risk, and life events.
  B. Family home visits: An important aspect of community health nursing's role in reducing health risks and promoting the health of populations has been the tradition of providing services to individual families in their homes.
    1. Purposes of home visits: Home visits provide opportunities for more accurate assessment of the family structure and behavior in the natural environment.
    2. Advantages and disadvantages: Home visits promote client control of the setting, are convenient for clients in terms of travel, and provide a natural, relaxed environment for the discussion of concerns and needs. Costs are a major disadvantage of home visits.
    3. Process for home visits: Five phases of a home visit can be delineated—initiation, previsit, in-home, termination, and postvisit.
  C. Contracting in family health risk reduction: Contracting is one way of formalizing and explicating the involvement of the family in risk reduction.
    1. Definitions and purposes: A contract can be defined as an agreement between the nurse and client that is focused on enhancing and supporting the client's active role in health care by defining who will do what to accomplish health-related goals.
    2. The process of contracting: Contracting is a learned skill on the part of both the nurse and the family. Three phases—beginning, working, and termination—can be identified with seven sets of activities. These activities are mutual exploration of problems or needs, mutual establishment of goals, mutual exploration of resources, development of a plan, mutual agreement on division of responsibilities, setting of time limits, and mutual evaluation, modification, and renegotiation or termination.
    3. Advantages and disadvantages: Contracting requires skill, time, and effort, as well as a willingness for mutual participation and responsibility.
  D. Enabling and empowering families: For families to become active participants in their health care, they need to feel a sense of personal competence, as well as a desire for and willingness to take action. Empowerment reflects three characteristics of the family seeking help: 1) access and control over needed resources, 2) decision-making and problem-solving abilities, and 3) acquisition of instrumental behavior needed to interact effectively with others to obtain resources.
    1. Empowerment requires a viewpoint that often conflicts with the perspective of many helping professions, including nursing. In empowerment the underlying assumption is one of a partnership between the professional and the client, versus one in which the professional is dominant.
    2. The nurse's approach to the family should be positive and focused on competencies rather than on problems or deficits. The interventions need to be consistent with family cultural norms and with the family's perception of their problem.
    3. The goal of an empowering approach is to create a partnership between the nurse and the family, characterized by cooperation and shared responsibility.

V. Community resources for health risk reduction in families: The community health nurse often mobilizes a number of resources to effectively and appropriately meet family health risk reduction goals.
  A. General types of resources: Governmental, voluntary, and proprietary organizations provide health and health-related resources and services to families.
  B. Identifying and accessing resources: Community health nurses assist families, not only in identifying resources, but also in being client

advocates in assisting families to learn to use resources.

Additional Critical Thinking Activities

1. Select one of the Year 2000 objectives and identify how Biologic Risk, Social Risk, Economic Risk, Life-style Risk, and Life-event Risk contribute to family health risk for that objective.
2. Select three to four families (hypothetically or from actual situations) representative of different ethnic and socioeconomic backgrounds. Complete a family genogram and ecomap for each family, and identify and compare major health risks.
3. Select one or more agencies in which community health nurses work, and examine the agency's and community health nursing's philosophies and objectives with emphasis on individual care, family care, illness care, risk reduction, and health promotion.
4. Identify three community health problems in your community and discuss the implications of these problems for the health of families. Identify three health problems common to families in your community and discuss the implications of the problems for the health and/or health care resources of the community.
5. Using an example of a referral for a home visit to follow up on a family with a ten-year-old child newly diagnosed with diabetes mellitus, role play the initial visit. Discuss how you would plan for the visit and what activities would follow the actual visit.
6. Based on either the above example or a clinical family, negotiate a contract with the client to achieve a risk reduction goal. Identify the phases of the contracting process and tell whether the contract is a formal or informal one.
7. For the community where you live or have clinical assignment, identify five agencies which provide health-related services to families. For each agency, discuss 1) what specific services are provided, 2) who is eligible for services, 3) how service is initiated, and 4) the cost of the services.
8. Based on your intervention plan for a clinical family, identify an appropriate community agency that offers services to assist with reducing a health risk for that family. With the family, develop a plan for the family to contact the agency, including a list of questions about services offered, eligibility criteria, how to initiate services, and costs.

Critical Analysis Questions

1. Identify the six areas of health risk factors for families, and give an example of each.
2. Name the four models of health identified by Smith, and give a brief definition of each.
3. Give an example of a normative event for a family. Identify whether it would be a Level I, II, or III change, and justify your classification.
4. List three family characteristics that have been identified as being related to family members' health behaviors.
5. List three characteristics of families seeking help that are inherent in a definition of family empowerment.
6. Identify three advantages of family home visits and two disadvantages.
7. What is the primary purpose of contracting?
8. What is the major difference between a contingency and a noncontingency contract?
9. What are the three phases of contracting? List one activity for each phase.
10. Name two governmental and two voluntary community agencies that provide health-related resources/services to families.

Answer Key

1. Biologic risk—a family history of diabetes mellitus.
   Social risk—living in a high crime neighborhood.
   Economic risk—loss of a job by the main wage earner.
   Lifestyle risk—high fat diet.
   Life events—birth of a child.
2. Clinical model—health is viewed as absence of disease.
   Role-performance model—health is viewed as effective performance of usual roles.
   Adaptive model—health is viewed as effective and fruitful interaction with the physical and social environment.
   Eudaimonistic model—health is viewed as the development of the individual's potential for general well-being and self-realization.
3. Birth of a child. Level I—what child-care tasks need to be done and who will do them; Level II—what are the roles of being a parent; Level III—what the value of children is in the family.
4. Flexible division of tasks; health training efforts by parents; active participation in the larger community; promotion of autonomy of family members; egalitarian power structure.
5. Access and control over needed resources; control over decision-making and problem-solving abilities; acquisition of instrumental behavior needed

to interact effectively with others to obtain resources.

6. Advantages: Convenience for the client; increased client control of the setting; natural, relaxed environment for discussion of concerns and needs. Disadvantages: Costs in terms of previsit preparation, travel to and from the home, and time spent with one client.
7. The primary purpose of contracting is to enhance and support the client's active role in health care by defining who will do what to accomplish health-related goals.
8. A contingency contract explicates a specific reward for the client based on completion of the client's portion of the contract. A noncontingency contract does not specify rewards. The implied rewards are the positive consequences of reaching of goals specified in the contract.
9. Beginning phase: Mutual data collection and exploration of needs and problems; mutual establishment of goals; mutual exploration of resources; mutual development of a plan.
   Working phase: Mutual division of responsibilities; mutual setting of time limits; mutual implementation of plan; mutual evaluation, renegotiation.
   Termination phase: Mutual termination of contract.
10. Governmental resources: Include Medicare, Medicaid, WIC, food stamps, and health department immunization clinics.
    Voluntary resources: Include Heart Association, Catholic Social Services, Meals on Wheels, Goodwill, and community clinics.

26 Family Nursing Assessment

Chapter Summary

Family nursing is defined as nurses and families working together to assure the successful adaptation of the family and its members' responses to health and illness. Family nursing occurs in all settings, especially community-based settings. The overall purpose of this chapter is to present strategies to practice family nursing in community-based settings.

Annotated Outline

I. Barriers to practicing family nursing: Two significant barriers to practicing family nursing are the narrow definitions of both family and health family used by health care providers and social policy makers. Other barriers are the following: (1) the common belief among nurses is that family is "common sense" and not a theory-based nursing; (2) a lack of good comprehensive family assessment models, instruments, or strategies exist in nursing; (3) the strong historical tie of nursing to medicine singles out the individual client as the focus of care; (4) the charting system is geared toward the individual client; (5) diagnostic systems used in health care are disease and individual focused; (6) health insurance has an individual client perspective; and (7) often the hours of services provided to families are at times of day when the whole family can not attend.

II. Definition of family and health families: The family has traditionally been defined using legalistic relational concepts such as blood ties, adoption, marriage, or guardianships. Family is broader than this narrow approach. Family is defined as "two or more individuals who depend on one another for emotion, physical, and/or economical support" (Hanson & Boyd, in press). Nurses should ask clients to identify whom they consider to be family and include these members in the health care planning.

A multidisciplinary approach to families refers to individual members, as well as to the family unit as a whole. Labeling a family as "dysfunctional" implies that nothing in the family system is working well and that they are a "bad" family. This catch-all phrase is non-specific and provides no direction or guidance to family members or health providers for creating interventions built on the family strengths. Families are neither all good nor all bad.

III. Family nursing: The family can be viewed from the following four perspectives: The first perspective is family as the context which places the individual family member in the foreground and the family in the background. The second approach is family as the client. The family is in the foreground and individuals are in the background. The family is seen as the sum of individual family members. The focus is on the ways that the individual members affect the whole family. The third approach is family as the system. The family is seen as the interactional and relational aspects of the family members. The fourth approach is family as a component of society. The family is viewed as the primary unit of society and as part of a larger system.

IV. Family nursing process: The family nursing process is a dynamic systematic organized method of critically thinking about the family. It is problem solving with the family to assist successful adaptation of the family to identified health care needs. The family nursing process is the application of the generic nursing processes grounded in knowledge of family nursing and family theory. It consists of the following steps:

A. Collection of a family nursing data base, including both identification of problem areas and family strengths. Data collection includes important pre-encounter data and information collected while making the appointment with the family. The nurse determines the appropriate place to meet with the family. Advantages for meeting in the home of the client are the following: (1) the opportunity to view the everyday environment of the family; (2) the increased likelihood of observing typical family interactions; and (3) the possibility that more family members may be present. Advantages for meeting in the clinic office of the health care professional are the following: (1) access to other professionals is available; (2) more structure is provided for the nurse; and (3) emotional distance the family may need to discuss problems is provided.

B. Diagnostic reasoning and generalization of specific family nursing diagnoses. The nurse makes clinical judgments about which problems can be resolved by nursing intervention, which need to be referred to other professionals, and which areas of concern the family is successfully adapting to on its own with interventions. Reflective questioning is used by the nurse to determine the more appropriate family nursing diagnoses.

C. Collection of prognostic nursing and medical data, and generation of data-supported nursing prognosis for each family nursing diagnosis. The nursing prognosis is a nursing judgment, based on the holistic view of the family and its members, which predicts the probability of the family's ability to respond to the current situation. The areas where changes can occur will be identified. The types of outcomes will be explored, and the trajectory of the course of events will be articulated by the nurse and family.

D. Treatment planning based on both family nursing diagnosis and prognosis, plus additional data on daily living and family resources or deficits as they affect planned nursing actions. The nurse and family work together to create a plan of action. A contract form is often used. The degree of involvement of each family member varies and needs to be negotiated. It is important to define who is responsible for what parts of the plan, including the role of the nurse. The plan of action should be built around the family strengths, as this increases the likelihood of the success of the plan.

E. Implementation of family-negotiated plans of action. The specific family and nursing interventions are carried out by the designated party to achieve the agreed-upon goals.

F. Evaluation of family/family members' responses to plans of action and to effects of family diagnosis, prognosis, and previous treatment. The evaluation is based on family outcomes and should be built into the plan of action.

G. Termination of the nurse-family partnership. The strategy includes a reduction in the frequency of sessions with the nurse, an invitation for follow-up, and referrals to resources. A summative evaluation meeting is planned with emphasis on the family strengths and progress.

V. Family nursing assessment; models and strategies: Assessing and intervening in family health is a systematic process requiring a conceptual framework and an approach that provides data as a foundation for action. Two family assessment models and approaches are presented: The *Family Assessment, Intervention Model and the Family Systems Stress Strength Inventory (FS^3I),* and the *Friedman Assessment Model and Short Form.*

The FS^3I is a systems model that uses family as client approach. The family members are asked to identify stressors and strengths they believe are affecting the family. The health care provider assesses the family members and the family as a whole, using a similar format. Based on this joint assessment, the nurse and the family determine interventions and create a family care plan.

The Friedman Assessment Model approaches the family from a structural-functional perspective. The family system is viewed through specific functions and structures that are known to exist in families. The specific functions explored are affective, socialization, and health care. The specific structures investigated are family developmental stage; family roles; family decision making; family values; family poser structure; family coping ability; and family communication structure.

The FS^3I measures specific dimensions of the family, which are identified by the family as needs, problems, stressors, and strengths. It presents a more microscopic view of the family. Friedman's Assessment Model is more broad and general. It provides a sweeping view of the family according to specific family functions and structures. It places the family in the broader family system perspective. Using the assessment tool jointly will provide a comprehensive family assessment.

VI. Genogram and ecomap: The genogram is a three-generational family tree format which depicts the family members and their relationships over time. It shows important family historical patterns and related health information.

The ecomap is a visual representation of the family unit in relation to the community around it. It is an organizational tool that shows the nature of the relationships between the family members and the subsystems with which it interacts. It shows the direction of energy flow from the family or into the family.

VII. Future implications for nursing and family policy: Family nursing will continue to be a significant aspect of health care reform in the United States as health care moves more toward community-based settings. To keep nursing in the forefront of these important health care system changes, nursing education must continue to include specific curricula on family nursing, nursing research needs to be family centered, and practicums and post-graduate education need to be conducted in community-based settings.

Family policy is governmental actions that have a direct or indirect impact on families. In short, all governmental actions, whether at the local, county, state, or national level, affect the family. The range of social policy decisions that affect families is vast; however, there is no specific national family policy in the United States. It will be crucial for nursing to be actively involved in family health policy legislation; they must lobby for overt family policy. The issues affecting families at the end of the 20th century are poverty, alcohol abuse, and family violence.

Additional Critical Thinking Activities

1. Define family.
2. Define family nursing.
3. Discuss how family assessment fits into community health nursing.
4. Identify five barriers to practicing family nursing in a community-based setting.
5. Describe how a family assessment is different from an individual client assessment.
6. Discuss the importance of family nursing diagnosis and prognosis as they relate to developing a plan of action with a family.
7. Explain why family assessment is the most critical aspect of the family nursing process.
8. What kind of difficulties could you experience when arranging for a family assessment interview?
9. Discuss factors to be considered when determining the place to conduct a family assessment interview. Include both pros and cons.
10. How would you select which family assessment tool to use?
11. Describe and compare the Family Stressor and Strength Inventory Assessment Tool and the Friedman Family Assessment Instrument.
12. Draw your own family genogram and ecomap. Discuss how they are used in family nursing.
13. Discuss the role of nursing as it relates to family policy.

Critical Analysis Questions

1. The definition of a family is:
   a. two or more people who are bonded together by legal blood relationships.
   b. a group of people with whom a person closely identifies.
   c. two or more people who depend on each other for emotion, physical, and/or economical support.
   d. two or more people that are related through adoption, guardianship, or marriage.
2. Which of the following is NOT a barrier to practicing family nursing?
   a. The traditional charting system in health care has been oriented to the individual.
   b. There are a lack of comprehensive family assessment tools.
   c. The nursing diagnostic systems are disease and individual focused.
   d. Insurance carriers recognize family as a unit, as well as the individual client.
3. Which aspect of the family nursing process is the most critical?
   a. assessment
   b. nursing diagnosis
   c. nursing prognosis
   d. planning and interventions
4. An ecomap assessment tool is important in a family assessment because it:
   a. depicts a three generation diagram of the family history.
   b. demonstrates how the family interacts with other systems.
   c. shows the identified family and the specific areas that are causing them problems.
   d. diagrams the current stressors the family is experiencing.

Answer Key

1. c
2. d
3. a
4. b

27 Children's Health

Chapter Summary

Nurses working with the child and adolescent population must understand the unique characteristics of how this group differs from others. The ongoing process of growth and development affects all interactions. It has a bearing on the assessment and management of physical growth, psychosocial development, nutrition, immunizations, and major health problems. An understanding of cognitive development determines how the nurse interacts with the child. The child is a part of a family and is dependent on the family for physical and emotional well-being. Family assessment and interventions are critical.

This chapter provides information on the principles of growth and development from birth through adolescence and on major health problems seen in this population. Family functioning is presented as a framework for nursing assessment and interventions. The chapter also focuses on the unique needs of children and families within the community, based on the *Healthy People 2000* objectives.

Annotated Outline

I. Needs of children and families: Unique factors distinguish this population from others.

A. Physical growth and development: A unique feature of this population is the ongoing process of growth and development, resulting in physical, cognitive, and emotional changes. Well-child assessments are scheduled on a regular, ongoing basis to monitor these processes. Nurses are responsible for assessment of growth; neuromotor development; feeding, sleep, and elimination patterns; and dental and skeletal assessments.

Health assessment tools include growth charts, developmental screening tools, and temperament and behavior assessments. Tools are developed for use with specific ages and are useful for parent teaching.

B. Nutritional needs: Good nutrition is essential for healthy growth and development, as well as for disease prevention in later life. Nursing assessment of the adequacy of a child's nutrition includes physical growth and dietary intake. Overall dietary recommendations for each age group are presented.

Infancy: The majority of brain growth occurs during this time. Parents need support and education to manage an infant's nutritional needs.

Childhood: Dietary intake is influenced by increasing independence and decreasing growth needs. Parents need information to offer a balanced, healthy range of foods.

Adolescence: Increasing growth needs and poor eating habits place this population at risk for poor nutritional health. Effective activities to educate and encourage better nutrition include group teaching and setting realistic goals.

C. Immunizations: Routine immunization has been successful in the prevention of selected diseases. The goal of immunization is to protect by using toxoids and vaccines to stimulate antibody formation. Antibodies are produced slowly and in small concentrations after the first injection; subsequent injections increase the rate and amount of response.

Recommendations regarding immunizations are made by the American Academy of Pediatrics and the U.S. Public Health Services Advisory Committee on Immunization Practices. Recommendations are designed to increase the number of children immunized.

Contraindications to immunizations include pregnancy, malignancy, immunosuppressive therapy or immunodeficient disease, sensitivity to components of the vaccine, or recent administration of globulin, plasma, or blood.

Legislation: The National Childhood Vaccine Injury Act deals with issues of informed consent and adverse reactions. Vaccines for Children provides free vaccines for eligible children.

D. Psychosocial development: The work of Erik Erikson focuses on the interaction of emotional, cultural, and social forces on personality development. Erikson believed that development is a continual process that occurs in distinct stages. Resolution of the crisis at each stage leads to new orientation to self and society.

Trust vs mistrust (infancy); Autonomy vs shame and doubt (early childhood); Initiative vs guilt (preschool and early school); Industry vs inferiority (school age); Identity vs identity diffusion (adolescence).

E. Cognitive development: Piaget's theory of development is used to understand the process of cognitive development. Schemes are actions and mental processes allowing the child to understand his environment. Cognitive development is the increasing complexity of the schemes. Nurses must understand the characteristics of cognitive ability at each stage to work effectively with the child and family.

Sensorimotor: Learns object permanence, causality, and symbolic play while moving from reflex to purposeful behaviors.

Preoperational: Magical thinking; inability to understand things from the perspective of others; can only focus on one aspect of a situation.

Concrete operations: Compensation, identity, and reversal enables understanding of time, space, number, and amount when applied to concrete entities.

Formal operations: Develops greater capacity for abstract thinking and can mentally perform deductive reasoning.

F. Major health problems: Injuries and accidents are the single most important cause of disease, disability, and death among children. Motor vehicle accidents are the leading cause of death; drowning, burns, poisonings, and falls contribute. Infants are at risk because of their small size and immature motor skills. Toddlers and preschoolers have a high level of activity and developing motor skills. School age children have the lowest rate; however, sports and athletic injuries are increased. Adolescents have the highest injury rate, largely due to motor vehicle deaths, drowning, and intentional injuries. Weapons and substance abuse also play an important role. The role of nursing in the prevention of accidents and injuries includes identification of risk factors, anticipatory guidance, environmental modification, and safety education.

Acute illnesses are primarily caused by infections. Most are self-limited and can be handled by the family on an outpatient basis. The nurse may be involved with the development of a home management plan, administration of therapy, and evaluation, as well as with teaching.

Sudden Infant Death Syndrome is the most common cause of death in the first year of life. Most deaths occur between one and five months of age. Few factors are useful to predict occurrence, but there seems to be an increased risk for preterm and low birthweight infants, those with upper respiratory tract infections, males, lower socioeconomic groups, infants whose mothers smoke, and infants who sleep in a prone position. Nursing interventions include teaching caretakers how to decrease risk factors.

Chronic health problems are varied among the pediatric population. There are many commonalties to guide nursing interventions: a need exists for routine health maintenance care, for ongoing medical care specific to the problem, and for coordination of care; skilled care procedures are often required; equipment needs are complex; educational needs are complex; safe transportation must be available; financial resources may be inadequate; and behavioral issues may exist.

Alterations in behavior are highly variable and may include eating disorders, attentional problems, substance abuse, elimination problems, conduct disorders, sleep disorders, and school maladaptation. Maladaptive behaviors may interfere with development of self esteem. Family-centered approach to management is needed.

II. Needs of children within the community: Nursing, through development and coordination of community-based services and through formation of public policies, promotes the well-being of children within the community. Programs based on the needs of specific at-risk populations are developed for the delivery of health care.

A. Strategies: Home-based programs are needed to extend the scope of services into the home. Services are based on the needs of the community and may include monitoring the health status of vulnerable populations, social support, or safety education.

Programs are needed to meet the needs of the homeless. This will decrease the impact of homelessness on the health of children. Families are the fastest growing segment of the homeless population. Children are at risk for Homeless Child Syndrome—a combination of health problems, environmental dangers, and stress. Outreach programs bring services to the homeless. The emphasis is on prevention and follow-up care, as well as on immediate problems.

Daycare/School are environments for children for a majority of the day. Nurses establish programs and serve as a resource for health care standards and health education.

B. Types of services

1. Health promotion—Nutrition programs based in schools, daycare centers; breast-

feeding support; parenting skills and support; anti-smoking.

2. Health protection—Injury prevention within the community: playgrounds, carseat programs, gun control, fluoride supplementation.
3. Preventive services— Sexually transmitted disease education programs, hearing and vision screening programs, immunization programs.

Additional Critical Thinking Activities

1. Attend a well-child clinic. Observe nurses taking histories to obtain information about nutritional adequacy, developmental growth, or the sleep and elimination patterns of the infant. What kinds of questions did the parent ask, and how did the nurse evaluate the effectiveness of the nursing intervention? Observe what kinds of immunizations were given and what kind of client education was performed regarding the immunization. Prepare a summary of your experiences for presentation to the class.
2. Administer the Denver II or DDST-R to:
   a. An 18-month-old child.
   b. A 3-year-old child.
3. Develop a program for day care workers on prevention, management, and control of common illnesses in the toddler and preschool age group. Detail your teaching plan, assessment of learning needs, teaching strategies, and evaluation measures. Prepare a short presentation for class discussion.
4. Develop and present a program on "How to brush your teeth" for a nursery school class of four-year-olds.
5. Identify a child abuse resource center, agency, or person in your area. Contact and obtain information on their program.
6. Develop and implement a program on bicycle safety for children aged eight to ten years through a local school.
7. Develop and implement a program on nutrition for 13- to 15-year-olds through a local school.
8. Identify the components of "suicide ideation." Identify the local resources available for referral for a teenager at risk for suicide.

Critical Analysis Questions

1. True or False? Patterns of sleep, eating, and elimination are frequently altered by growth spurts.
2. True or False? An initial immunization series does not need to be restarted if interrupted.
3. True or False? Vitamin and mineral supplementation is not necessary for breast-fed infants.
4. According to Erikson, ______________ affect(s) the psychosocial development of children.
5. True or False? Children who are concrete thinkers are able to understand that properties of an object remain the same, even if the physical appearance changes.
6. Identify two methods of assessing the quality of nutrition.
7. The most reliable tool for assessing sexual maturity is ______________.
8. The leading cause of death in the pediatric population is ______________.
9. Identify four groups of infants who are at risk for SIDS.
10. Identify two effects of exposure to "second-hand smoke" on children.
11. Nursing anticipatory guidance for all age groups of children should focus on ______________.
12. The major psychosocial task of adolescence is ______________.
13. The screening tool designed to assess the maturation level of four- to five-year-olds is ______________.

Answer Key

1. True
2. True
3. True
4. Emotion, social, and cultural forces
5. True
6. Growth, dietary recall
7. Tanner Scale
8. Motor vehicle accidents
9. Low birthweight, preterms, males, low socioeconomic status, maternal smoking, upper respiratory tract infection, prone sleeping
10. Increased otitis media and upper respiratory tract infections
11. Prevention
12. Development of Identity
13. PRESS

28 Women's Health

Chapter Summary

Women's health primarily focuses on women's psychosocial and physiological well-being, functional abilities, and experiences of symptoms and health problems. This broad emphasis of women's health is in distinct contrast to viewing women in terms of their reproductive health or their role in parenting children. Although the importance of women's health began gaining national recognition during the last two decades, questions continue to be raised about the health and well-being of American women. While progress has been made in treating women, who comprise 52% of the population, continuing issues related to women's health exist. These issues include questions related to areas of health care neglect, shortcomings of health services available to women, and the need to understand the key health problems of women. The purpose of this chapter is to explore the health needs of women and the role of the community health nurse in meeting those needs.

Annotated Outline

I. Status of women: While women have made some strides in their efforts to achieve economic equality during the last decade, progress has been slow.
   A. Women comprise half of the world's population and head one-third of all households in the world; yet the majority of individuals who live in poverty are women and children.
   B. In the United States, two-thirds of all poor adults are women. The majority living below the poverty level are single mothers with children.
   C. Employed women are more likely to work in lower paying service sector jobs.

II. Development of women: The work of classic human developmental theorists, such as Erikson, Freud, Piaget, and Kohlberg, is based on research conducted on males.
   A. Emerging research of women is expanding our understanding of human development.
   B. Chodorow and Gilligan have found that a female's identity is not found through independence and separation, but instead in the relationships that she forms with others.

III. Health of women: Women have a longer life expectancy than men. Women experience more morbidity and use health services at higher rates than men. The three major causes of mortality in women are heart disease, cancer, and cerebrovascular disease. The three major chronic conditions women experience are heart conditions, arthritis, and hypertension; these conditions increase with age.
   A. Heart disease: Heart disease is the leading cause of death among women over 50 and the second leading cause of death among women 35-39 years of age.
      1. While women are less likely to have heart attacks than men, they are more likely to die from one.
      2. Cessation of smoking is the most important factor in decreasing the morbidity and mortality of heart disease in women. For women who smoke and take oral contraceptives, the risk of heart disease increases significantly.
      3. Postmenopausal women are at risk for heart disease, due to decreased levels of estrogen. Hormone replacement therapy reduces the risk of death from heart disease by 50%.
   B. Cancer: Cancer is the second leading cause of death for women. The most common types of cancer in women are lung, breast, colorectal, ovarian, and pancreatic. Many women have a great deal of fear and incorrect information about the incidence, diagnosis, and treatment of cancer.
      1. Lung cancer is the leading cause of cancer deaths among women, surpassing breast and colorectal cancer. Most lung cancer is preventable; smoking causes the majority of lung cancer.
      2. Breast cancer is the second leading cause of death from cancer among women. Breast cancer increases significantly for women over 50 years of age. Although breast cancer occurs most frequently in women of higher socioeconomic status, economically disadvantaged women have the highest mortality rate. Early detection of breast cancer (including a combination of mammography, clinical breast examination, and breast self-

examination teaching) is the most important strategy to increase breast cancer survival.

3. Ovarian cancer causes more deaths than any other gynecologic cancer, accounting for 6% of all cancers in women. Postmenopausal women have the highest incidence and mortality rates from ovarian cancer. A major risk factor is family history. Other risk factors include nulliparity, late first pregnancy, infertility, late menopause, high-fat diet, higher socioeconomic status, and occupational exposure to talc and asbestos. The periodic pelvic examination is the only reliable screening test available.
4. About one-third of gynecologic cancers include uterine cancers (cervical and endometrial). Endometrial cancer occurs most commonly in postmenopausal women. Risk factors include nulliparity, late menopause, early menarche, obesity, high socioeconomic status, and a family history of breast cancer. With early detection, appropriate treatment, and adequate follow-up, cervical cancer is one of the most preventable diseases. Major risk factors for cervical cancer include low socioeconomic status, a history of multiple sexual partners, early onset of sexual activity, and use of oral contraceptives. Moreover, sexually transmitted viral diseases, such as herpes and human pappilloma, have recently been recognized as playing a possible role in the development of cervical cancer. The principal screening test for cervical cancer is the Pap test. All women should be educated about the importance of having regular gynecologic exams.

C. Human Immunodeficiency Virus (HIV): HIV is a major health problem and cause of death among women.

1. The highest HIV seroprevalence rates in women are found in women of childbearing age. Injection drug use is the main risk factor for women, accounting for over 50% of cases.
2. Over 70% of women with HIV are black or Hispanic. While membership in an ethnic group is not a risk factor, this over-representation is believed to be linked to the disproportionate numbers of minority members engaged in high risk behaviors. The majority of HIV-infected women are clustered within urban areas, where poverty and drug abuse are prevalent.
3. Generally, women with HIV have many more co-existing problems than men have, including malnutrition, other sexually transmitted diseases, substance abuse, lack of social support, and poor access to health care.
4. HIV is often a family illness. Many of these families experience many other difficulties: poverty, isolation, poor education, unemployment, inadequate housing, and drug use.

D. Women and weight control: Often women of normal weight and even less-than-normal weight view their bodies as too large.

1. The prevalence of obesity and the associated risks of obesity in the development of diabetes, hypertension, cardiovascular disease, and other medical problems make this condition a major health problem among women.
2. Women may also suffer adverse social and psychological consequences of obesity, including social and economic discrimination. More women enter weight treatment programs for their perceived loss of attractiveness rather than for health concerns.
3. In the last twenty years, there has been a noticeable increase in reports of disordered eating. While many girls and women are dissatisfied with their current shape and weight, only a small number of these actually develop serious eating disorders. The most common eating disorders seen in women are anorexia nervosa and bulimia.

E. Arthritis: Arthritis is the most prevalent chronic condition experienced by women. The most common form of arthritis is degenerative joint disease or osteoarthritis. Women with arthritis often suffer from chronic pain and activity restriction.

F. Osteoporosis: Osteoporosis is a major health problem for postmenopausal and elderly women.

1. The most common fractures associated with osteoporosis are compression fractures of the vertebrae and hip fractures. Hip fractures are the leading cause of loss of independent living for women.
2. Prevention of osteoporosis includes maintaining a desirable weight, maintaining an adequate intake of dietary calcium, phosphorus, and vitamin D, and participating in regular weight-bearing exercise. Premenopausal women should be encouraged to take 1000 mg of calcium daily; postmenopausal women need calcium supplementation of 1500 mg a day and a vitamin D supplement.

G. Urinary Incontinence (UI): Between 15 and 64 years of age, up to 25% of women report experiencing urinary incontinence. It is believed that the incidence of UI is greatly under-reported, since many women believe that losing continence is just the normal result of childbearing or growing older.

1. While the risk for the development of UI increases with age, young, healthy nulliparous females may experience UI. Activities that provoke the highest degree of UI involve jumping, high impact landings, and running.
2. The consequences of UI can be devastating. It creates an economic burden, a loss in self-esteem, a sense of guilt, and isolation. UI in the elderly is the major factor contributing to the initiation of institutional care.
3. Many women attempt to manage the problem without seeking professional help. The vast majority of women are never asked questions about UI during a routine physical examination. Women can pursue a number of behavioral activities that can prevent or minimize UI.

H. Depression: Depression is a major mental health problem for women. A number of factors may contribute to the development of depression, including unhappy intimate relationships, history of sexual and physical abuse, reproductive events, multiple roles, ethnic minority status, low self-esteem, poverty, and unemployment.

IV. Reproductive health: Women often enter the health care system because of reproductive issues or problems.

A. Family planning: While women have a wide array of effective contraceptives from which to choose, more than half of the six million annual pregnancies in the United States are unplanned and about half end in abortion.

1. The goal of contraceptive counseling is to ensure that women receive appropriate instruction to take charge of their own reproductive choices.
2. Many women have a great deal of wrong information regarding the relative risks of contraceptive methods. For example, women often overestimate the cancer risks of oral contraceptives.

B. Preconceptional counseling: Preconceptional counseling includes education, assessment, diagnosis, and interventions to address risks prior to conception. The goal of preconceptional care is to reduce or eliminate risks for both the woman and infant.

1. A great number of risks can be identified and corrected prior to conception.
2. Preconception assessment should include discussion of a woman's family, medical, reproductive, nutritional, and social history. During assessment, areas deserving attention can be identified.

C. Prenatal care: Prenatal care is a variable strongly associated with improved birth outcomes.

1. A number of factors may increase the motivation of pregnant women to seek prenatal care: transportation assistance, telephone or mailed reminders, child care, cash payments, layette gifts, and posters.
2. Lifestyle problems, such as inadequate nutrition, smoking, substance use, poor maternal health, psychological distress, and violence, are important contributors to high infant mortality.

V. Women at midlife: The years between 35 to 65 are commonly referred to as midlife.

A. During the midlife, women can be encouraged to make additional lifestyle changes to avoid ill health during later years. Women should be encouraged to stop smoking, reduce obesity, reduce dietary fat, increase dietary fiber, adopt a sensible exercise regimen, minimize sun exposure, decrease alcohol and caffeine consumption, avoid abuse of medications, seek screening exams, and adopt a stress management program.

B. While menopause is a universal life transition for women, women are poorly prepared for this stage of their lives.

VI. Transitions in aging: Older adults, of which women are the majority, are the fastest growing segment of the population.

A. Caregiving has defined the lives of many women. This continues as women age and care for ill partners. The demands of spousal caregiving are often the most difficult for women because of their own age, fading health, and lack of resources.

B. Women have a greater life expectancy than men. It is estimated that half of the additional life expectancy of women is spent in a state of disability. The cost of these years of disability further depletes the already limited resources of elderly women.

VII. Women's use of health services: For many women, caring for family members is informal care that they provide in addition to paid employment.

A. The wages lost by women to fulfill their role as caretaker of the family's health are immeasurable.

B. Access to medical care is inextricably linked to health insurance. Women lack health insurance for various reasons. Many women work part-time or are employed in low-paying jobs that do not provide insurance coverage.

C. The health behaviors of women are influenced by their access to health care; in turn, their access to health care is influenced by their level of education and income.

D. Despite women's pivotal role in providing care, very few women participate in public decisions regarding health care.

VIII. Programs for women's health services: Programs for women's health should offer comprehensive screening and education for women in one convenient setting.

IX. Special populations: Three groups of women warrant special consideration because of the uniqueness of their lives: lesbians, women in prison, and single mothers.

A. Although many of the health care needs of lesbian women are the same as those of heterosexual women, there are some special considerations. Lesbians are at low risk for vaginal infections, sexually-transmitted diseases, and HIV.

B. Many lesbian women neglect their health care needs. Lesbian women complain that health care providers assume their heterosexuality.

C. While women represent only a small percentage (5.5%) of the total state prison population, this number is drastically increasing. The upsurge in the female prison population is directly attributed to drugs and drug-related crimes. Many women in prison are poor, minority, single mothers.

D. Most single mothers do the work of two with resources for one. The synergistic effect of the multiple responsibilities of home and a job can lead to depression and stress.

E. A growing population of single-mothers-by-choice is characterized by a woman who is older, well-educated, and financially able.

X. Health policy: With the exception of reproductive health, policy makers have paid little attention to the needs of women. Until the 1990s, women's health issues were absent in public policy and medical research.

A. With the passage of two pieces of legislation, the Family and Medical Leave Act of 1993 and the Women's Health Equity Act of 1990, many of the needs specific to women will be addressed.

B. The Family and Medical Leave Act provides job protection and continuous health benefits to eligible employees who need extended unpaid leave.

C. As a result of the Women's Health Equity Act, women's health has emerged as a field of discussion, study, and research in many schools of nursing and medicine.

D. Although women's issues are at the forefront of public policy today, there is still much work to be done. It is because women are the primary family caregivers at both ends of the age continuum that a national child care policy and a policy on aging is of particular concern.

Additional Critical Thinking Activities

1. Conduct a health assessment on a set of mother-daughter clients in which the daughter is between 18 and 40 years of age. Compare and contrast the health concerns of each.
2. Design a teaching plan for an older woman that reflects a maximum level of health promotion.
3. Evaluate health promotion and prevention services that target a special population (e.g., lesbians, women in prison, single mothers). Identify additional services that are needed.
4. Attend a community meeting that focuses on the health care needs of childbearing women. Identify the barriers to optimum health care that are addressed.
5. Conduct a focused interview with a woman about stressors she experiences. Determine the major stressors in her life; the various ways stress is manifested; and the coping strategies she uses.
6. Analyze a week of health-related newspaper articles that focus on women. What ages and concerns are addressed? What health care advances are proposed or announced?

Critical Analysis Questions

1. Discuss the traditional and expanded scope of women's health.
2. Identify four factors that contribute to the "feminization of poverty."
3. Discuss Chodorow and Gilligan's research findings regarding female identity formation. Compare these findings to the classic theories of adult human development.
4. Identify the leading causes of death in women.
5. Compare the differences between men's and women's experiences with heart disease.
6. Identify the most important factor in decreasing the morbidity and mortality of heart disease in women.
7. The most prevalent chronic condition experienced by women is:
   a. osteoporosis.
   b. depression.
   c. arthritis.
   d. urinary incontinence.
8. Identify the risk factors associated with osteoporosis in women. Develop a plan of care to prevent osteoporosis in a premenopausal woman.

9. Identify two reasons lesbian women neglect their health care needs; discuss ways that the community health nurse can encourage lesbians to seek health care.
10. Discuss factors that contribute to caregiver burden.
11. Discuss a key legislative act that has an impact on the lives of women as caregivers. Identify two areas where public policy for women are lacking.

Answer Key

1. Traditionally, women's health has focused on the medical treatment of menstruation, childbirth, and menopause, and on the role of women in parenting. The expanded scope of women's health focuses on women's psychosocial and physiological well-being, their functional abilities, and their experiences of symptoms and health problems. The health of women is recognized through the biological, social, and cultural dimensions of their lives. Menstruation, childbirth, and menopause are viewed as normal female development.
2. Factors include a gender wage gap; the number of single female-headed households; the teen birth rate; a welfare system that provides a subsistence below the poverty level; a lack of adequate affordable child care; a lack of enforcement of child support payments; budget cuts in social programs; and women who assume the principal caretaker role in the family.
3. Chodorow (1978) and Gilligan (1979, 1982) found that females develop their identity through the relationships that they form with others. These findings are in stark contrast to traditional theories of human development which espouse that adults must first separate and become autonomous from others in order to achieve identity formation.
4. The leading causes of death in women are heart disease, cancer, and cerebrovascular disease.
5. Coronary artery disease develops 10 to 20 years later in women than in men. Women with heart disease are more likely to present with complaints of chest pain, while men typically present with acute myocardial infarction. Many women delay seeking treatment because their pain is not intense or because they are often misdiagnosed by health care providers. Because of the late onset of symptomatic heart disease, women who require cardiac surgery are much older than their male counterparts. Advanced age at the time of surgery may explain why women have higher operative mortality rates than men. Post-operatively, women are less likely to participate in cardiac rehabilitation than men. Women are less likely to follow discharge instructions; they often allow family responsibility and level of fatigue to guide their post-operative activity.
6. Smoking cessation
7. a
8. Risk factors for osteoporosis include both uncontrollable and controllable factors.
   a. Uncontrollable risk factors associated with osteoporosis:
      - age (50 years and over)
      - race (Caucasian or Asian)
      - bone structure (petite or slim frame)
      - being menopausal
      - early onset of menopause
      - family history of osteoporosis

      Controllable risk factors associated with osteoporosis:
      - inadequate intake of calcium
      - inadequate amount of exercise
      - smoking
      - excessive alcohol use

   b. Early prevention of osteoporosis should begin with adolescent girls. Prevention efforts include maintaining a desirable weight, participating in regular weight-bearing exercises, and maintaining adequate intake of calcium (1000 mg daily for premenopausal women), phosphorus, and vitamin D. Athletic women should be counseled about preserving bone density by avoiding excessive exercise that results in amenorrhea.
9. a. Two reasons lesbian women may neglect their health care needs:

      Many lesbian women delay health care to avoid an encounter with a health care provider.

      Many lesbian women believe that they are at little risk for an abnormal Pap test; consequently, they delay regular gynecologic screening and breast examination.

   b. Ways that the community health nurse can encourage lesbians to seek health care:

      Lesbians are more likely to seek health care services when health care providers are open and nonjudgmental. The community health nurse can create a nonthreatening environment for lesbian women. The nurse can avoid assuming everyone is heterosexual by asking women their sexual status. The nurse can teach lesbians the importance of regular gynecologic screening and breast examination. Lesbians should also be taught that, although the risk of vaginal infections, sexually transmitted diseases, and HIV is low, women who have ever had heterosexual intercourse are at risk of cervical cancer.
10. a. Many women juggle the roles of wife, employee, and caregiver to children, parents, and in-laws with little assistance from spouses, employers, and government.

b. The additional time that women spend fulfilling their roles as caregivers can lead to increased stress and self-neglect.
c. For the many women who quit their jobs or work part-time to care for a family member, the interruption in employment often leads to a decline in family income, and loss of insurance coverage and retirement contributions.
d. Many older women who care for their ill husbands are particularly vulnerable to caregiver burden because of their own age, fading health, and lack of resources.

11. a. The key legislative act that has an impact on the lives of women as caregivers: The Family and Medical Leave Act that passed in 1993 provides job protection and continuous health benefits (if applicable) to eligible employees who need extended unpaid leave for personal or family health conditions, including the birth or adoption of a child.
  b. Areas where public policy influencing women are lacking: The enactment of a national child care policy would provide assistance to working parents.

  Currently, older couples must spend much of their assets in order for Medicare to pay for the cost of nursing home care for their spouses. Revamping current Medicare law would alleviate the financial burden that many older women endure when they must place their husbands in nursing homes.

29 Men's Health

Chapter Summary

Men's health, as a separate and distinct practice of care, is in an early developmental level. Men's health goes beyond care of the prostate and genitals and dealing with issues of sexual dysfunction and associated disease. Today's focus is on the entire person, requiring a holistic approach. The data is quite convincing; men are physiologically the more vulnerable gender. More male infants die at birth. More men die of cardiovascular, liver, and chronic pulmonary diseases, as well as from cancers and suicide. Furthermore, a man has a shorter predicted lifespan. Many explanations exist for such differences in gender health outcomes: genetics, risk-taking behaviors, stressors, ignoring warning signs, and many other explanations.

This chapter will discuss men's health by reviewing developmental stages of men, identifying men's health problems and needs, and exploring the nurse's role in maintaining and promoting men's health in the community.

Annotated Outline

I. How men define health
   A. While men and women have similar ideas of health, men have a much different perspective. They see health as being individualized.

      Men tend to avoid getting help for as long as possible. This leads to more serious health problems. Men use medical specialties less frequently than women.

II. Development
   A. Psychosocial: Two psychosocial stages affecting men are young and middle adulthood. Each stage has its distinctive tasks.
   B. Moral: Kohlberg identified three stages: Preconventional Morality, Conventional Morality, and Universal Principles.

III. Men's health and mortality in the world: The United States men's life expectancy for all ages is one of the lowest in developed countries. Males in the United States are expected to live 71.8 years, compared to 76 years for Japanese men.

IV. Gender difference
   A. Shorter life expectancy: Men have a shorter life expectancy than women. In 1993, the age adjusted death rate for men of all races was 1.7 times higher than that of women.
   B. Riskier behavior: Men engage in more risk-taking behavior than women. This is particularly true of behaviors involving physical challenges or illegal behavior.

V. The leading causes of men's deaths
   A. Heart and cardiovascular diseases: Heart disease is the leading cause of death in men. The main risk factors associated with heart disease are smoking, sedentary lifestyles, improper diet, and obesity.
   B. Cancer: Malignant neoplasms are the second leading cause of death in men.

      The most significant cancers affecting men are prostate, testicular, and skin cancer. Earlier detection is essential for successful treatment.

      1. Prostate cancer is the most common cancer among United States men. The risk for prostate cancer increases with each decade after age 50. An annual digital examination is recommended for men over age 40.
      2. Testicular cancer is the most commonly found solid tumor in the 15-35 age group. Men should perform a monthly testicular self-examinnation (TSE).
      3. Skin cancer is the most common of all cancers. Men's death rates are much higher than women's death rates. Being exposed to prolonged sun contributes immensely to the high incidence of cancer in men. Prevention includes decreasing exposure to direct sunlight, applying sunblock solutions, and wearing protective clothing while in the sun.
   C. Accidents
      1. Men are at higher risk for fatal occupational injuries than women. In 1992, men accounted for about 90% of all fatally injured workers. Transportation and assault/violent acts were the two leading causes of occupational fatalities.
      2. Men accounted for nearly two-thirds of the nonfatal occupational work-related injuries.
   D. Pulmonary Diseases: Chronic obstructive pulmonary disease is the fifth leading cause of death in men. Men have a 1.33 times greater chance of dying from pulmonary diseases than

women. The incidence of emphysema is more than twice as high for men as for women. Respiratory cancer death rates are 1.8 times higher in men as in women.

Smoking is a definite pulmonary disease risk factor. Smokers who quit before age 40 have pulmonary functions similar to people who never smoked. Education is an important factor concerning gender differences in smoking.

E. HIV/AIDS: AIDS is the seventh leading cause of death in men for all ages. There is a vast difference in death rates between men and women.

The World Health Organization reported that 60% of HIV transmission is heterosexual.

F. Suicide: Suicide is the eighth leading cause of death for men. The suicide rate for men is 20.1 compared to 4.7 for women per 100,000 population. Suicide can be prevented. Nurses can often identify men at risk for suicide.

G. Homicide: Homicides are the tenth leading cause of death in men of all ages. The homicide death rate for men is 16.9 compared to 4.4 for women per 100,000 population. Nurses must be able to identify signs and symptoms of violent behavior and must know how to intervene.

VI. Men's health practice in everyday life: Men and women have different views on the most important health needs. Men evaluate their health experiences by what they have accomplished and by their overall physical shape and conditioning. An important health outcome is for men to focus on their total health and on their strategies for staying healthy.

VII. Legislation affecting men's health: Major legislation affecting men's health over the last decades were Medicare, the Workman Compensation Act, the Americans with Disability Act, the Family and Medical Leave Act, and the Veteran's Administration health plans.

VIII. The community health nurse's role in men's health: The community health nurse must use nursing knowledge and skills to assess, diagnosis, plan, implement, and evaluate the care of men. Four nursing roles are important to maximize men's health:

1. The nurse educator provides knowledge and skills to enable men to learn new behavior or change unhealthy behavior.
2. The patient advocate ensures that men's long term health care needs are met.
3. The case manager does more than coordinate; the nurse problem-solves and manages men's health care services.
4. The men's health care nurse practitioner provides comprehensive men's health care.

Additional Critical Thinking Activities

1. Instruct students to search local newspapers for men's health care issues. Have them bring the articles to class, highlight the key points, and engage in a roundtable discussion.
2. Survey the community's resources for intervening in the leading causes of men's death. What are the agencies' missions, goals, personnel, budget, and other resources to optimal men's health?
3. Schedule students for observations in ambulatory clinics. Focus on the communication patterns between male clients and physicians. Write a five minute process recording about the interaction between the doctor and the male client. Evaluate the communications.
4. Interview men about their life style and health risk factors. Conduct an assessment and identify the leading contributors to men's mortality. Develop a teaching program to reduce the risk factors.
5. Develop and implement a program for the early testicular cancer detection for a class of junior high school males.
6. Identify a men's health care nurse practitioner in your region or state. Observe the nurse's advance practice role.

Critical Analysis Questions

1. Describe how men define health.
2. List the three leading causes of death for all ages in men.
3. List four risk factors associated with heart and cardiovascular disease.
4. Discuss the most prominent death rate differences between the genders.
5. In 1993, men's life expectancy in the United States was:
   a. 72 years.
   b. 70 years.
   c. 65 years.
   d. 76 years.
6. Describe how men's risk-taking behaviors affect their health.
7. Which men's age group has the highest infection rate for HIV?
   a. 5-14
   b. 25-44
   c. 45-64
   d. 65 and older
8. Name three major cancers affecting men's health.
9. Name four factors associated with African-American male youth violence.
10. Explain the conception of how men look at themselves compared to how women do.

11. Discuss how the Family and Medical Leave Act affects men.
12. You are planning a health fair for young adult men. Your focus is early cancer detection. Explain the steps for testicular self-examination (TSE).
13. What is the role of the men's health nurse practitioner?
14. How can nurses be advocates for men and their health care needs?

Answer Key

1. Men view health as being physical, mental, and emotional. Men see health as being individualized. What one man believes is healthy may be far different for other men. Men tend to avoid getting help for as long as possible, which may lead to further, more complicated health problems. Men who earn high incomes perceive themselves as being healthier; however, this may not be the case.
2. The top three leading causes of death in men are (1) *Heart and Cardiovascular Disease:* This disease accounted for 32% of all men's mortalities in 1991. Young men (25-44) have a 2.7 times higher incidence and middle-aged men (45-64) have a 2.6 times higher incidence of heart disease than women. (2) *Cancer:* Malignant neoplasms are the second leading cause of death for men of all ages. They accounted for 24% of all men's deaths. The most significant cancers affecting men are prostate, testicular, and skin cancer. (3) *Accidents:* Accidents are the third leading cause of death for men of all ages. In 1992, men accounted for about 90% of all fatally injured workers. Men accounted for about two-thirds of non-fatally injured workers.
3. The four main risk factors associated with heart and cardiovascular disease are smoking, sedentary lifestyles, improper diet, and obesity. Individuals can control each of these factors.
4. The age-adjusted death rate for men of all races was 1.7 times that of women. The most prominent death rate differences between genders are found in deaths due to accidents, pulmonary diseases, HIV, suicides, homicides, and alcoholism-related liver diseases. Women have higher death rates in cerebrovascular disease, pneumonia, and diabetes.
5. a
6. Men engage in more risk-taking behavior than women. This is especially true in behaviors involving physical challenges or illegal behavior. Men drink more alcohol than women, causing higher accidents, more liver cirrhosis, and a higher incidence of some types of cancer. Men's jobs are more hazardous, leading to higher occupational fatality rate. Men are also exposed to more industrial carcinogens.
7. b
8. Prostate, testicular, and skin cancer.
9. Social, economical, cultural, environmental.
10. The concept of body maintenance image has two components: "inner" and "outer." Inner refers to optimal functioning, performance, and capacity to do things. Outer refers to appearance, movement within social space, and having the potential to be heard and be touched.
    Men use the inner phenomenon more than the outer. Men evaluate how they performed during the day, what they accomplished, and how their physical shape contributed to their performance. Women focus more on the outer phenomenon.
11. The Family and Medical Leave Act offers men the opportunities to meet family responsibilities. They are eligible to take a 12-week leave for the birth of a child, to care for an ill child or spouse, to adopt or accept a foster or adoptive child, or to recover from a serious health condition. When a man's leave is over, he is entitled to return to work in the same or equivalent position with the same or equivalent pay scale and benefits.
12. The TSE is performed during a warm bath or shower. Roll each testicle between the thumb and fingers. Check for shape, size, texture, position, and tenderness.
13. The men's health nurse practitioner (MHNP) is an advance practice role that focuses on delivering comprehensive men's healthcare. Assessing and managing minor health problems as well as managing acute and chronic conditions, conducting histories and physical examinations, ordering and interpreting diagnostic studies, prescribing medications and treatments, providing health maintenance care, promoting positive health behaviors and self care, and collaborating with physicians and other health professionals are some of the MHNPs functions and roles.
14. The goal for the advocacy role is to inform and support men in their health care decisions. The nurse needs to become knowledgeable about the health care options and to support the individual's decisions.

30 Elder Health

Chapter Summary

The population of the United States in the age group 65 years of age or older is growing more rapidly than the population as a whole. Health care providers are becoming more knowledgeable not only about elders, but also about how to accurately assess this population. In order to deliver the most appropriate care, it is vital that providers understand the typical elder as well as the uniqueness of an individual elder. Increased life expectancy is accompanied by increased chronicity and physical changes, as well as by social and economic changes.

This chapter describes elders as a group, discusses the major health problems that affect elders, explains how to assess elders to obtain information for the management of their care, describes the role of the community health nurse, discusses long-term care for elders, and explains health care delivery issues.

Annotated Outline

I. Demography: The average life expectancy in the United States has increased from 47 years at the turn of the century to 75 years in 1987.
   A. Geography and elders: The majority of elders live independently; only 5% live in an institution.
   B. Economics and elders: Even though the income of elders has increased over the years, many are still vulnerable economically, especially if they have to pay out-of-pocket health care expenses.
   C. Educational level and elders: The older population is less educated than the younger population. It is predicted by the year 2000, the median number of school years completed by elders will be 12.4.

II. Myths and theories of aging: Many myths portray elders in an unfavorable light. The theories of aging are not always acceptable for explaining the uniqueness of elders.
   A. Myths: Ageism is the term for prejudice toward elders. It perpetuates stereotypes of elders that many people have. Ageism can also result in isolation of elders.
   B. Theories: Many theories of aging have been postulated, and not all are accepted. Some of the theories summarized include the disengagement theory, activity theory, continuity theory, exchange theory, and wear-and-tear theory.

III. Developmental tasks of aging: Erikson and Havighurst's stages of development are discussed, as well as Butler's life review.

IV. Major health problems of elders: The incidence of chronic conditions rises with increasing age. Other conditions are also problematic for elders. The causes of death for elders are portrayed.

V. Role of the community health nurse: Community health nurses, in achieving the goals of prevention of disease and maintenance of health, are involved in client and community education, counseling, advocacy, assessment, and management of care. Achieving this involves all three levels of prevention.
   A. Health assessment of elders: An accurate and comprehensive assessment includes identifying problems that elders encounter. Without a comprehensive assessment, the community health nurse cannot plan appropriately for an elder. A comprehensive health assessment includes obtaining a health history, which includes a nutritional, functional, and psychosocial assessment. A physical examination is fundamental to a comprehensive assessment, and the community health nurse can assist in making appropriate referrals.
   B. Intervention strategies involve the community health nurse making appropriate referrals to other providers of care or to community agencies, based on the data obtained from the comprehensive assessment. The community health nurse is well qualified to act as case manager of care for elders.

VI. Long-term care: Long-term care can be delivered in an institutional setting, or it can be delivered in the community. Long-term care has become a significant portion of the health care system in the United States.
   A. Federal programs: The Social Security Act and Medicare have influenced the health care of elders. The cost of long-term care is escalating,

and government programs are being strained economically.

B. Nursing homes: The nursing home industry has exploded and has resulted in the Medicaid budget being stretched to the limit. Nursing homes are organized in a hospital-like environment and focus on custodial care rather than meaningful social activities, psychological care, or rehabilitative services.

C. Community-based long-term care: Home care refers to care that is provided in homes or in community and home-like settings. There is no significant government funding for home services, and large numbers of elders are not able to obtain home-based care at all.

D. Family caregiving: The role of informal caregiving has increased, due to the cost of other forms of care. It places great demands on the family caregivers, yet most view institutionalization as a failure.

VII. Health care delivery issues: There has been a shift in emphasis from responsibility in meeting humanitarian needs to that of reimbursement. Meeting the needs of elders will require emphasis on primary and preventive care involving multidisciplinary teams, service in the home, long-term care, and gerontological education.

Additional Critical Thinking Activities

1. From the clinical application in the chapter:
   A. Identify an example of a theory of aging.
   B. Identify an example of ageism.
   C. Derive at least two nursing diagnoses.
2. Interview an elder and determine how he would rate his health on a scale of one to ten. Also ask the elder how he perceives that his health influences other aspects of his life. Ask the elder to compare his current health status with his health status twenty years ago.
3. Observe both an elder and a younger individual in a community setting, and compare the observed physical characteristics of each.
4. Select a relative who is 65 years of age or older and:
   A. List his health problems, if any.
   B. Observe his activity level.
   C. Ask the relative to keep a 24-hour dietary recall history.
   D. Keeping the United State Guide to Clinical Preventive Services screening recommendations for persons 65 and older in mind, devise a screening plan for the relative. Also include secondary and tertiary prevention measures, where appropriate.
   E. What theory of aging best fits your relative? Why?
5. Interview two persons not in health-related study or work environments, and ask them to describe a "typical" elder.
6. Describe your perception of a typical elder, and compare that to the information obtained in #4. Are examples of ageism apparent in either?
7. Visit a senior center in your community, and report what you observed in terms of physical characteristics of the elders participating at the center, the activities in which they were engaged or planned to be engaged, the food served, and the safety features observed. Ask residents to describe collectively how they feel that elders are perceived by others.
8. Describe the community services available for elders in your community; then describe problems that elders may encounter when attempting to access those services.

Critical Analysis Questions

1. List at least three demographic facts pertaining to elders.
2. Define ageism and describe how it influences elders.
3. Describe the exchange theory of aging.
4. Mr. Winters is a 77-year-old widower who lives alone in the house he and his wife shared for 40 years. Their children live out of state, but the daughter telephoned the local health department to ask that a community health nurse visit her father. Mr. Winter's daughter reports that her father says he has been fatigued for a month or more and is having difficulty getting chores done. The community health nurse visits Mr. Winters in his home. While there, the most appropriate action that the community health nurse could take is to:
   a. perform a physical examination.
   b. perform a comprehensive assessment.
   c. administer the SPMSQ.
   d. obtain information from a systems review.
5. The community health nurse discovers that Mr. Winters is not sleeping well, that there have been several robberies in the neighborhood lately, and that his weight has decreased about ten pounds over the last two months. The nurse also observes that Mr. Winters has a shuffling gait and that he stumbled over the threshold of the kitchen door. The community health nurse should also assess for:
   a. depressive symptoms.
   b. environmental hazards.
   c. nutritional status.
   d. all of the above
   e. none of the above
6. In talking further with Mr. Winters, the community health nurse discovers that Mrs. Winters has

been dead seven months and that Mr. Winters is having a hard time adjusting to the loss of his wife. He can't bring himself to sit at the kitchen table where they used to eat because he says he can still see her sitting in her usual chair, so he eats in a chair in front of the television. The most likely diagnosis, based on the information you have, is:

a. malnutrition.
b. confusion.
c. depression.
d. b and c
e. a and c

7. What else should the community health nurse assess in Mr. Winter's home to aid in prevention of falls?
8. Compare and contrast Alzheimer's type of dementia to multi-infarct dementia.
9. The most common causes of death for elders are ischemic heart disease, malignancies, cerebrovascular disease, and diabetes mellitus. Devise a health promotion plan for an elder who has no evidence of disease at this time.

Answer Key

1. Life expectancy has increased from 47 years in 1900 to almost 75 years in 1987. Elders are better off economically but are still vulnerable, as 15.2% of elders have incomes of no more than 1.5 times the poverty level. The majority of elders live alone, elders are less educated that younger persons, and African-Americans are the largest minority.
2. Ageism is a term for prejudice about older persons. Ageism fosters stereotypes of elders that can result in social isolation.
3. The exchange theory of aging views elders with esteem as a result of their experience and knowledge. The elder exchanges this knowledge for a position of respect from younger persons.
4. b
5. d
6. e
7. The community health nurse should assess for scatter rugs, proper lighting, floors with slick spots, easy reaching of items in the kitchen, grab bar availability, even sidewalks, and firm non-skid shoe soles.
8. Alzheimer's type of dementia is a gradually progressive dementia that affects more women than men, especially if over 75. The cause is not known. There is much diversity with both symptoms and the progression. Multi-infarct dementia results when a person has either a sustained or recurrent cortical or subcortical strokes. It is difficult to differentiate between the two, as some may have aspects of both.
9. The health promotion plan should include such things as assessment of nutritional status, level of activity, and functional status, and should encourage smoking cessation (if needed), following the recommended screening guidelines, and obtaining the correct immunizations.

31 The Physically Compromised

Chapter Summary

As a result of increasingly sophisticated medical care, of the aging of the United States population, of federal legislation and funding, and of greater acceptance by citizens, people who are physically compromised are more likely to be living in the community, to be cared for at home, to be attending school or working, and to be participating in the life of the community.

Community health nurses are in a key position to provide the leadership for improving the quality of life for this population. Discussed in this chapter is the use of the nurse's knowledge, skill, and concern, which enables her to coordinate and provide family-centered care for those of all ages with special needs.

Annotated Outline

I. Definitions and concepts: Several terms and concepts pertaining to being physically compromised are defined, and their interrelationships are discussed.

II. Scope of the problem: Complex and far-reaching problems are associated with disabilities. The size of this population is increasing due to medical advances, the aging of the United States populations, and other factors. The exact prevalence and incidence of disabilities across the lifespan are unknown. However, this is a serious community health problem.

III. Effects of being physically compromised

A. The community health nurse needs to consider the effects on the affected individual, his family, and his community.

B. Effects on children are influenced by such factors as the child's previous health, his developmental stage, the condition and its treatment, and other factors.

C. Effects on adults may result from the impact of the disability on the adult's roles, as well as from financial strains, availability of social support, resiliency, and other factors.

D. Effects may include inappropriate behaviors, developmental stagnation or regression, cognitive losses, nutritional deficits, and inability to function in anticipated roles.

E. Effects on the family may include strain, fatigue, feeling "trapped," anxiety, and depression. Sleep and appetite disturbances are also common among primary caregivers. Other family members can be affected in a variety of ways.

F. Effects on the community may include the need for additional or different services, the reallocation of resources, additional support from informal groups, and mandated architectural changes.

IV. Special populations

A. Rural: Those who live in rural areas are often likely to be at greater risk for disabilities than are non-rural dwellers. They are also more likely to have less access to care due to geographical distances and limited insurance.

B. Low income: Those with limited income are at greater risk as a result of such economic factors as less access to health care, likelihood of practicing all levels of prevention, and lifestyle factors.

C. Occupational/worksite: The extent of disability in the workplace is unknown, but is generally believed to be under-reported. Worksite disability may result from job-related illnesses or injuries. Other issues related to occupational disability are concerned with the Americans with Disabilities Act of 1990 and with appropriate accommodations in the workplace for those who are disabled.

V. Special issues related to being physically compromised

A. Abuse: Abuse of children and the elderly is well documented in the literature, although there is limited information about abuse of disabled young adults. Children may become disabled following abuse, be abused after disability, or both. The nurse needs to be aware of any of her own state's laws concerning abuse of the disabled.

B. Health promotion: Many health promotion needs of those who are physically compromised are similar to those of the general population. However, it is an area that is typically not dealt with by health care providers of the physically compromised. This is an especially important function of the community health nurse for these clients.

VI. Healthy People 2000 objectives: Almost all the objectives can be viewed as significant for the state of being physically compromised, particularly at the primary prevention level. However, Objective 17 is especially pertinent for this chapter.

VII. Health Cities: Concepts of Health Cities are clearly related to those objectives from Healthy People 2000 that deal with environmental aspects of health. Also, the involvement of all major organizations and groups in a community in identifying problems, establishing priorities, and developing interventions implies inclusion of those who are physically compromised in the broader life of their community.

VIII. The role of the community health nurse: All the roles of the community health nurse may be appropriate with the physically compromised client and his family at various times. These roles include caregiver, educator, counselor, advocate, referral agent, primary care provider, case manager, coordinator, collaborator, casefinder, and change agent.

A. Legislation: Federal legislation of special significance for those with disabilities are P.L. 93-112, P.L. 94-142, and P.L. 101-336. State legislation and rules and regulations at all levels of government may have implications for the community health nurse working with this client population.

Additional Critical Thinking Activities

1. Interview a nursing staff member of a setting that provides care for those who have Alzheimer's disease or other dementias of aging. Ask the nurse his/her role in working with others who care for those clients and with the family in assisting them to adapt to the needs and problems of their affected family member. Present the results in a written paper for a class presentation.
2. Interview a leader and/or member of a family support group for any chronic health problem. Ask these participants about the process that group members go through in dealing with the medical diagnosis and needs of the family member. Ask about the advantages and disadvantages of involvement in a support group; find out what kinds of questions and issues emerge during discussions. Present your findings in a written report for presentation to the class.
3. Visit an elementary school in the community in which children are mainstreamed into the classrooms with all other students and, using each approach, answer these questions:

   Questions:

   A. What are the advantages to the developmentally disabled child?
   B. What are the advantages to the other children?
   C. What are the disadvantages to each group?
   D. What alternatives might exist?

   Approach:

   A. Observation.
   B. Discussion with teacher and/or teacher's aide.
   C. Discussion with children.
   D. Discussion with parents of developmentally disabled children and with parents of other children.
   E. Participation in classroom activity with children.
4. Sit in a quiet place free from interruptions and reflect on the following:
   A. The first time I remember seeing a person who was disabled, I thought . . .
   B. The first time I remember seeing a person who was disabled, I felt . . .
   C. If I had a family member who was physically compromised, I would . . .
   D. If I were to have a family member who was physically compromised, I would have to make the following modifications in my home (either where you live or the home in which you were raised).
   E. I know someone with a relative who is disabled, and his or her life is enriched by this person because . . .
   F. I know someone with a relative who is disabled, and his or her life is hampered because . . .
5. Locate a community setting where you can observe and participate in interactions with disabled people. What alterations have been or should be made in the following areas so that their needs are met?
   a. Physical facilities.
   b. Nutrition (type of meals).
   c. Type of instructions (directions, assistance).
6. Select a federal or state program that provides services to the handicapped. Determine how persons qualify, what services are available, how clients are identified, and what (if any) services are available for the support of the entire family. Present your findings in written form for presentation to the class.
7. Interview a physically compromised adult. Determine the contact that this person has had with health professionals and his or her satisfaction with the services provided. Ask the client what he or she would recommend for any additional or different services. Present your findings in a written report.
8. Interview a family with a disabled member and ask them what needs they have that they perceive

are different from other families'. What assistance have they received from health care providers that has been useful or has not been useful? What are their suggestions for working with similar families?

Critical Analysis Questions

1. Which one of the following statements is most accurate?
   a. The community health nurse who works with a client with type I diabetes mellitus knows that concepts related to disabilities and impairments may apply to her client.
   b. Functional limitations resulting from a physical condition are essentially the same as handicaps.
   c. Developmental disabilities are those that result from physical impairments which occur before the individual is 22 years old.
   d. Disabilities may lead to impairments or to functional limitations.
2. There are several causes of becoming physically compromised. Categories of these causes include all the following *except*:
   a. chronic diseases.
   b. perinatal complications.
   c. injuries.
   d. developmental disabilities.
3. The Healthy People 2000 objective dealing with surveillance is important in relation to those who are physically compromised because:
   a. this enforces compliance with the 1990 Americans with Disabilities Act.
   b. the information will be used to determine life insurance rates for the general United States population.
   c. there is limited data about the extent and kinds of disabilities in people of all ages in this country.
   d. the community health nurse needs the data to implement individual care plans in her caseload.
4. All the following type causes of developmental disabilities are likely to occur prenatally *except*:
   a. central nervous system infections.
   b. placental insufficiency.
   c. chromosomal defects.
   d. inborn errors of metabolism.
5. Detrimental effects of an impairment on a child may result from the condition itself, from effects of the treatment, or from the child's relationships with others. Which of the following conditions are most likely to have negative effects on children as a result of treatment?
   a. blindness, deafness
   b. cerebral palsy, lead toxicity
   c. cleft lip and palate, infantile seizures
   d. leukemia, asthma
6. The community health nurse meets with a neighborhood group that is concerned about the housing of developmentally delayed adults in their neighborhood. None of these residents have prior experience with such clients. Which of these effects on the community of the physically compromised is the nurse dealing with?
   a. increased need for other services; e.g., transportation
   b. discomfort/fear due to lack of knowledge of disability
   c. need/demand to reallocate resources
   d. need to comply with legislation
7. The community health nurse who counsels a family with a physically compromised adult member needs to remember that:
   a. such issues as financial strains, parenting skills of the affected adult, and conflicting role demands on the primary caregiver may have more negative effects on the family than does the client's illness or medical diagnosis.
   b. primary caregivers are more likely to regard respite care as unnecessary and undermining of their roles and authority in the family.
   c. there are typically no significant differences between low-income women and those with higher incomes in relation to their own perceptions of stress and adequacy of the social support they receive.
   d. there is no significant gender difference in determining who is most likely to be the primary caregiver for a disabled family member.
8. Which one of the following statements about abuse and those who are disabled is accurate?
   a. Sexual abuse is less likely to occur in adults and children who are mentally retarded than in the general population.
   b. In children, abuse may result in disabilities, or abuse may occur after children are disabled.
   c. In adults, abuse is more likely to cause disabilities than to occur after the onset of disabilities.
   d. The community health nurse needs to focus on the potential victims and abusers, not on their environments, in order to prevent abuse of those with disabilities.
9. Which of the following is *not* a reason that people with low incomes are at greater risk for the onset and progress of disabling conditions?
   a. They have less access to health care throughout their lives.
   b. They have no significant differences in health risk from lifestyle.
   c. They are less likely to participate in all levels of prevention.

d. They are often unemployed, even when they are able and are hoping to work, thereby lacking access to health insurance.

10. A community health nurse in a rural area finds that a family uses advice from a neighbor on an adjoining farm to try to alleviate the wife's severe rheumatoid arthritis, rather than the nurse's suggestions. The value most likely demonstrated here is:
    a. independence.
    b. hardiness.
    c. practicality.
    d. self-reliance, wariness of "outsiders."
11. Define three of the following terms:
    a. developmental disability
    b. disability
    c. impairment
    d. functional limitations
    e. handicap
    f. chronic disease, or illness
    g. physically compromised
12. Discuss why the attitude of the nurse is essential to work effectively with families in which one member is physically compromised.
13. Briefly describe the role of the nurse in providing support to families who have a member who is physically compromised.
14. Situation: Cindy Green is a six-month-old infant born with spina bifida. Her condition was diagnosed at birth and, while still a newborn, she had a shunting procedure to prevent the development of hydrocephalus and closure of the meningomyelocele. She was referred to the public health clinic for follow-up care.
    Which action(s) would be most appropriate for the community health nurse initially?
    a. Give mother instructions for handling the infant.
    b. Make a developmental assessment of the child.
    c. Refer the mother and child to the state crippled children's service.
    d. Assess the readiness of the mother to learn about the child's care.
15. Follow-up care for Cindy should include which of the following?
    a. routine physical and developmental assessments
    b. enrollment in a normal day care program, when the family desires this service
    c. placement in a state institution for the handicapped
    d. interdisciplinary or multidisciplinary evaluation
16. Mrs. Green asked the nurse if she thought Cindy should be given immunization injections. Which of the following answers reflects the best nursing judgment?
    a. "Since Cindy will not be around many other children now, just wait and start them in six months."
    b. "Yes, Cindy needs the same immunizations as other children because she is subject to having the same diseases."
    c. "She will need the DPT and polio, but the measles vaccine might be dangerous for her."
    d. "Yes, Cindy will need them, but we will not start the series until she has had her first birthday."
17. Evaluate the advantages and disadvantages of at least two of the following pieces of legislation that affect people with disabilities:
    a. Title XIX of the Social Security Act.
    b. Rehabilitation Act of 1973.
    c. Education for All Handicapped Children Act.
    d. Americans with Disabilities Act of 1990.

Answer Key

1. a
2. b
3. c
4. a
5. d
6. b
7. a
8. b
9. b
10. d
11. See chapter content.
12. The family responsibility for these clients is tremendous, and nurses must recognize the toll that the physically compromised take on their energy, time, and emotional and fiscal resources. Nurses may be repelled by people who are physically compromised and might avoid them because they are different; the nurses need to recognize their attitudes when possible so they are able to deal effectively with these clients and the families.
13. Include the family in a plan of care. Help the family deal with grief and other feelings associated with the diagnosis. Assist families in moving through the stages leading to acceptance of the diagnosis. Plan effective strategies with the family for helping them cope.
14. d
15. d
16. b
17. See Legislative section.

32 Vulnerability and Vulnerable Populations: An Introduction

Chapter Summary

Certain population groups are more vulnerable to the effects of risk factors than is the population as a whole. This is due in part to the cumulative effects of multiple risks that make it more difficult to be resilient in the face of stressors. These populations are generally underserved and have been targeted by Healthy People 2000 and Healthy Communities Model Standards for goals and interventions that are based on their unique needs. The vulnerable populations that are described in this chapter are the poor and homeless, pregnant adolescents, migrant workers, the severely mentally ill, substance abusers, those who have been abused, people with communicable diseases, people with AIDS and hepatitis, and people with sexually transmitted diseases. Vulnerability is a multidimensional concept. It involves limited personal control over health, victimization, disenfranchisement, disadvantaged status, powerlessness, and health risk. Low socioeconomic status, age and health-related causes, and past life experiences predispose individuals to vulnerability. Without appropriate social supports and interventions, outcomes of vulnerability are likely to be negative, including poor health status, chronic stressors, hopelessness, and a perpetuating cycle of vulnerability. On the other hand, community nursing interventions that empower members of vulnerable populations and help them break the cycle of vulnerability can lead to positive outcomes. Community nursing assessment must account for the unique needs of vulnerable populations. Interventions and evaluation strategies must also be tailored to the special needs of these groups. This chapter introduces the concept of vulnerability and overall community health nursing roles and strategies for working with vulnerable populations.

Annotated Outline

I. Perspectives on vulnerability
   A. Definition: Vulnerability means that an individual or group is more susceptible to the effects of risk factors than the population as a whole. Vulnerable populations are more likely to develop health problems when exposed to risk factors and are more likely to have poor outcomes. Essentially, they have a lower threshold for risk than those who are more resilient in the face of risks.
   B. Description of vulnerable population groups: Vulnerable population groups include the poor and homeless, pregnant adolescents, migrant workers, severely mentally ill, substance abusers, those who have been abused, people with communicable diseases, people with AIDS and hepatitis, and people with sexually transmitted diseases.
   C. Trends: Just as in colonial America, the current trend is toward providing more care in the community rather than in institutional settings. There is also a trend toward providing more outreach and case finding for vulnerable populations in order to make health care more accessible and more culturally competent for these groups. More community-based agencies are providing comprehensive services so that care for vulnerable individuals and families is more responsive to their needs as opposed to being organized around the needs of health care professionals. Finally, there is a trend to provide services where people live and work, such as in the home, in schools, in occupational settings, and in migrant camps and migrant work settings. Mobile vans are often used to provide outreach services.

II. Public policies affecting vulnerable populations
   A. Landmark legislation: Legislation that has affected vulnerable populations can be categorized as that which directly or indirectly subsidized care for vulnerable populations, that which provided funds for building health care facilities, and that which has changed the way that health care is reimbursed (toward a more prospective model).
   B. Implementation issues: Once a law has been passed, it must be implemented to achieve its intended effects. Often, implementation leads to unintended effects that can result in people following "the letter of the law," but not complying with the spirit of the law. Distribution effects are those outcomes which influence people other than those intended by policy makers. One example was the outcome of deinstitutionalizing the severely mentally ill.

These individuals do receive most of their care in the community, but the care they receive is often fragmented because there are often few incentives for coordinating services across agencies. Nonfinancial barriers to access, such as attitudes, also represent unintended implementation issues for providing care to vulnerable populations.

C. Health care reform: States and individual health care agencies are reforming the way health care is provided. One major shift is toward managed care. This may affect care for vulnerable populations because these groups are more expensive to care for, thereby making them less attractive enrollees for managed care programs. Medicaid and Medicare are moving toward providing managed care services for their enrollees. ANA proposes that health services for vulnerable populations should account for the interrelationships between health, income, housing, sanitation, and social support.

III. Conceptual bases of vulnerability: Vulnerable populations are highly susceptible to harm. Personal, social, and environmental variables contribute to vulnerability. Limited control, victimization, disenfranchisement, disadvantaged status, powerlessness, and health risk are some of the concepts that contribute to an understanding of vulnerability.

A. Limited control: According to the health field concept, individuals share control and responsibility for their health status with the larger society. Vulnerable groups are exposed to certain socioeconomic and environmental conditions that are beyond their control.

B. Victimization: Vulnerable groups may be victimized and blamed for their problems. Social control factors, such as eligibility criteria for health and welfare programs, may contribute to victimization.

C. Disenfranchisement: Vulnerable groups are often socially isolated and thus relatively invisible to many. Not only does this contribute to a potential lack of social support, but it also makes it less likely that society will actively seek to create health and social programs for those who are disenfranchised.

D. Disadvantaged status: The limited political power of these groups contributes to their relative disadvantaged status in relation to the design of health programs.

E. Powerlessness: Members of vulnerable populations do not have the necessary resources to have sufficient power to easily change the social constraints that influence them.

F. Health risk: Vulnerable populations often suffer from multiple, cumulative risks. They seem to be more sensitive to the effects of risk factors than others.

IV. Predisposing factors

A. Socioeconomic status: Poverty, both in its absolute and its relative sense, predisposes people to vulnerability. The United States Federal government sets the official poverty level which influences eligibility for certain health, social, and economic programs. Poverty is, in fact, relative to buying power and is more widespread than the Federal poverty level would suggest. The near-poor and those who are un- and under-insured suffer from the effects of relative poverty. Reliance on a market model for health services tends to lead to attitudes that have been labeled "Social Darwinism." Social Darwinism implies that those who can afford to purchase health services are somehow "worthy" of receiving these services, and those who cannot afford them are to blame for their situations. Social isolation is also an aspect of socioeconomic status that can predispose people to vulnerability.

B. Age-related causes: The very young and the very old are more vulnerable than others, in part because they are less able to adapt physiologically than others. Developmental stressors also interact with socioeconomic and health risks to make people more vulnerable at certain ages than at others. For example, adolescents have developmental tasks that place additional stress on their ability to cope with health risks and that interact with these risks.

C. Health-related causes: Presence of certain diseases compromises the ability to respond effectively to additional risks. For example, elderly individuals may have comorbidities, or multiple chronic illnesses, that stress their immunocompetence and interfere with their functional status.

D. Life experiences: Negative experiences early in life may make people less resilient to health risks. Research suggests that those who have been abused early in life or who have suffered severe trauma are often more vulnerable to later stressors. Those who develop an internal locus of control are better able to cope with such stressors than are people with an external locus of control.

V. Outcomes of vulnerability

A. Poor health outcomes: Vulnerable populations are more likely than others to suffer negative outcomes from health problems.

B. Chronic stressors: Vulnerability leads to the presence of chronic stressors, adding yet another burden with which these groups must cope.

C. Hopelessness: The chronic nature of these problems often leads to feelings of hopelessness.

D. Cycle of vulnerability: Without effective intervention, predisposing factors lead to poor health outcomes, which in turn worsen the predisposing factors. This leads to a cycle of vulnerability that is difficult to break out of without assistance.

VI. Assessment issues: This section discusses guidelines for assessment of both vulnerable individuals and families. Two key principles are to assess only those areas for which the nurse has a purpose or reason for needing the data, and to assess all necessary parameters at one time. Vulnerable clients should not be subjected to unnecessarily intrusive assessment if no reason exists for gathering the data. (This is not unique to vulnerable clients, but is more difficult for such clients to cope with.) Also, vulnerable clients may not be able to return for follow-up, nor may they be able to seek specialized services from other agencies. For these reasons, assessment should be both targeted and comprehensive. Standardized assessment tools may not be appropriate for use with vulnerable populations. Such tools should be evaluated for any modifications that may be necessary before adopting them for use with these populations.

A. Nursing conceptual approaches: Community health nurses will find it useful to select a nursing theory to use as the basis for their work with vulnerable populations. Roy's Adaptation Theory, Orem's Self-Care Theory, and Neumann's Systems Model are particularly well suited to community health nursing practice with vulnerable populations.

B. Socioeconomic considerations: Because socioeconomic variables are such important factors that predispose people to vulnerability, assessment should include evaluation of the adequacy of the individual's or family's social supports and economic self-sufficiency.

C. Physical issues: Assessment of individuals should include relevant physical parameters, based on that person's risk factors.

D. Biological (genetic) issues: Family history is an important component of a targeted, comprehensive assessment. This is consistent with the health field approach described earlier in the chapter.

E. Psychological issues: Psychological issues such as perception of stressors and locus of control should be included in the assessment of vulnerable individuals and families.

F. Lifestyle issues: Lifestyle issues, including smoking, diet, exercise, and presence of stressors, as well as high-risk behaviors, such as sexual practices and substance abuse, should be incorporated into assessment.

G. Environmental issues: Environmental hazards should also be addressed, including presence of asbestos, lead-based paint, noise, carbon monoxide, loose throw rugs, space heaters, guns and ammunition, and hazardous behaviors, such as smoking in bed.

VII. Planning and implementing care for vulnerable populations

A. Community health nursing roles: Community nursing roles when working with vulnerable populations include case finder, health teacher, counselor, direct care provider, monitor and evaluator of care, case manager, advocate, health program planner, and participant in developing health policies.

B. Outreach and case finding: Outreach and case finding are especially important for vulnerable populations, because members of these groups may not choose to seek health care. They may not know what services exist or how to obtain those services. They may be discouraged by cultural, financial, or bureaucratic barriers to care. Vulnerable individuals and families also may not know what types of services could potentially be helpful for them.

C. Client empowerment: One of the most important community health nursing interventions is to increase client health-related skills so they can become effective providers of self-care and effective consumers of health services. Community health nurses may have to begin by fostering the client's sense of self-worth and by facilitating problem-solving skills.

D. Levels of prevention and strategies for promoting a healthy lifestyle: Healthy People 2000 delineates health promotion and illness prevention goals for the United States. Community health nurses should work with vulnerable clients to develop realistic and attainable health promotion and illness prevention goals. Illness prevention interventions may focus on primary, secondary, or tertiary prevention.

E. Year 2000 National Health Objectives and Healthy Communities 2000 strategies: The Year 2000 Objectives include modified goals for special population groups, because the baseline indicators for these groups are often so poor. Health Communities 2000 suggests strategies for targeting health promotion and illness prevention strategies for special population groups.

F. Comprehensive services: It is often best to provide comprehensive, "one-stop" services for vulnerable populations because members of these groups may find it unmanageable to return for repeated visits. Comprehensive services are more responsive to client needs than are more specialized services, which may be efficient for health professionals, but appear fragmented and unfriendly to clients.

G. Resources for vulnerable populations: Community resources may often be found in local phone books. These include health departments, community mental health centers, voluntary agencies such as the American Red Cross, food and clothing banks, missions and shelters, nurse-managed neighborhood clinics, social service agencies, and church-sponsored health and social service assistance. The personal coping skills and informal social support networks of vulnerable individuals and families are important resources as well.

H. Case management: Community health nurses often provide case management for members of vulnerable populations. In addition to providing direct care, they often link clients with services available in the community. Effective linkage involves not only making referrals, but helping clients make the most out of the referral and following up on the outcomes of the referral.

VIII. Evaluation of nursing interventions with vulnerable populations: Evaluation should be based on goals and objectives mutually established with clients. It may include the nature of clinical outcomes, client satisfaction with care, and cost of services.

IX. Clinical application: The concepts and ideas in the chapter are applied to the case of a pregnant, homeless woman.

Additional Critical Thinking Activities

1. Together with several classmates, role play a scenario of a low income family planning and shopping for groceries for a week. Compare the prices for the groceries necessary for this menu between a grocery in a low income area in your community and a large chain grocery in a more affluent area.*
2. Pretend that you are a 20-year-old single mother with two small children. You are on welfare and receive Medicaid. You have recently been diagnosed with a bipolar disorder and are taking Lithium. One of the children is five years old and the other is a six-month-old infant. The five-year-old was born with myelomeningocele and has had numerous surgeries. The three of you are going to spend the day going to utilities and other places, paying bills by cash. After you pay your bills, you must take the children to the health department for well-child check-ups. Take a trip on the mass transportation system with your classmates to do this, imagining what it would be like. Stop at the health department and interview one of the nurses, asking how clients make appointments for well-child visits, how long the average waiting time is once they arrive at the health department, and how often referrals are usually made as a result of the visit. Would this mother likely qualify for Women, Infants, and Children food vouchers? What kinds of help are available in your community for low income children with physical and developmental disabilities? At the next class session, discuss what the experience was like and what you were feeling. What potential health needs do you think this family has? What other community resources might be useful for this family? How might you intervene with this family?**
3. Make a list of places frequented by the homeless in your community. This list might include the unemployment office, a mission, a shelter, a soup kitchen, the Salvation Army, and so on. Pretend you are newly homeless (e.g., you may have just lost your job) and are new in town. With your classmates, spend the day walking from place to place, trying to obtain the resources you will need. At the next class session, discuss how you felt, the problems you may have had, and any new insights you may have regarding the needs of this group.***
4. Interview a hospice nurse who cares for patients with AIDS about the needs that these clients and their loved ones experience. Ask the hospice nurse which services the hospice is able to provide (e.g., pastoral counseling, social services), and which community resources are used most often. Report back to your class and discuss the types of community services needed by people who are HIV+ before they begin experiencing symptoms and as the disease progresses. Are there any service gaps in your community? What kinds of programs might community health nurses develop to fill these gaps?
5. Send an E-mail message to an electronic nursing network and initiate a discussion of the needs of vulnerable populations. What kinds of things are community health nurses doing to meet the needs of these groups in the United States? What about other countries? Request input into the conversation from nurses in Canada, the United Kingdom, Norway, Australia, and other countries. Does the type of health system in place in the country seem to make a difference in the way vulnerable populations are cared for? Discuss with your classmates the health implications of national health insurance versus a private market model of health services for vulnerable populations.

* Thanks to Katherine Parker, Instructor at Midway College, Midway, Kentucky, and Mary Alice Pratt, Professor Emeritus, University of Kentucky College of Nursing, Lexington, Kentucky, who originally developed this exercise and generously shared it.
** Thanks to Katherine Parker, Instructor at Midway College, Midway, Kentucky, and Mary Alice Pratt, Professor Emeritus, University of Kentucky College of Nursing, Lexington, Kentucky, who developed the original exercise on which this activity is based and generously shared it.
*** Thanks to Delwyn Jacoby, who was Assistant Professor, University of Kentucky College of Nursing, Lexington, Kentucky, at the time she developed this exercise, for generously sharing it.

Critical Analysis Questions

The first five questions refer to the case described below.

Shannon Hansen, RN, BSN, is employed as a case manager in a neighborhood clinic that serves a large number of teens who abuse drugs and alcohol. A significant number of them are HIV+, and many of the teenage girls are pregnant at any one time.

1. Knowing that the teens she works with are vulnerable, what should this suggest to Shannon as she evaluates the health risks in this group?
   a. They may be more sensitive to the effects of multiple risk factors than other teens who are not so vulnerable.
   b. She should not assume that their risks will be any different from other teens'.
   c. She should use a standardized risk assessment tool with these teens.
   d. She should focus her risk assessment of the teens on substance abuse, HIV, and adolescent pregnancy rather than on more common issues such as adolescent developmental needs, exercise, or diet.
2. Shannon links clients with services and coordinates these services for her clients. She knows that, for vulnerable populations, one of the potential problems with moving more services from the hospital into the community is:
   a. the quality of services may decrease.
   b. costs of care may increase.
   c. access to care may be limited because of fragmented services provided by multiple agencies.
   d. the services that clients receive may not match their needs as well as before.
3. One of Shannon's clients, 14-year-old Tammy Morgan, recently gave birth to a boy weighing 1437 grams. Tammy was discharged from the hospital shortly after the birth, but the baby stayed in the Neonatal Intensive Care Unit. Tammy found it difficult to visit her baby because she was staying at a local women's shelter, and the shelter was not on a bus line convenient to the hospital. Which of the following actions would be *best* for Shannon to take *initially*?
   a. Shannon should counsel Tammy on why she needs to find permanent housing for herself and the baby.
   b. Shannon should help Tammy problem-solve around how to find transportation to the hospital so she can bond with the baby.
   c. Shannon should ask the director of the shelter to take Tammy to the hospital to visit her baby.
   d. Shannon should teach Tammy about infant nutrition and well-baby care so Tammy will be ready to care for the infant after discharge.
4. Douglas Frankel is another of Shannon's clients. He is 19 years old and has just learned that he is HIV+. Douglas has recently moved to this city and has few friends. He worries that his employer will demote him or possibly even fire him if the news of his HIV status gets out. Douglas told Shannon that most of the people he works with think that people who get AIDS somehow deserve it. Which of the following dimensions of vulnerability does Douglas seem to be experiencing?
   a. disenfranchisement and victimization
   b. powerlessness and limited control
   c. disadvantaged status and health risk
   d. limited control and disadvantaged status
5. Shannon has noticed that a number of her clients share Douglas' fears about losing their jobs or friends due to beliefs that people with AIDS deserve their illness. Which of the following community-focused interventions would be *best* for Shannon to initiate?
   a. She should organize a support group for people with AIDS to discuss their feelings about these fears.
   b. Shannon should organize a meeting of community agency representatives to teach them about AIDS.
   c. Shannon should discuss the problem with other staff at the clinic and encourage each of them to let their clients ventilate their feelings and concerns.
   d. She should organize a series of educational public service announcements that focus on HIV risk factors and that target myths about HIV transmission.

The following five essay questions focus on issues discussed in this chapter.

6. Explain how public attitudes toward vulnerable populations have changed over time, and how attitudes influence social supports available for members of vulnerable populations.
7. Explain why outreach, case finding, and comprehensive services are important for ensuring access to health care services for vulnerable population groups.
8. Explain how community health nursing interventions can help interrupt the cycle of vulnerability, using the example of working with victims of domestic violence.
9. William Butler, RN, works with severely mentally ill adults in a community mental health center. Many of his clients must be referred to multiple agencies for the services they need, such as vocational rehabilitation, medical doctors, legal agencies, and housing (e.g., board and care homes). Describe the factors William should take into account when making referrals and helping his clients follow through effectively on the referrals.
10. Explain the semantic, instrumental, and principled approaches to providing culturally sensitive health care. Analyze the ethical dilemmas associated with relying on these approaches when designing culturally sensitive AIDS prevention strategies.

Answer Key

1. a
2. c
3. b
4. a
5. d
6. Answer should include awareness of ambivalence toward those who are "worthy" of help versus "victim blaming." The best answer will provide historical evidence of the correlation between public attitudes and community services for vulnerable populations. For example, in colonial America, the public believed that disadvantaged members of society should be cared for in their own communities. Community members provided care and support for the mentally ill and disabled members of society. During more conservative political times, a market model dominates public opinion and people believe that those who don't work hard somehow deserve their situation and that the public should not be expected to pay for their care. This results in decreased government funds available for vulnerable populations and increased reliance on local philanthropy. The market model and closely related attitudes of Social Darwinism are in direct opposition to the health field concept, which conceptualizes health as the result of the interrelationships between individual behavior, biology, environment, and health services.
7. Answer should focus on the difficulties that members of vulnerable population groups often have with obtaining access to services as they are commonly organized; e.g., dispersed over multiple facilities, each requiring that clients go to the facility to obtain service, and often requiring that client appointments be organized by specialized problems. Also, answer should include some discussion of cultural and other nonfinancial barriers to care organized within the confines of existing agencies, such as language barriers, transportation barriers, and attitudinal barriers. Outreach and case finding represent active efforts by health care professionals to go to people in need of services, rather than expecting people to come to them. Outreach and case finding offer opportunities to overcome cultural, transportation, and attitudinal barriers. Providing comprehensive, "one-stop" services is more client-focused because it is easier for clients to receive services for multiple needs at one time. Also, comprehensive services reduce the possibility that clients will be lost to follow-up.
8. Answer should include discussion of the way that the factors that predispose people to vulnerability lead to poor health outcomes, and how these poor outcomes themselves intensify the predisposing factors, leading to a spiral effect toward poor health. Appropriate, effective community health nursing interventions are aimed at interrupting this cycle by identifying the relevant predisposing factors and reducing those factors. Community health interventions may be aimed at client empowerment, working with the community to improve social and economic circumstances of vulnerable groups, to identify hazardous lifestyle factors such as abuse, and to develop interventions to reduce abuse. Community health nurses may help victims of domestic violence break the cycle of vulnerability, first by assisting them to develop strategies to get out of the abusive situation (e.g., by referral to a shelter). Then, community health nurses should reinforce the victim's sense of self-worth and should emphasize that the victim did not cause the abuse and does not deserve to be abused. It may be necessary to refer the individual for specialized counseling and for further social and economic assistance.
9. William must know the services provided by these agencies and their eligibility criteria, so his referrals will be appropriate and clients will not needlessly be turned away. He must know the kind of

information the agency will need from him and from the client. He must help the client develop a strategy for following through with the referral; e.g., helping his client problem-solve transportation issues and any problems getting away from work, if he is employed. Further, he should instruct the client on what to expect from the referral and the kinds of questions the client might ask to get the maximum benefit from the referral. Following the referral, he should follow up with the client and the agency, if necessary, to ensure that the client's goals are being met by the referral.

10. Answer should include a description of each approach, using Bayer's (1994) definitions and an example of how to use each approach in AIDS prevention education. Discussion of ethical principles should focus on the potentially divergent demands of cultural autonomy versus paternalism, and of the potential for decreasing the spread of a public health problem (utilitarian values) versus assuming that the dominant culture offers the best approach for illness prevention (ethnocentrism).

33 Poverty and Homelessness

Chapter Summary

Poverty and homelessness affect the health and well-being of individuals, families, and communities. In 1993, the United States Bureau of the Census reported that approximately 39.3 million or 15.1% of the population lived in poverty. The media has brought to our attention the plight of the poor and homeless. The condition of poverty and homelessness, however, is very difficult for most Americans to fully understand. It is an individual, and often isolating, condition. The community health nurse's concept of poverty is shaped and influenced by many variables, including personal beliefs, values, and knowledge of poverty; the life stories of those who experience poverty; and social, political, cultural, and environmental factors.

Poverty and homelessness directly affect the health of individuals and families across the lifespan. The poor and homeless have higher rates of illness and chronic disease, higher rates of morbidity and mortality, shorter life expectancy, and more complex health problems. Health care is often acute and episodic with very little emphasis on preventive care. Certain population groups, such as women, infants, children, and the elderly, are at even greater risk for poor health outcomes.

Community health nurses have a critical role in the delivery of care to persons who are poor or homeless. Nurses' respect for the worth and dignity of the human person, as well as their emphasis on a wholistic approach to people, provides a foundation for intervention. In order to provide effective nursing interventions, the community health nurse needs to understand the epidemiology, health problems, and risk factors associated with poverty. The nurse must first identify individual health care needs and barriers to care, and must then coordinate and provide essential health care services.

This chapter weaves together the voices and stories of those who live in poverty and homelessness and provides information on the ways in which poverty and homelessness affect the health status of individuals, families, and communities. It also outlines strategies that community health nurses can use to promote the health of their poor and homeless patients.

Annotated Outline

I. Understanding the concept of poverty: The concept of poverty is difficult to grasp from solely a didactic approach. The concept of poverty necessitates considerable reflection and analysis. The opportunity for the student to visit a homeless shelter, to speak with a homebound elderly person, or to see the effects of poverty on children deepens the nurse's experience and understanding.
   - A. Personal beliefs, values, and knowledge: The personal beliefs, knowledge, and values that one holds can influence the understanding of the concept of poverty. Nurses must recognize the personal beliefs, values, and knowledge that serve as foundational principles for their practice.
   - B. Patients' perceptions about poverty and health: Poor people are not a homogenous group. Listening to the stories of those who are poor can instruct nurses on what it means to be poor. Many persons that we define as poor may not define themselves as poor.
   - C. Social, political, cultural, and environmental factors
     1. Social: The lack of common definitions of poverty complicates our understanding of poverty. Poverty can be defined as a lack of resources, a power issue, or a lack of income. The federal government uses two terms to discuss poverty: the poverty thresholds and the poverty guidelines. The poverty thresholds are issued by the United States Census Bureau and are used primarily for statistical purposes. The poverty guidelines are issued by the Department of Health and Human Services and are used to determine financial eligibility for services.
     2. Political: A historical and political review reveals changing attitudes and an interest in the plight of the poor.
     3. Cultural: The meaning of poverty differs greatly by culture.
     4. Environmental: Some of the causes of poverty include decreased earnings; increased rates of unemployment; changes in the labor force; a shift to female-headed households; inadequate education and job skills; inade-

quate antipoverty programs; low benefits from AFDC; and increased number of births out of wedlock.

II. Poverty and health: Impact across the lifespan
   A. Childbearing women and poverty: Poor pregnant women are more likely to receive late or no prenatal care, and to deliver low-birth weight babies, premature babies, or babies born with birth defects. Poverty also affects skills, knowledge, self-esteem, and academic performance.
   B. Children and poverty: Child poverty rates in the United States remain twice as high as adult rates. Poverty affects the physical, emotional, spiritual, and intellectual health of children. Some effects of poverty include infant mortality, prematurity, low birth weight, birth defects, chronic diseases, injuries, developmental delays, poor nutrition, and delayed or incomplete immunizations. Poor children also experience more frequent health problems and poor academic performance. The younger the child, the more potential for risk.
   C. Poverty and the elderly: The rate of elderly persons living in poverty has decreased as a result of policy changes and improvements in Social Security and Supplemental Security Income. The poor elderly suffer from high rates of chronic illnesses, higher morbidity rates, shorter life expectancy, and more complex health problems. Isolation and loneliness compound their health risk.
   D. Poverty and the community: Poverty affects both urban and rural communities. Characteristics of poor neighborhoods include high rates of unemployment, economic deterioration, increased rates of crime, racial discrimination, substance abuse, and police brutality. Housing and education conditions are substandard. Persons living in poor communities are often members of minority groups and are often members of single parent families.

III. Understanding the concept of hopelessness
   A. Personal beliefs, values, and knowledge: The nurse's personal beliefs, values, and knowledge about hopelessness influence their relationships and their ability to intervene with persons who are homeless.
   B. Patients' perceptions about homelessness and health: Those who live on the street are the poorest of the poor made visible to us. Yet, so often they become faceless, nameless, and invisible. Researchers studying the experience of being homeless report that several themes emerge: lack of boundaries, self-respect, self-determination, and privacy; difficulty maintaining connections and relationships; fatigue/despair; and frequent relocations.
   C. A portrait of the homeless: Homelessness involves a lack of adequate and permanent shelter and is a potentially transient condition. Accurate estimates of the number of homeless persons are difficult to obtain. The traditional population of middle-aged homeless men is being joined by families, children, single women, substance abusers, adolescent runaways, and the mentally ill. Families with children represent the fastest growing segment of the homeless population.
   D. Causes of homelessness: People move into homelessness gradually and after all other options have been exhausted. Numerous factors contribute to the increasing number of homeless persons: increased number of poor persons; decreased numbers of affordable housing; loss of employment or income; a crisis requiring money; gentrification of neighborhoods; deinstitutionalization of the mentally ill; and alcohol and drug abuse.

IV. Homelessness and its impact on health: Health care is often episodic and crisis-oriented. Specific problems include hypothermia, infestations, peripheral vascular disease, hypertension, respiratory infections, tuberculosis, AIDS, trauma, and mental illness.
   A. Homelessness and at-risk populations
      1. Pregnant women: Homelessness makes it difficult to maintain adequate nutrition, control hypertension, control gynecologic disease, and receive adequate prenatal care.
      2. Homeless children: Homeless children suffer from more frequent and complex health problems. Well-child care and immunizations are often inadequate or absent. Inadequate nutrition can lead to delayed growth and development, failure to thrive, or obesity. Homeless children experience high rates of school absenteeism, academic failure, and emotional and behavioral maladjustments.
      3. Homeless elderly: Chronic medical conditions include tuberculosis, hypertension, arthritis, stroke, and malnutrition. Acute medical conditions include injuries, burns, frostbite, and hypothermia.
   B. Federal programs for the homeless: The Stewart B. McKinney Assistance Act of 1987 marks the federal government's official involvement in the needs of the homeless. The Act created the Interagency Council on the Homeless to coordinate and direct federal homeless activities. Homeless families are eligible for services through the WIC program and the AFDC program. Grants through several foundations have established Health Care

for the Homeless Projects which provide community-based health care services.

V. The role of the community health nurse: The community health nurse has a critical role in the care of persons who are homeless or poor. Nurses must reach out to this population and meet them where they are. Trust, respect, compassion, and concern are essential in the delivery of care. The nurse must use a coordinated multidisciplinary approach that takes into consideration the many stressors and barriers to care that this population endures. Advocacy, coordination of services, therapeutic communication skills, teaching, counseling, collaboration, prevention, and political advocacy are also important strategies of care.

Additional Critical Thinking Activities

1. Discuss with your classmates the poem entitled "On Hearing the News of a Patient's Death," Figure 33-1. Ask one classmate to read the poem aloud while the others imagine the characters and scenes in the poem. Identify and discuss the persons in the poem. What are your personal reactions to the poem? What emotions does the poem stir in you? How does it make you feel? Explore with your classmates creative outlets for expressing some of the various emotions you experience when working with persons who are homeless or poor.
2. Examine health statistics and demographic data to identify the rate of poverty and homelessness in your geographic area. What resources and agencies are available in your area to support these populations? What services are available through the federal government, the state, and the local community? Identify specific geographic boundaries, and survey the area to identify community resources, soup kitchens, health centers, food banks, and clothing distribution centers. How do persons who need these services access them? Have various class members make appointments with key persons in the community to learn more about available services eligibility requirements, and the methods used to evaluate the services.
3. Identify nurses in your community who are working with homeless or vulnerable groups. Invite the nurses to a class session. Organize a panel discussion. Ask the nurses to describe the population they work with; have them describe a typical day. What are the rewards and challenges of working with these high risk populations? How did the nurses first become involved with their work? How do they deal with the frustrations and challenges of their work? How do they remain hopeful in the midst of despair and suffering? What advice do they have to offer the class?
4. Imagine yourself as a community health nurse working in a homeless shelter or making a home visit to a family that lives in an impoverished neighborhood. What previous experience have you had with these situations? What are you anticipating? Write down your fears, anxieties, and apprehensions as you anticipate this work. Discuss your writing with your classmates.
5. Discuss the issue of welfare reform. What is meant by the welfare system in America? What is your understanding of who is on welfare? Who is eligible for welfare? How do people apply for welfare? Do you believe in reforming, restructuring, or abolishing the welfare system? Discuss current legislative proposals dealing with welfare reform. What is the financial and personal cost involved in reforming the welfare system? Identify the senators and representatives in your district. Where do they stand on the issue of welfare reform? How do you propose the welfare system should be restructured?
6. Identify homeless shelters in your area that provide services to families. Ask to visit and meet with the director and staff. Ask what health needs have been identified. Offer to do a teaching session on an identified health need. Once a topic is identified, write an outline, objectives, and a teaching plan that could be utilized to present health information to homeless families.

Critical Analysis Questions

1. Marisa is a four-year-old child who attends a Head Start program. The school nurse diagnosed scabies and recommended that Marisa's father seek treatment for his child. Four days later, Marisa had not yet been seen in a health clinic. When questioned about the delay in seeking treatment, Marisa's father replied that he had not been able to bring Marisa for care because he did not have transportation, and he had numerous appointments with the social worker to apply for housing assistance. How would you explain Marisa's father's behavior?
   a. His behavior is noncompliant.
   b. His behavior is resistant and noncooperative.
   c. His behavior reflects a difference in priorities than the school nurse's.
   d. His behavior is negligent.
2. Financial eligibility for assistance or services under a particular federal program is determined by the:
   a. number of persons living in a household.
   b. poverty thresholds.
   c. employment status of the head of household.
   d. poverty guidelines.

3. In recent decades, the number of people living in poverty is increasing in which of the following groups?
   a. women and children
   b. adolescents and young adults
   c. middle-aged men and the elderly
   d. adolescents and the elderly
4. Felicia is a homeless adolescent who is in her 34th gestational week. She has not received any prenatal care. Felicia's baby is at increased risk for which of the following:
   1. low birth weight
   2. prematurity
   3. birth defects
   4. infant death
   a. 1, 2, 3
   b. 1, 3
   c. 1, 2
   d. 1, 2, 3, 4
5. The fastest growing segment of the homeless population is:
   a. adolescent males.
   b. substance and alcohol abusers.
   c. the chronically mentally ill.
   d. homeless families.
6. John is a 46-year-old male who is living in a homeless shelter. As a result of living in close quarters in the shelter, he is most at risk for which one of the following conditions?
   a. hypothermia
   b. hypertension
   c. tuberculosis
   d. AIDS
7. The federal government officially became involved with meeting the needs of the homeless with the passage of which act?
   a. the Kerrs-Mill Act
   b. the Social Security Act
   c. the Stewart B. McKinney Assistance Act
   d. the War on Poverty Act
8. Many persons who are poor or homeless are frustrated and disappointed with the health care and social care systems. Which of the following is critical to the development of a therapeutic relationship?
   a. scheduling frequent home visits
   b. creating a trusting environment
   c. coordinating services with other health care providers
   d. referring families for counseling
9. Carla is a 14-year-old mother living on public assistance. You are the community health nurse who is making an initial visit to her home following the birth of her son. One of the most important interventions that you can provide on the first home visit is:
   a. to refer Carla and her baby to WIC for supplemental foods.
   b. to refer Carla and her baby to the American Red Cross for child safety and education.
   c. to nurture and support Carla and her baby.
   d. to discuss birth control and infection prevention with Carla.
10. The American welfare system is in actuality a series of complicated systems. Most discussion on welfare focuses on the program known as:
    a. Aid to Families with Dependent Children (AFDC).
    b. Supplemental Security Income (SSI).
    c. Women, Infants, and Children (WIC).
    d. Food Stamps.

Answer Key

1. c
2. d
3. a
4. d
5. d
6. c
7. c
8. b
9. c
10. a

34 Teen Pregnancy

Chapter Summary

Teen pregnancy has become an area of greater public concern as the resources used to provide the special support needed become less available and more costly. The number of teens becoming pregnant has remained high, and increases are seen among the teens least prepared to parent; those under age 15. The reasons that teens become pregnant are often multiple, and in some cases, the pregnancy is deliberate.

Improvements have been made in teen birth outcomes as prenatal care becomes better utilized and young women are more willing to receive care. However, the long-term effects for the young mother and child continue to be deleterious. For example, failure to complete high school will contribute to long-term financial dependency on the teens' families or social support systems. Adolescents are not prepared to parent effectively, and this can place their children at risk for poor cognitive development, as well as for abuse and neglect.

Annotated Outline

I. The adolescent client: Teens have limited experience with independently seeking health care services. Reproductive health concerns are often the reason for an initial visit. Teen behavior during an interview may be difficult to interpret, as these encounters are stressful for the young person.
   A. The interview begins with the chief complaint: The nurse must give indications that the concern is taken seriously, even when it is not felt to be in the best interest of the client; e.g., if a teen presents desiring a pregnancy.
   B. Teens often lack an adequate vocabulary for discussing reproductive health: The nurse should be familiar with local slang expressions and should assist the young person in learning more appropriate terms. This discussion may allow the nurse to recognize misconceptions about normal anatomy and physiology, and to educate accordingly.
   C. Debate exists over whether teens should make reproductive health care decisions without their parents' knowledge: Even through federal laws protect one's right to contraceptive services, other obstacles (such as costs, transportation, and scheduling) can exist that prevent teens from receiving treatment. Abortion services and the adolescents' ability to consent independently will vary by state. The nurse can anticipate these issues for the adolescent and, while honoring confidentiality, may work with this young person and her family to overcome communication problems.

II. Trends in adolescent sexual behavior and pregnancy: Births to teens comprise 24 percent of all first births in the United States. Rates are highest among black teens, followed by Hispanic teens and white teens. A disproportionate number of births to teens occur in the southern states. Forty-one percent of pregnancies to teenagers end in elective abortion and twelve percent in spontaneous abortion. There has been a trend of decreasing abortion rates and increasing birth rates. The United States leads developed nations in teen pregnancies, teen births, and teen abortions.

III. Background factors in teen pregnancy: Characteristics of teens giving birth are changing. Three-quarters of these teens are poor and often see limited value in delaying a pregnancy. Most teens report that a pregnancy was unintended, yet their behaviors do not match this opinion. Teens often feel invincible and do not believe they will become pregnant. If they do become pregnant, they do not believe they could experience negative outcomes.
   A. Sexual activity and use of birth control: The sexual debut is earlier. By 9th grade, 40% of teens are sexually active, and by 12th grade, 72% are sexually active. Birth control use among teens has improved, with 65% of young women reporting birth control use at first coitus. Yet half of all first time teen pregnancies occur within the first six months of initiating intercourse. The earlier a teen initiates intercourse, the less likely birth control will be used. Knowledge about sexuality, birth control, and pregnancy will vary because school curricula are not standardized.
   B. Peer pressure/partner pressure: Teens are more likely to be sexually active if their friends are sexually active. Some young men may feel that

fathering a child would make them feel more manly.

C. Sexual victimization: Adolescent women who have a history of being sexually abused are at risk for earlier initiation of voluntary sexual intercourse, are less likely to use birth control, are more likely to use drugs and alcohol at first intercourse, and are more likely to have older sexual partners. The youngest women are more likely to experience coercive sex.

D. Family structure: Adolescents from families in which divorce, remarriage, and single parenting exist are more likely to have intercourse.

E. Parenting influences: Teenagers of parents who are neglectful are more sexually experienced, followed by teens whose parents are very strict and controlling. Parents who discuss sexuality, birth control, and pregnancy with their teens can have a positive influence on delaying sexual initiation and on using birth control effectively.

IV. Young men and paternity: One in fifteen males becomes a father during the teen years. More than half of the fathers in teen births are between the ages of 20 and 24. Establishing paternity, or fatherhood, can be done at the time of the baby's birth. States may vary on the procedure among non-married couples. Young men often want to be involved in a young woman's pregnancy and the birth of their child. Over time, the teen relationship may dissolve, but contact with the child could continue. Involvement of the young father will have a positive affect on his child's development and will provide greater personal satisfaction for himself and greater role satisfaction for the young mother.

V. Early identification of the pregnant teenager: Young women may ignore early signs of pregnancy, hoping that it will just go away. The community health nurse must be sensitive to subtle cues that a teenager may offer. Counseling should be provided at the time of pregnancy testing. The nurse and the client can explore pregnancy options, such as abortion, adoption, and parenting. Referrals for prenatal and support services, if desired, should be initiated at the counseling visit.

VI. Special issues in caring for the pregnant teen: Problems associated with teen pregnancy can often be averted when nursing interventions are in place. Teens need particular assistance in the following areas:

A. Initiation of prenatal care: Inadequate prenatal care has been negatively associated with health risks to both the mother and fetus. Half of all pregnant teens delay entering prenatal care until after the first trimester. Barriers to seeking care include cost, denial of the pregnancy, fear of telling parents, transportation, dislike of providers' care, and attitudes among clinic staff toward pregnant teens.

B. Low birth weight infants/preterm delivery: Teens are more likely than adult women to deliver babies weighing less than 5 1/2 pounds or to deliver before 37 weeks gestation. These babies are harder to care for, which challenges the limited skills of the young mother.

C. Nutrition: A teen may begin a pregnancy with her own nutrient growth needs, as well as poor dietary habits and limited reserves of essential vitamins and minerals. This requires a substantial change in her diet to accommodate the needs of the growing fetus. Younger teen mothers have the greatest needs and may need to gain more weight than older teens. Iron deficiency is a particular problem which can contribute to prematurity, low birth weight, postpartum hemorrhage, and other serious complications.

D. Infant care: Teens benefit from education about infant care and stimulation. The nurse can include the young father and the teen mother's family in educational efforts. Particular attention should be placed on understanding child development and adopting realistic expectations for their children. The nurse can observe the young mother's ability to respond appropriately to her infant's cues, and she can offer positive reinforcement, which will help the young woman gain confidence in her role.

E. Repeat pregnancy: Twenty-four percent of teens will have a second birth within 24 months, and the younger the teen, the greater the risk of an early second pregnancy. Family planning can be discussed during the pregnancy, and a method can be decided upon. The nurse should work with the young woman to look at her risk of repeat pregnancy realistically.

F. Schooling and educational needs: Pregnant teens need encouragement to continue school. Special arrangements can be made for homebound instruction in the case of medical complications during the pregnancy, as well as during the six week postpartum period. Teens who return to school after delivery are more likely to delay a second birth. Acquiring and affording day care is a significant problem.

VII. Teen pregnancy and the community health nurse

A. Home-based interventions: Young women at risk for pregnancy may be identified in families currently visited by the community health nurse. Home visiting during the pregnancy allows for assessment of the environment. It also allows for family members to be included in educational sessions and promotes family communication.

B. Community-based interventions: The nurse can participate in broad-based coalitions that target teen pregnancy issues specific to the local community. The nurse can also be a valuable asset to the schools as a consultant or participant in the family life program. School-based clinics are emerging throughout the country, and the community health nurse may participate in the services offered.

VIII. Clinical application: The case study reviews the identification, support, education, and collaboration involved in working with a pregnant teenager.

IX. Summary: This chapter reviews the causes and consequences of teen pregnancy and parenting and points out interventions that the community health nurse can employ to improve mother-baby outcomes.

Additional Critical Thinking Activities

1. Interview several pregnant and parenting teenagers. Determine their reasons for becoming pregnant and their level of satisfaction/dissatisfaction. Note any differences in family and/or partner support.
2. Compile a directory of local programs that provide assistance to pregnant teenagers. Look specifically at programs designed to encourage school continuation and vocational training. Determine whether resources are adequate for the numbers of pregnant and parenting teens in the community.
3. Attend a meeting of a coalition or task force that addresses local teen pregnancy issues. Observe the membership for organizational and cultural diversity.
4. Develop an education program for young fathers. Include topics on physiology of pregnancy, role of the coach in labor and delivery, infant care and development, and establishment of paternity. Identify ways to recruit young men into this program.
5. Interview the nurse in the local high school (either the school nurse or the community health nurse). Ask the following questions:
   A. Is teen pregnancy a problem? Describe.
   B. What are the obstacles to school attendance for the pregnant and parenting teenager?
   C. What school programs have been successful for either the pregnant teen or for prevention of sexual activity and/or pregnancy?
   D. Does teen pregnancy affect the rest of the student body?

Critical Analysis Questions

1. When interviewing the adolescent client, which of the following is true?
   a. Discussions about sexuality should always be done with a parent present.
   b. The client may have difficulty disclosing sexual information.
   c. Encouraging birth control use is always useful.
   d. Information on normal anatomy and physiology is always useful.
   e. b and d
2. Pregnancy rates are highest among which teenagers?
   a. teens living in poverty
   b. teens living in the southern states
   c. older teens
   d. all of the above
3. What percentage of teens choose adoption?
   a. 5%
   b. 1%
   c. 10%
   d. 30%
4. Inconsistent use of birth control can reflect which of the following?
   a. teens as risk takers
   b. dissatisfaction with available methods
   c. ambivalence about becoming pregnant
   d. all of the above
5. True or False? Teens are more likely to be sexually active if they have friends who are sexually active.
6. Which two parenting styles can adversely affect a teenager's initiation of sexual activity and pregnancy risk? (Select two.)
   a. parents who discuss sexuality with their children
   b. parents who have high demands for their children to act maturely
   c. parents who are demanding and controlling
   d. parents with low expectations for their children
7. List three circumstances that can increase the risk of pregnancy for a young woman with a history of sexual victimization.
8. The establishment of paternity means:
   a. child support.
   b. fatherhood.
   c. visitation rights.
   d. promise of marriage.
9. Which of the following statements is *false*?
   a. Teens generally have realistic attitudes about weight gain in pregnancy.
   b. Frequent snacking and fast food restaurants can not provide a solid nutritional foundation for pregnancy.

c. Young women with a gynecological age of two years or less have increased nutrient requirements during pregnancy.
d. Weight gain is one of the strongest predictors of infant birth weight.

10. List three interactions a young mother could employ with her infant to promote maternal-infant bonding.
11. A repeat pregnancy may be averted in the teenager who:
    a. marries the father of the baby.
    b. returns to school after delivery.
    c. begins birth control pills immediately after delivery.
    d. experiences severe financial struggles after the child is born.
12. Homebound educational instruction is available for the pregnant teenager who:
    a. has been severely socially stigmatized by the pregnancy.
    b. is recommended by school personnel because of poor role modeling to other students.
    c. experiences medical complications or has delivered.
    d. has delivered and cannot work out child care arrangements.
13. Which statement best describes the family dynamics in teen pregnancy?
    a. Initially there is a crisis stage, but the birth of the baby gives way to great acceptance and cooperation.
    b. Family support for a teen parent can have a positive influence on her and her infant.
    c. Families in crisis that experience a teen pregnancy have little hope for restoration and healing.
14. Which community-based interventions can benefit from nursing participation?
    a. broad-based coalitions
    b. school-based clinics
    c. family life education
    d. church groups
    e. all of the above

Answer Key

1. e
2. d
3. a
4. d
5. True
6. c and d
7. If pregnancy results from forced intercourse; she is more likely to use drugs and alcohol at first intercourse; and past abuse affects a young woman's ability to exert control over future sexual experiences.
8. b
9. b
10. Make eye contact with the baby; talk often to the baby; do not prop the bottle but instead hold the baby comfortably in your arms to feed.
11. b
12. c
13. b
14. e

35 Migrant Health

Chapter Summary

A migrant farm worker is defined as a laborer whose principal employment involves moving from farm to farm, planting or harvesting agriculture and attaining temporary housing. Migrant farm workers and their families are a vulnerable population, characterized by unique social, economic, and health risks that lead to disenfranchisement, victimization, and helplessness.

Annotated Outline

I. Migrant health problems
   A. Health and health care: Migrant farm workers have a 25% higher infant mortality rate than the national average and a life expectancy of 49 rather than 75 years. They also have an increased rate of parasitic and infectious diseases.
   B. Work conditions: Migrant farm workers are faced with adverse working conditions, including pesticide exposure, increased physical demands, and unfair wage practices. Although some state and federal policies are in place to protect migrant farm workers, they may be rarely enforced. The vast number of farms covered by a single government inspector makes upholding the standards for workers' safety and fairness virtually impossible.
   C. Pesticide exposure: Migrant farm workers are exposed not only to the immediate effects of working in fields foggy and wet with pesticides, but also to the unknown effects of chronic pesticide exposure. Some of these may include skin rashes, conjunctivitis, infertility, liver damage, and cancer.
   D. Housing: The worker's home is usually tied to his job. Therefore, when his job ends, he becomes simultaneously unemployed and homeless. Costly and cramped living conditions are common and contribute to many health problems.
   E. Women: Women are often expected to work in the fields and still provide care for their children and meals for their families. They report isolation, depression and anxiety, sexual harassment, and rape. Some programs fund education of migrant women to serve as a link between existing health care agencies and farm worker families.
   F. Child and youth: Many migrant children suffer from malnutrition, infectious diseases, dental caries, inadequate immunizations, pesticide exposure, or accidents. Children often attend many different schools in the same year and miss several days due to travel. In some areas, federally funded summer programs exist to supplement education for migrant children.

II. Barriers to migrant health care
   A. Lack of knowledge
   B. Lack of income
   C. Lack of state and federal support
   D. Location of health services
   E. Hours of health services
   F. Lack of child care
   G. Mobility and tracking
   H. Discrimination
   I. Documentation
   J. Lack of bicultural/bilingual health care staff

III. Social and cultural considerations in migrant health care
   A. Work ethic and gender roles: The male head of the family is often in charge of finances and transportation. He often makes the final decision of whether to secure health care services, whereas the wife/mother usually makes the determination that health services are needed.
   B. Family: "Familialism" is common and refers to the concept that family needs take precedent over individual needs.
   C. Health values: Health is seen as a harmonious relationship between the social and spiritual aspects of being. Use of curanderas is common.
   D. Interactive styles: "Personalismo" is a health care provider with a similar background, culture, and language to the patient. "Simpatia" refers to the need for polite, respectful, and nonconfrontational communication between the health care provider and the patient. "Collectivism" is defined as the practice of family and friends being involved in the assessment and management of the patient.

IV. Health promotion and illness prevention: Farm workers often do not view illness as a problem unless it prevents them from working. In seeking health care, the expectation is a complete recovery with a rapid return to work. Outreach workers provide a vital link between traditional health care and migrant families, via home and work place visitation.

V. Role of the community health nurse: The community health nurse can be a catalyst for change and may employ the nursing process to assess farm worker needs continually, to direct members in search of health services, and to evaluate the success of their efforts.

VI. Legislative issues: The Migrant Health Act of 1962 provides primary and supplemental health services to migrant farm workers and their families. The National Council on Migrant Health meets triennially to advise, consult with, and make recommendations concerning the organization, operations, selection, and funding of migrant health centers.

Additional Critical Thinking Activities

1. Interview health care workers and determine their definition of migrant farm worker. Health care workers could include social workers, nurses, physicians, and registered dietitians. Compare and contrast their definitions.
2. Interview community leaders to determine the presence of migrant farm workers in your area. Compare and contrast information about migrant farm workers by interviewing teachers, clergy, and politicians versus migrant outreach workers, Wage and Hour personnel, Department of Labor personnel, and Migrant Head Start program employees.
3. Consult your library to review vital statistics and census track data to confirm the presence of migrant workers documented in your area. Are there any contradictions between documented statistics and your interview in activity 2? Why is it difficult to account for (much less track) migrant farm workers?
4. Determine eligibility for Medicaid and Aid to Families with Dependent Children services. You may consult the county health department and the state office. Do migrant workers in your state qualify?
5. Design a clinic to provide health care to migrant workers in your area. What services would you provide? What hours would you operate?

Critical Analysis Questions

1. A ________________ is best defined as a laborer whose principal employment involves moving from farm to farm, harvesting agriculture, and attaining temporary housing.
   a. seasonal farm worker
   b. migrant farm worker
   c. transient worker
   d. share cropper
2. The average life expectancy of the migrant farm worker in the United States is:
   a. 72 years.
   b. 61 years.
   c. 55 years.
   d. 49 years.
3. A variety of symptoms/diseases in migrant farm workers (including skin rashes, conjunctivitis, and even cancer) are highly correlated with:
   a. crowded living conditions.
   b. poor field sanitation.
   c. pesticide exposure.
   d. automated machinery.
4. The largest primary residence (home base) for migrant farm workers in the United States is:
   a. southern Florida.
   b. southern Texas.
   c. southern California.
   d. southern New Mexico.
5. Proportionally, the cultural group most likely to drop out of the "migrant stream" and establish residency quickly is:
   a. American Black.
   b. non-Hispanic White.
   c. Southeast Asian.
   d. Mexican American.
6. Which of the following characteristics of migrant farm workers and their families place them at higher risk for acquiring/transmitting tuberculosis?
   a. poor sanitation
   b. unregulated pesticide exposure
   c. temperate field work
   d. crowded living conditions
7. Migrant farm workers typically seek health care:
   a. when they can no longer work.
   b. after home remedies have failed.
   c. when they find a clinic with evening hours.
   d. when a curandera is not available.
8. A nurse who is respectful and nonjudgmental of the dynamics of the migrant worker family demonstrates understanding of the concept of:
   a. simpatia.
   b. collectivism.
   c. familialism.
   d. personalismo.

9. Viral hepatitis is ____________ times more likely to occur in migrant farm workers than in other United States aggregates:
   a. 3
   b. 10
   c. 30
   d. 300
10. True or False? Most migrant farm workers are Medicaid eligible.
11. True or False? Over 50% of migrant farm workers utilize health services funded by the Migrant Health Act.
12. True or False? President John F. Kennedy signed the Migrant Health Act in 1962, following a 15-year lapse without any federal policy for migrant health services.
13. Unscramble the letters to form words; then unscramble the circled letters to finish the phrase at the bottom of the puzzle.

N	I	I	S	P	A	C	H

(_) _ (_) _ (_) _ _ _

T	R	I	G	M	A	N

_ _ _ (_) (_) _ _

R	E	A	R	F	M

(_) _ _ (_) (_) _

E	N	V	O	L	C	I	E

(_) _ (_) _ (_) _ _ _

P	E	T	I	T	A	I	S	H

(_) _ _ _ (_) _ _ _ (_)

WHAT THE MIGRANT FARM WORKER BRINGS TO THE AMERICAN DINNER TABLE:

_ _ _ _ _ _ _   _ _

"_ _ _ _ _"

Answer Key

1. b
2. d
3. c
4. b
5. c
6. d
7. a
8. a
9. d
10. False
11. False
12. True
13. HISPANIC, MIGRANT, FARMER, VIOLENCE, HEPATITIS, HARVEST OF SHAME

36 Mental Health Issues

Chapter Summary

Challenges in the mental health field pertain to issues of care for people with problems that range from severe, disabling mental disorders, to mental health problems that are less incapacitating, but that are also long-term in nature. Other factors that contribute to nursing challenges include the scope and chronicity of mental illness, and the uncertainty about specific cause, cure, and treatment for most severe mental disorders. Limited resources compound the problems and present challenges in community mental health work.

Types of services and treatment in various countries are influenced by cultural beliefs and generally parallel economic development. Yet, two universals exist: services for people with mental disorders are inadequate in all countries, and the impact of mental illness on families, communities, and nations is profound. Therefore, specialized knowledge and skills about severe mental illness and mental health problems are necessary for effective community nursing practice. Helpful information includes knowledge about the organization of mental health services from historical perspectives, as well as trends in current health care demands and delivery. Knowledge about populations at risk for psychiatric-mental health problems and insight about illness outcomes in terms of biopsychosocial consequences are even more important. Finally, it is necessary to refine and broaden nursing process skills in treatment planning to include the impact of mental illness on families and on the community.

This chapter focuses on the development of community mental health services, current health objectives for mental health and mental disorders, the role of the nurse, and use of the nursing process in community settings while working with clients who have mental health problems or disorders. Frameworks and concepts useful in community mental health nursing practice are also presented. Because other chapters in this book are devoted to risk groups like the homeless population and those with substance abuse problems, the focus of this chapter is on populations who have long-term, severe mental disorders and on groups who are vulnerable to mental health problems. *Severe mental disorders* are determined by diagnosis and by criteria that include degree of functional disability (American Psychiatric Association [APA], 1994), whereas *mental health problems* are difficulties related to an individual's inability to negotiate the daily challenges of life without experiencing undue social isolation, emotional distress, or behavioral incapacity (Department of Health and Human Services [DHHS], 1990).

Annotated Outline

I. Evolution of community mental health care
   A. Historical perspectives: Early treatment of people with mental disorders was cruel and inhumane. Beliefs were based on superstitions, and treatment was attributed to witches and magicians. People with mental disorders were mistreated, and many were placed in jails. Humane treatment and reform of primitive conditions was influenced by Philippe Pinel (1759-1820) in France and Benjamin Rush (1745-1813) in America.
   B. Humanitarian reform: During the humanitarian reform movement, the efforts and actions of Dorothea Dix focused attention on criminals, people with mental disorders, and victims of the Civil War. She fostered the belief that people with mental disorders needed health and social services. Because of her efforts, which included political action, hospitals were constructed, hospital and nursing standards were established, and mental health care was altered in America and Europe.
   C. Hospital expansion, institutionalization, and the mental hygiene movement: Humanitarian reform resulted in the proliferation of hospitals, including the construction of large psychiatric institutions that were usually built in rural areas. Because of the locations of the psychiatric hospitals, the individuals who were admitted were essentially separated from their families and communities. For the most part, the psychiatric hospital populations consisted of individuals with severe mental disorders and of the elderly with dementia. These populations expanded beyond proportion, partly because many were never discharged. Overcrowded, unsanitary hospital conditions and exploitation of patients were reported by Clifford Beers, an individual who knew about the conditions be-

cause he had been hospitalized for psychiatric disorders on more than one occasion. His advocacy efforts and writings influenced the founding of the National Committee for Mental Hygiene and led to the mental hygiene movement. During the mental hygiene movement, attention was focused on prevention, early intervention, and the influence of environmental and social factors on mental illness; an important concept that took shape was the idea of a multidisciplinary team approach to treatment in community settings. These developments increased understanding about the scope of mental illness, which was later reinforced when many men screened for military service during World War II were found to have neurological and psychiatric mental health disorders.

D. Federal legislation for mental health services: The first legislation influencing mental health services was enacted prior to World War II, when the Social Security Act was passed in 1935. Following the war, additional legislation was passed because of the demand for services. This was due, in part, to increased awareness that environmental conditions and stress had a bearing on mental health.

E. Post-World War II legislation: After World War II, The National Mental Health Act was passed, and the National Institutes of Mental Health was designated to administer education and research programs for community mental health approaches to treatment. While education and research programs developed readily, community services expanded slowly. Instead, the medical model, psychotherapy, and psychiatric units in general hospitals developed, while treatment that was long-term in nature, for individuals with severe mental disorders and the elderly with dementia, continued to be provided in large state hospitals. The Mental Health Study Act of 1955 resulted in the *Action for Mental Health Report* that emphasized the importance of reducing the size of the hospitals and of shifting services for severe mental disorders to community health clinics.

F. Legislation for community mental health centers: Public awareness of mental illness and mental retardation early in the 1960s resulted in legislation that formalized the community mental health centers concept. The Community Mental Health Centers Act provided matching funds to states if they developed programs that included short-term and partial hospitalization, aftercare, emergency services, outpatient treatment, rehabilitation, and vocational counseling. State programs developed in diverse ways. At the same time, large numbers of individuals were discharged from state psychiatric institutions before adequate community services were developed.

G. Deinstitutionalization: The cost of institutional care was a major reason for moving patients out of the state hospitals. However, earlier discovery of psychotropic drugs that resulted in better management of patients with severe mental disorders also influenced the movement. Factors that contributed to the failure of deinstitutionalization included inadequate services for transitions from hospitals to community settings; placement of patients in unsupervised settings where they could not maintain suitable living conditions; lack of education and support services for family members; and lack of education for many staff members in community settings. Civil rights activism addressed issues related to lack of services as well as to discrimination.

H. Civil rights legislation for people with mental disorders: The Americans with Disabilities Act (ADA) mandated that people with physical and mental disabilities be brought into the mainstream of American life. Mainstreaming involved (1) employment, (2) public accommodations, and (3) public services programs and activities. This meant that state and local governments were obliged to integrate programs that were suitable for people who had special problems like mental health disorders. The ADA also specified that individuals with mental health disorders had a right to equal employment opportunities. Violations of the law are considered equal to violations of the Equal Protection Clause of the Constitution.

I. Consumer advocacy: *Consumer* refers to persons who are current or former recipients of mental health services. Prior to the 1980s, consumers and family members in general lacked self-advocacy skills and effective avenues for advancing their ideas about needs for mental health services. Consumers were often ineffective because programs fostered passivity; family members were ineffective because they knew little about treatment. Self-advocacy is important because it fosters self-confidence, promotes participation in treatment, and may influence public policy. Consumer and family member organizations, like the National Alliance for the Mentally Ill (NAMI), were formalized early in the 1980s. There was evidence of their self-advocacy ability during the health care reform debate of the mid-1990s, when consumer and family affiliates joined with professional groups to promote parity for mental health services in health care reform.

II. Current and future perspectives in mental health care

A. National objectives for mental health services: Current perspectives about mental disorders and mental health in the United States are outlined in *Healthy People 2000* (Department of Health and Human Services, 1990) and in the National Institutes of Mental Health (NIMH) objectives for severe mental disorders. Target populations for persistent mental disorders (e.g., autism, schizophrenia, and major depression) include children, adolescents, and adults. Target populations for mental health problems (e.g., stress and emotional disorders) essentially include all ages across the life span. The objectives also highlight the seriousness of violence in the society. The national objectives can be useful for guiding community mental health practice.

B. Model standards for implementing national objectives: Guidelines for implementing the *Healthy People 2000* objectives are available in *Healthy Communities 2000: Model Standards*. The overall goal of the healthy communities standards emphasizes prevention, maintenance, and/or restoration of mental health and independent functioning. Historically, these types of services have been lacking. Community mental health nurses can attempt to encourage or reverse that trend by using the standards in practice. Specific examples include using the standards in community assessments with other groups or agencies who provide mental health services. Other examples are illustrated in the discussion about vulnerable populations in Chapter 36, Mental Health Issues.

C. The scope of mental illness: Mental illness is prevalent in all segments of society, both nationally and internationally. In the United States, an estimated 23 million noninstitutionalized adults have cognitive, emotional, or behavioral disorders, excluding alcohol and substance abuse problems. Useful classifications for discussion of the scope are severe mental disorders and mental health problems.

D. Severe mental disorders: Severe mental disorders strike at the human qualities of thought and behavior. Examples of severe mental disorders include schizophrenia and major depression. Of the four million people in the United States who have a severe mental disorder, 900,000 live in institutions, and the rest live in communities. Factors that contribute to the large number living in the community include continuing deinstitutionalization, reduced hospital admissions, and fewer days spent in the hospital. Many of those who live in the community live in substandard housing and have difficulty maintaining themselves. Many of the homeless population have a severe mental disorder. Important sites of nursing services include shelters, soup kitchens, and other places where people seek shelter.

E. Mental health problems of high-risk populations: One view of mental health is that it is the empowerment force that motivates the individual in the pursuit and fulfillment of life's goals. Threats to mental health create stress and undermine the individual's ability to function. Internal factors, like biopsychosocial makeup, and external factors in the environment, like assets of communities, influence mental health. Both untoward incidents and anticipated life events influence the individual's ability to function. Death of a family member can be used to illustrate the phenomenon. Bereavement reactions to an anticipated death of a family member include loss of appetite, sadness, and difficulty making decisions. Conditions of the situation can increase risk for mental health problems in bereavement. Examples include guilt, if the family member dies as a result of suicide, and stigma associated with AIDS-related death. Because there are multiple threats to mental health, considering specific age groups is useful.

Children and adolescents: Approximately 12% of the 63 million children under age 18 have a mental disorder. Risk factors include maternal deficits during the prenatal period, environmental conditions associated with neglect and violence, and lack of consistent caregivers. Conditions typically diagnosed during childhood include depression, anxiety, attention-deficit disorder, mental retardation, Downs syndrome, and autism. Common problems of adolescence include conduct disorders, eating disorders, substance abuse, and depression. Suicide and attempted suicide are common problems during adolescence; suicide is the second leading cause of death among adolescent males between the ages of 15 and 19.

Adults: In 1990, approximately one in five adults, or 41.2 million Americans, had a mental disorder. Conditions included severe and persistent mental disorders like schizophrenia and major depression. In addition, multiple sources of stress threaten the mental health of adults. Examples are multiple role responsibilities, job insecurity, unstable relationships, and environmental and intrafamilial violence. The incidence of homicide and suicide among adults in the United States suggests the profound nature of these problems for individuals, as well as for their family survivors. The impact of mental illness on family members is revealed in research findings about caregivers. Findings suggest that threats to mental health include lack of social support, chronic strain, burden, high levels of distress, heightened anxiety, and depression.

Older adults: The population over age 65 is steadily increasing. Many maintain highly functional lives, but others have mental health deficits because of normal sensory losses and failing physical health. Common physical problems include arthritis, osteoporosis, stroke, terminal illness associated with cancer, cardiovascular disease, and respiratory conditions. Another factor that contributes to mental health status includes life changes related to work roles and loss of family and friends due to death. Loss of these types of social networks can result in deprivation, isolation, and depression. Suicide, one outcome of depression, is not uncommon among older adults. In the United States, men between the ages of 65 and 74 are in the highest risk category for suicide.

Low income, ethnic, and minority groups: All socioeconomic and cultural groups have mental health problems. Ethnic and minority groups deserve special mention because historically they have lacked access to adequate, culturally sensitive services. Poverty contributes to mental health conditions because it undermines both physical and mental health. Also, substandard living conditions contribute to infectious disease, including tuberculosis and, when combined with risk behaviors, HIV infection. Environmental hazards also contribute to risk for accidental deaths, while violence takes a toll on individuals and family members. Though members of minority groups are represented in all socioeconomic groups, many live at or below the poverty line. Therefore, they are at risk for problems previously mentioned. African-Americans make up the largest minority group in the United States, followed by Hispanic-Americans. The third largest minority group is made up of Asian and Pacific Americans, who speak over 30 different languages and have diverse cultures. Diversity is also a characteristic of the fourth largest minority group—Native American and Alaska native populations. When conducting community assessments, it is important to identify the needs of special populations and to determine types of services available for addressing mental health problems, including prevention. Locations of assessments should include but not be limited to the following: pre-schools through post-secondary education systems, work sites, senior citizen housing and services, and organizations and systems that attract particular cultural and ethnic groups.

III. Role of the nurse in community mental health: The scope and standards for psychiatric mental health nursing practice were redefined in 1994. Functions suggest the overlapping roles of practitioner, educator, and coordinator.

A. Practitioner: Objectives of the practitioner role are to help the client maintain or regain coping abilities that promote functioning by using the nursing process to guide the diagnosis and treatment of human responses to actual or potential mental health problems. Role functions at the basic practitioner level include case management, counseling, milieu therapy, and psychobiological interventions. In the community, practice is based in a variety of settings including the home, schools, community mental health centers, and public health departments. Other settings are places where those with severe mental disorders live or seek shelter—personal care homes, nursing homes, boarding houses and hotels, short-term shelters, and soup kitchens.

B. Educator: The educator role involves the use of the teaching-learning process to enhance understanding about the various dimensions of mental illness in working with individuals and groups. The educator role is foundational to functions like health maintenance, health promotion, and community action. Both formal and informal teaching is important. One example of a formal teaching activity is educating elders about over-medicating. An example of informal teaching is to enhance positive coping skills with clients.

C. Coordinator: Coordination of care is a basic principle of the multidisciplinary team approach in community mental health services. Objectives of the coordinator role include promoting the client's well-being by promoting independence and self-care in the least restrictive setting. The phenomenon of homelessness suggests that there is a lack of coordination, as well as a lack of services, in most communities. Therefore, at minimum, basic functions of the coordinator role include case finding, referral, and follow-up to evaluate system breakdown and deficits. Other functions include intake screening, crisis intervention, and home visits. To approximate the objectives and functions of the coordinator role, the nurse works with a variety of professional and para-professional workers, family members, and community volunteers. Like the practitioner and educator roles, an aim of the coordinator is to enhance the quality of life for the client, significant others, and the community.

D. Frameworks: Theories and concepts that help to explain relationships or the dynamics of mental illness are used to guide nursing process activities. An aim of nursing process activities is to enhance principles of the mental health movement. The principles foster people's right to mental health services, including services in the least restrictive environment.

E. Theories: Systems theory is a useful framework for community mental health practice because it emphasizes the importance of relationships of the parts or elements of a unit to the whole. A holistic view of systems can be applied in a variety of ways. One example is the subsystem of cultural groups in a community; another is the family system of individuals and their support systems in the community. Other theories that are useful include those that enhance understanding of biological systems, personality, and lifespan development.

F. Prevention: Health promotion and illness prevention are fundamental to community mental health practice, as are the previously described national health objectives. Primary, secondary, and tertiary prevention are useful concepts for practice. *Primary prevention* refers to the reduction of health risks; *secondary prevention* refers to activities aimed at reducing the prevalence or pathology of a condition; *tertiary prevention* refers to restoration and enhancement of functioning. Examples of primary prevention include education and lifestyle management classes. Secondary prevention activities include providing group or individual psychotherapy. Tertiary prevention includes monitoring illness symptoms and coordinating transition from the hospital to the home.

G. A Vulnerability-Stress Model: Liebermann et al. (1993) proposed the Vulnerability-Stress-Coping-Competence Model of major mental disorders to promote understanding of mental illness and to enhance rehabilitation of the client in the community. The model helps to explain that individuals with mental disorders have psychobiological vulnerabilities because of the interplay of genetics and stressful life events. Biological vulnerabilities may inhibit development of social skills early in life. Social skills deficits combined with stressful life events can overwhelm a person's coping ability. Protective factors, another concept of the theory, are important moderators of vulnerability and stress. Coping and competence are essential protective factors. Family members, natural support systems, and professional treatment can help develop a person's coping and competence. Other protective factors are rehabilitation programs, housing programs, and case management. Relapse management is also central to many of these programs and activities.

H. Relapse Management: Murphy and Moller (1993) suggested that managing relapse is a major goal of intervention in community mental health practice. The relapse management concept is compatible with vulnerability-stress models of mental illness. The Moller-Murphy Symptom Management Assessment Tool (MM-SMAT) was developed to provide consumers, family members, and professionals with a common framework for managing neurobiological disorders like schizophrenia, bipolar disorder, and major depression. Categories of the MM-SMAT focus on the frequency, intensity, and duration of symptoms related to health, environmental, and behavioral triggers that may lead to illness relapse. Examples of triggers are poor nutrition, poor social skills, and poor symptom management. Interventions are aimed at fostering coping skills related to illness triggers to offset relapse of symptoms. Medication management is an important intervention for offsetting relapse. While discoveries and scientific advances related to psychopharmacology have improved the lives of people with mental illness, neuroleptics are not without controversy. Controversies include side effects that may involve serious central nervous system manifestations. Clozapine is a relatively new antipsychotic drug that has improved the lives of many people who did not respond to the more traditional neuroleptics. While fewer nervous system side effects are associated with clozapine, there is risk for agranulocytosis. Monitoring blood levels is necessary for treatment when clozapine is used, but this drives up the cost of care and may reduce access to treatment for many. Perhaps the greatest controversy in psychopharmacology is whether or not to prescribe medications without incorporating other relapse management approaches.

IV. Application of the nursing process

A. The clinical example is based on a three generation family. One member of the family is diagnosed with schizophrenia and is at risk for HIV infection because of lifestyle factors. Another is at risk for mental health problems because of role strain related to caregiving. Primary, secondary, and tertiary interventions are discussed, emphasizing the importance of family and community in relapse management activities with the client. Evaluation of the case reveals limited housing for the client and lack of respite programs for family members. These deficits become targets in planning for community mental health services.

Additional Critical Thinking Activities

1. Through a local veterans group, meet with an individual who was active in World War II and with one who was in the Vietnam conflict to discuss conditions and experiences that affected their mental health. Pay particular attention to services that were available to them, both during and after their military service, and to ways the experience influenced their lives, as well as that of family members. Describe findings in a written report.
2. Assess the status of mental health services in your community with members of your local mental health system, public health department, and a consumer group. Identify (1) availability of primary, secondary, and tertiary mental health services; and (2) current legislative activity to address service deficits. Compare your findings with national health objectives and community strategies that are referred to in Chapter 36. Summarize your findings in a written report.
3. In your community, identify services/agencies that are available for victims of abuse across the life span. Visit with a representative of one of the agencies to discuss the situations of individuals who seek services. Based on your findings, write up a case study, develop a comprehensive treatment plan for the primary client, and outline prevention activities for other family members who may be at risk for mental health problems.
4. Consider the list of services/agencies for learning activity number 3. Identify groups who are vulnerable for abuse and who do not have access to services. Construct short- and long-term plans for addressing the deficit by proposing ways to integrate services in existing agencies/organizations and by projecting new programs.
5. Assign student groups to conduct mental health service assessments in settings for populations at points along the lifespan. Include preschools, elementary and high schools, work sites, and senior citizen centers. Have each group identify specific risks for the particular developmental stage of the population that they are assessing. Specifically, have them observe environmental factors that could influence mental status of the population. Identify nursing interventions for practitioner, educator, and coordinator nursing roles.
6. Assign groups of students to role play case studies similar to the one described in the Clinical Application section of Chapter 36. Have each group identify (1) theoretical/conceptual frameworks for nursing process activities; (2) functions of the three nursing roles that are described in Chapter 36; (3) nursing interventions for each role; and (4) evaluation activities.
7. Have students read four of the articles from the references listed for Chapter 36 and write summary reports for each article.

Critical Analysis Questions

1. Match the dates with the events:
   _____ 1990
   _____ 1955
   _____ 1986
   _____ 1975
   a. Mental Health Study Act: Resulted in transformation of state hospital systems.
   b. Americans with Disabilities Act: Prohibited discrimination and promoted employment for people with disabilities.
   c. Developmental Disabilities Act: Addressed the rights and treatment of people with developmental disabilities.
   d. Protection and Advocacy for Mentally Ill Individuals Act: Legislated advocacy programs for the mentally ill.
2. Prior to humanitarian reform, treatment of people with mental disorders involved:
   a. custodial care.
   b. hospitalization.
   c. superstitious beliefs.
   d. family support.
3. The individual who contributed the most to the development of hospitals as the site of care in the United States was:
   a. Clifford Beers.
   b. Florence Nightingale.
   c. Philippe Pinel.
   d. Dorothea Dix.
4. During the hospital expansion era, most psychiatric institutions were located:
   a. near small communities with access to families and social activities.
   b. in rural areas removed from family and social activities.
   c. near urban areas with access to families and low paying jobs.
   d. in urban areas without access to families and jobs.
5. An early consumer who advocated the improvement of mental health services was:
   a. Clifford Beers.
   b. Benjamin Rush.
   c. Dorothea Dix.
   d. Philippe Pinel.

6. Which of the following best describes the focus of the mental hygiene movement?
   a. cruel, inhumane treatment and incarceration in jails
   b. mental health clinics for treatment of severe mental disorders
   c. construction of hospitals for the severely mentally ill
   d. prevention and early intervention in community services
7. Which of the following best describes legislation for mental health services?
   a. In general, states legislated adequate services and required little assistance from the federal government.
   b. Historically, legislation has shifted from federal to state levels, where services developed in diverse ways.
   c. Historically, the federal government has legislated for specific services that states developed in similar ways.
   d. In general, legislation shifted from state to federal levels, resulting in adequate services in most states.
8. Which of the following statements about deinstitutionalization is the most accurate?
   a. It represented a dramatic change in the locus of care and resulted in unexpected service gaps.
   b. It was a well-planned movement, brought about by scientific discoveries, that resulted in improved access.
   c. It resulted in improved quality of life for consumers because they were taught to advocate for themselves.
   d. It was a movement promoted by family members because consumers did well on psychotropic drugs.
9. Which of the following was a guiding principle of the community mental health movement?
   a. People with mental disorders had a right to jobs and services in the setting they desired.
   b. People with mental disorders had a right to treatment in the least restrictive environment.
   c. People with mental disorders had a right to refuse treatment if adequate services were not available.
   d. People with mental disorders had rights similar to those who had physical disabilities.
10. A resource for the community mental health nurse that was often overlooked prior to 1980 was:
    a. political and legislative groups.
    b. physicians and psychiatrists.
    c. consumer and family groups.
    d. social workers and psychologists.
11. A practical and basic way for the community mental health nurse to use national health objectives and the complimentary model standards for healthy communities is to use them:
    a. to influence legislators.
    b. to teach consumers and family members.
    c. to assess community services.
    d. to develop care plans.
12. When developing a nursing diagnosis with the severely mentally ill, a reference that is a must for all community mental health nurses is:
    a. the ANA standards of practice.
    b. the DSM IV.
    c. national health objectives.
    d. nursing textbooks.
13. It is important to consider cultural and ethnic groups in community assessments for mental health services because historically:
    a. they have lacked culturally sensitive services.
    b. they have not been able to afford services.
    c. they did not have services in their country of origin.
    d. they did not need them because family members helped.
14. The group at highest risk for suicide is:
    a. adolescent girls.
    b. older women.
    c. middle-aged men.
    d. elderly men.
15. Which of the following best depicts the role of the practitioner in tertiary prevention?
    a. teaching a client about the importance of nutrition
    b. referring a family member to a stress management class
    c. case management of a client discharged to a personal care home
    d. directing client self-care via the home health aide
16. The Vulnerability-Stress-Coping-Competence Model discussed in Chapter 36 helps to explain that:
    a. developmental theories are important in understanding mental illness.
    b. psychobiological deficits, lack of social skills, and difficult life events can overwhelm the client.
    c. triggers for relapse are based on neurobiological impairments that make the client vulnerable.
    d. stress causes vulnerability that is difficult to offset with protective factors that promote competence.

Answer Key

1. b, a, d, c
2. c
3. d
4. b
5. a

6. d
7. b
8. a
9. b
10. c
11. c
12. b
13. a
14. d
15. c
16. b

37 Substance Abuse in the Community

Chapter Summary

Heavy tobacco, alcohol, and other drug use have been linked to numerous forms of morbidity and mortality.

Substance abuse is a major target for community health nurses to address. This has become apparent as attention has increasingly been focused on prevention.

In one way or another, substance abuse affects all ages, races, sexes, and segments of society. Directly or indirectly, few people are immune to the hazards of substance abuse, either through direct consumption or through indirect avenues such as sidestream smoke, increased accident potential for abusers, and family disruption when one or both parents or a child abuses alcohol or other drugs.

The purpose of this chapter is to examine ways to minimize health disruptions that are directly or indirectly attributed to substance abuse.

Annotated Outline

I. Understanding the problem

A. Historical perspective: Some form of psychoactive drug use has been endemic to virtually all cultures since the beginning of man. Prohibition has been attempted with alcohol and other drugs with questionable success. Under prohibition, drug use becomes a criminal offense, and thus the health care delivery system is hampered due to no quality control with the drugs available and to avoidance of the health care system by the users. Educational efforts have been effective in reducing the use of tobacco and abuse of alcohol.

B. Attitudes and myths: Attitudes are developed through cultural learning and personal experiences. The American society has developed the belief that there are "good" (legal) drugs and "bad" (illegal) drugs, and attitudes have developed that are based on this premise. Use of prescription drugs and over-the-counter drugs can be just as harmful or addictive as use of alcohol, tobacco, or illegal drugs. Addicts are often viewed as immoral, weak-willed, or irresponsible people who should try harder to help themselves. Many attitudes are based on myths.

To be therapeutic, community health nurses must develop a trusting, nonjudgemental relationship with the client. To develop a therapeutic attitude, the nurse must realize that any drug can be abused, anyone can develop drug addition, and that drug addiction can be successfully treated.

C. Social conditions: The fast pace of life, competition at school or in the workplace, and the pressure to accumulate material possessions contribute to the daily stressors. Professional marketing by pharmaceutical, alcohol, and tobacco companies entice the public to use their products to feel better. With the high technology of telecommunication, people grow up believing that most of life's problems can be solved quickly and easily through the use of a drug. For persons with a lower socioeconomic background, with minimal educational and employment possibilities, psychoactive drug use may offer a way to numb the pain or to escape from their hopeless reality. The black market associated with illicit drug use puts otherwise law-abiding citizens in close contact with criminals, prevents any quality control of the drugs, increases the risk of AIDS and hepatitis to a level secondary to needle sharing, and hinders the health care professionals' accessibility to the abuser or addict. The community health nurse needs to approach the problem of substance abuse as a real health problem, rather than as a moral or criminal problem.

D. Definitions: Over the years, the term "drug" has come to include only illegal drugs when discussing drug use and abuse. The term "substance" is currently being used to broaden the scope to include alcohol, tobacco, legal drugs, and even foods. *Substance abuse* is the use of any substance that threatens a person's health or impairs his social or economic functioning. More recently, the phrase "alcohol, tobacco, and other drug (ATOD) problems" is being used instead of substance abuse to emphasize that alcohol and tobacco are our leading drug problems. *Psychoactive drugs* are those drugs that affect mood, perception, and thought. *Drug dependence* is a state of neuroadaptation caused by regular administration of a drug, in which continued use of the drug is necessary to prevent withdrawal symptoms. *Drug addiction* is a pattern of drug abuse characterized by an overwhelming preoccupation with the use of the drug and with securing its supply, and by a high tendency to relapse if the drug is removed. *Alcoholism* is simply addiction to alcohol. The disease concept of alcoholism/addiction under the biopsychosocial model identifies this as a chronic, progressive disease in which a person's use of a drug(s) continues despite the problems it causes in any area of life—physical, emotional, social, economical, or spiritual. Many theories exist on the etiology of addiction, and there is no consensus on specific causes.

II. Psychoactive drugs: In addition to the specific drug being used, two other major factors will influence the particular drug experience: set and setting.
   A. Depressants
      1. Alcohol: Alcohol abuse ranks third following coronary diseases and cancer as the major cause of death in the United States, killing approximately 125,000 persons each year. At least 70% of Americans consume alcohol, and of those, approximately 10% will become alcoholic. Alcohol costs the country billions of dollars in lost productivity, property damage, medical expenses with alcohol-related illnesses and accidents, family disruptions, alcohol-related violence, and neglect and abuse of children. Chronic alcohol abuse exerts profound negative metabolic and physiologic effects on all of the body's organ systems.
      2. Barbiturates: Commonly known as sleeping pills or downers, the short-acting barbiturates are similar to alcohol in their CNS effects and are frequently abused. They are not as toxic to the body's organ systems as alcohol; however, the tolerance to the effects on mood develop faster than the physical tolerance to the lethal dose, resulting in greater risk of accidental overdose.
      3. Benzodiazepines: These drugs were introduced in the 1960s and were heavily marketed toward housewives for everyday stress. Doctors often misprescribe these drugs for long-term therapy, rather than treating the underlying stress. This can lead to dependence.
      4. Opiates: This group includes natural and synthetic drugs that are the most effective drugs for pain relief. There are approximately 500,000 heroin addicts in the United States and more than two million persons who use the drug occasionally. Tolerance and physical dependence develop quickly. The negative consequences primarily result from their illegal status: lack of quality control (varied strength and purity), unsafe administration (e.g., dirty needles), and the high cost on the black market, leading to crime to support the addiction.
   B. Stimulants
      1. Caffeine: This is the most widely used psychoactive drug in the world. High doses can lead to insomnia, irritability, tremulousness, anxiety, and headaches.
      2. Cocaine: In 1985, there were approximately 22.2 million lifetime users of cocaine in the United States, with an estimated 5.75 million current users (people who used it within the last month). The intranasal route has been a popular drug among the "rich and famous," but the cheaper "crack" form has become quite popular among the black population. The smokeable and intravenous forms of cocaine are much more rapid and powerful in their effect, and thus more dangerous and addictive than the intranasal use. High doses can cause extreme agitation, hypothermia, hallucinations, cardiac arrhythmias, convulsions, and possibly death.
      3. Amphetamines: Although these drugs are very similar to cocaine, the effects last much longer and the drugs are cheaper. These drugs are popular among truck drivers and college students. "Ice," a smokeable form of crystallized methamphetamine, was introduced in the late 1980s as an alternative to crack because it can be easily manufactured and the effects last up to 24 hours.
      4. Nicotine: One in five deaths in the United States is attributed to cigarettes. In 1991, the Centers for Disease Control estimated that 434,000 deaths per year are caused by complications of cigarette smoking. 1993 medical costs related to smoking were estimated at $50 billion. Currently, the prevalence of cigarette smoking has dropped to 31.7% for men and 26.8% for women. Most of the decline has occurred among the better educated and the white populations. Sidestream smoke contains greater concentrations of toxic and carcinogenic compounds than the mainstream smoke. Diseases and conditions associated with smoking include cancer, cardiovascular and pulmonary problems, and perinatal effects.
   C. Marijuana: Marijuana is the most widely used illicit drug in the United States. Estimates of

regular users range from 20 to 30 million Americans, and as many as 60% of those between the ages of 18 and 25 have tried marijuana at some point in their lives. There is no typical marijuana user, as use cuts across all demographic lines. Marijuana has very little toxicity; however, because of its illegal status, there is no quality control, and a user may consume contaminated marijuana. Adverse reactions may include anxiety, disorientation, and paranoia. The greatest physical concern for chronic users is the possible damage to the respiratory tract. The medicinal value of marijuana has been acknowledged, and legal action is being pursued to have marijuana moved from Schedule I to Schedule II of the controlled Substances Act, so that physicians may prescribe it.

D. Hallucinogens: Also called psychedelics (mind vision), these drugs are capable of producing hallucinactions. The set and setting will greatly influence the mental effects experienced by the user. Many of these drugs have been used for centuries in religious ceremonies and healing rituals, and have been used by many cultures to produce euphoria and to act as aphrodisiacs.
   1. LSD: Lysergic acid diethylamide is the most well-known drug in this category and is very potent—as little as 25 mcg in a single dose will last 10 to 12 hours. Adverse reactions include depersonalization, hypertension, panic, psychosis, and flashbacks.
   2. PCP: Phencyclidine is a potent anesthetic and analgesic with CNS depressant, stimulant, and hallucinogenic properties. By the early 1970s, 25% of the psychedelic drugs consumed in the United States were PCP. Adverse reactions include combative behavior, inability to talk, a rigid robotic attitude, confusion, paranoid thinking, catatonia, coma, and convulsions. Unlike the other hallucinogens, addiction can develop with this drug.

E. Inhalants: This group of psychoactive drugs includes gases and solvents.
   1. Organic solvents: The majority of the users are between the ages of 10 and 20. The effects are similar to alcohol, but have a rapid onset and last a short time.
   2. Volatile nitrites: Amyl nitrite is the most common and is most often used by urban male homosexuals. It is frequently used during sexual activity to intensify the experience and prolong the orgasm.
   3. Nitrous oxide: Also called "laughing gas," nitrous oxide is supplied in tanks and is also found in whipping cream aerosol cans (released by spraying the can upside-down). Administration can be dangerous when inhaling directly from pressurized tanks, because the gas is very cold and can cause frostbite to the nose, lips, and vocal cords. Also, if not mixed with oxygen, the user may die from asphyxiation.

III. Primary prevention

A. Promotion of healthy lifestyles and resiliency factors: Assisting clients to achieve optimal health includes identifying interventions other than or in addition to the use of drugs whenever possible. Assertiveness skills and decision-making skills help clients increase their responsibility for their health and increase their awareness of various options available. Stress reduction and relaxation techniques, along with a balanced lifestyle, can address many nagging health problems (such as sleeping difficulty, muscle tension, lack of energy, and mood swings) more directly and effectively than psychoactive drugs. Community health nurses can identify community resources and can assist in the development of programs that help clients develop a balanced lifestyle, that provide education or job training, and that offer drug-free recreational/leisure activities.

B. Drug education: The problems of substance abuse extend much further than abuse of psychoactive drugs. It has been estimated that prescription drugs are involved in almost 60% of all drug-related emergency room visits and 70% of all drug-related deaths. Approximately 25% of hospital admissions of elderly people result from problems related to noncompliance and drug reactions. Community health nurses can teach their clients that no drug is completely safe and that any drug can be abused. Nurses can be most effective in drug education by teaching clients guidelines/rules to use when deciding whether or not to use a drug. This will reduce the harm caused by indiscriminate drug use. These guidelines encourage a patient to know what the drug is, how and where it works, the dosage, possible interactions with other drugs and foods, possible allergic reactions, and risks of tolerance and dependence. Basic drug education programs for young people should include content on self-esteem, decision-making skills, assertiveness skills, stress management, recreational activities, and factual information about drugs.

IV. Secondary prevention

A. Assessing for substance abuse problems: Assessing for substance abuse problems should be routine with all basic health assessments. The client's reason for the drug use and the pattern of drug use should be determined. It should also be determined if there are any socioeconomic problems secondary to substance abuse. A history of withdrawal symptoms will help determine the presence of physical dependence, and a progression in drug-use patterns and related problems will alert the nurse to the possibility of addiction. Denial is a primary symptom of addiction.

1. Drug testing: Drug testing can be done by testing a person's urine, blood, saliva, breath, or hair. Drug testing in the workplace secondary to documented impairment may be helpful in substantiating the cause of the impairment. It can also be used in the work setting with recovering addicts to ensure continued abstinence. Urine testing is the most common method of drug screening; however, it only indicates past use of a drug, not intoxication. Alcohol, the most common drug of abuse in the workplace, is not identified in a urine drug screen.
2. Employee assistance programs (EAPs): These programs identify health problems among employees and offer counseling or referral to other health care providers as necessary. Nurses are frequently utilized to develop and run these programs.

B. High-risk groups

1. Pregnant women: The use of any drug during pregnancy should be discouraged unless medically necessary, because of the risk of negative effects on the fetus. Nicotine and alcohol are among the top three drugs used during pregnancy. Fetal alcohol syndrome (FAS) has been identified as a leading cause of mental retardation in the United States. Negative consequences from cocaine use are being observed more frequently. Pregnant women may not receive help for their substance abuse problems because of ignorance, poverty, lack of concern for the fetus, lack of available services, or fear of criminal prosecution for illegal drug use.
2. Youth: The younger a person is when beginning intensive experimentation with drugs, the more likely dependence will develop. Almost 90% of adolescents 18 and under have consumed alcohol, making it the most popular drug used by teenagers. Cigarette smoking among teens is up to 62% by 12th grade; 57% have used marijuana, and 6% tried cocaine. The greatest single variable influencing substance use among adolescents is peer pressure.
3. Elderly: The elderly represent 12% of the United States population and consume approximately 25% of all prescribed drugs. Factors such as slowed metabolic turnover of drugs, age-related organ changes, enhanced drug sensitivities, a tendency to use drugs over long periods of time, and a more frequent use of multiple drugs all contribute to greater negative consequences from drug use among the elderly.
4. Intravenous drug users: In addition to the problem of addiction, intravenous drug users are at risk for other health complications. There is a great risk of overdose, contamination by other chemicals, and emboli secondary to particles present in the solution. AIDS, hepatitis, and other blood-borne diseases can be transmitted through shared needles, as well as infections and abscesses secondary to dirty needles and poor techniques. For addicts unwilling to treat their addiction, the community health nurse can provide education on the use of bleach to clean needles or can assist in needle exchange programs.

C. Codependency and family involvement: Codependency is a companion illness in which the "codependent" is addicted to the addict. Codependents try to meet the addict's needs at the expense of their own. Codependency may underlie many of the medical complaints and much of the emotional stress seen by health care providers. Enabling is the act of shielding the addict or preventing him from experiencing the consequences of the addiction. Thus, the addict is "enabled" to continue to use. Whether or not the addict is willing to get treatment, the community health nurse can assist family members in identifying the problems and can provide counseling and information on available support services.

V. Tertiary prevention

A. Detoxification: This is the process of clearing the drug(s) from the person's body and the managing of withdrawal symptoms. Withdrawal symptoms vary depending on the drug used, and can range from uncomfortable to life-threatening. Drugs such as alcohol and barbiturates can produce life-threatening withdrawal symptoms, and medical management may be necessary to ensure a safe withdrawal. A general rule in detoxification is to wean the person off the drug by gradually reducing the dosage and frequency of administration.

B. Treatment for addiction: Addiction treatment focuses on the addiction process. Health care providers must help clients recognize the addiction as a chronic disease and must assist them to make lifestyle changes that will halt the progression of the disease process.

1. Controlled use/medical management: For those addicts unwilling or unable to completely abstain from psychoactive drugs,

other drugs have been utilized to assist the client in abstaining from their drug of choice. Methadone has been used for treatment of heroin addiction by producing a cross-tolerance and decreasing the craving for heroin. Methadone is taken orally and thus eliminates the dangers of IV use. Naltrexone is used for opiate addiction. It is an opiate antagonist that blocks the effects of opium-derived compounds and prevents the psychological and physical reinforcements of opiates if a person should slip and use an opiate. Disulfiram (Antabuse) may be prescribed for the recovering alcoholic as a deterrent to drinking because of the negative effects that occur when alcohol is consumed by a person on disulfiram.

2. Total abstinence: Total abstinence is the recommended treatment for drug addiction. Treatment may be inpatient or outpatient, generally depending on the stage of the illness. Education about the disease, counseling, and group interaction are provided to assist clients in making the necessary lifestyle changes. In addition, education and counseling are provided for the family of the addict. Treatment is becoming more specialized to meet the needs of various client populations. Relapses may occur during recovery.
3. Smoking cessation programs; Smoking cessation is a difficult process, but research shows that the development of a plan in collaboration with the smoker will be most effective.

C. Support groups: The success of Alcoholics Anonymous (AA) has led to the development of other support groups such as Narcotics Anonymous (NA) for narcotic addicts, and Pills Anonymous for polydrug addicts. AA/NA consists of a 12-step program of recovery to guide alcoholics/addicts and provides a social network that offers support, encouragement, and fellowship. Al-Anon, Alateen, and Adult Children of Alcoholics are self-help groups that have developed for the family members of alcoholics. Women for Sobriety and Rational Recovery are newer support groups with less of a spiritual focus.

Additional Critical Thinking Activities

1. Review at least four popular monthly magazines and at least two hours of prime-time television to identify the following:
   A. Advertisements for over-the-counter medication for common complaints such as headaches, colds, fatigue, insomnia.
   B. Public service messages against drug use, such as the "Just Say No" federal government campaign.

   Utilizing examples from your research, provide evidence of the ambivalent values we have in the United States toward drug use in our everyday lives. Analyze your findings and present them in written form.
2. A tenth grade teacher at a local high school has asked you to present an inservice seminar for teachers on (a) early detection of drug use and (b) appropriate intervention to be taken if abuse is suspected in a student. You will only have one 30-minute session with the teachers. Outline a teaching plan for this request, including learner needs, motivational considerations, ethical considerations, and evaluation measures of program effectiveness. Include a method for involving teachers in the presentation.
3. Assess three different popular magazines that are read by teenagers to identify articles dealing with alcoholic parents. Use examples from your research to summarize current information for teens. Include an assessment of the information.
4. You have been asked to provide a 15-minute presentation at the first faculty meeting for elementary school teachers on the detection of children who are living with an alcoholic. The principal is concerned that there have been an increased number of alcoholic families in her district, and she would like to inform teachers about the importance of early intervention. Sketch a brief teaching plan, learner assessment, and teacher motivational activities. Specify what you would include in your presentation and how you would evaluate the effectiveness of your teaching.
5. Develop a plan for your local school district, utilizing the techniques listed in your test that have been found to be successful in primary prevention of drug use among youth. As a community health nurse, specify whom you would initially involve, how objectives and activities would be determined, and how you would evaluate the effort's effectiveness. Outline your plan in a written report.
6. Review your community for positive ways of coping with stress and anxiety as an assessment of your community's risk for substance abuse. Produce examples and write two recommendations for ways to promote healthy coping in your community.

Critical Analysis Questions

1. True or False? Attitudes toward alcohol and other drug abuse tend to be more severe than toward smoking.
2. True or False? Nurses tend to view addicts as having a health problem, yet feel that addicts could help themselves if they would try harder.
3. True or False? In terms of financial aid for the war against drugs, the federal government places education ahead of law enforcement and treatment.
4. Explain the danger of clients accepting the belief that over-the-counter and prescription drugs are "good" drugs.
5. Approximately how many persons die each year from the effects of alcohol?
   a. 6,500
   b. 12,000
   c. 125,000
   d. 500,000
6. True or False? A typical alcoholic is the skid row bum.
7. Identify three costs associated with alcohol abuse.
8. Define tolerance.
9. Drug, set, and setting are the three primary factors that determine what effects a drug will have on an individual. Set and setting are particularly important in which group?
   a. depressants
   b. stimulants
   c. narcotics
   d. hallucinogens
10. True or False? The greatest national health risk from heroin is the threat of overdose.
11. True or False? Smoking or intravenous use of cocaine is highly addictive because the effects are so immediate and intense.
12. True or False? The best method of diagnosing addiction is by determining the amount, frequency, and type of drug ingestion, along with the length of use.
13. True or False? Urine testing is a current method used in the work setting to determine intoxication by various drugs.
14. Identify three groups at risk for alcohol/other drug problems.
15. True or False? Cocaine is a central nervous system depressant and helps people relax.
16. List three healthy alternatives to drug use for managing stress.
17. True or False? Cigarette smoking is the single most preventable factor contributing to illness, disability, and death in the United States.
18. Define sidestream smoke.
19. Abrupt withdrawal from which of these groups of drugs would be most life-threatening?
   a. amphetamines
   b. barbiturates
   c. opiates
   d. hallucinogens
20. Define and differentiate between the terms "substance abuse" and "addiction."
21. True or False? Education has been effective in decreasing the use of/addiction to cigarettes among the American population.
22. List five rules that clients should follow when deciding whether or not to use a drug.
23. When taking an alcohol and/or other drug use history of a client, what are two open-ended questions you could ask, *in addition to* inquiring about the type, amount, frequency, route, and duration of drug use, to better assess the client's potential or actual problems with drug use?
24. Define primary, secondary, and tertiary prevention as they relate to substance abuse/addiction, and give examples of nursing implications for the community health nurse in each area.
25. Define the term "enabler" as it relates to addiction.

Answer Key

1. True
2. True
3. False
4. They do not realize possible risks of many medications and expect to fix many of their minor health problems quickly with a pill rather than by changing their behavior. They are not aware of possible drug interactions.
5. c
6. False
7. Lost productivity, property damage, medical expenses with alcohol-related illnesses and accidents, family disruptions, alcohol-related violence, neglect and abuse of children.
8. The need to continually increase the dosage of a substance to achieve the desired effect.
9. d
10. False
11. True
12. False
13. False
14. Those with a family history of drug problems, youth, elderly, pregnant women, and those with severe personal problems.
15. False
16. Exercise, relaxation techniques, balanced diet, adequate sleep, drug-free leisure activities.
17. True
18. The smoke that comes from the lit end of a cigarette and goes into the atmosphere to be inhaled by others in the area.
19. b

20. Substance abuse is the use of any substance which threatens a person's health or impairs his social or economic functioning, while addiction extends beyond that definition. Addiction is a pattern of drug abuse characterized by an overwhelming preoccupation with the use of a drug (craving) and with securing its supply, and by a high tendency to relapse if the drug is removed.
21. True
22. Determine the drug being taken, how and where it works, dosage, possible drug interactions, possible allergic reactions, and the possibility of drug tolerance or dependence.
23. Questions inquiring about drug-related health, family and/or social problems, work, the law, finances, or spiritual issues.
24. Primary prevention targets clients before a problem develops, and the nurse can educate clients towards the dangers of indiscriminate drug use, substance abuse, and addiction, as well as giving alternatives to drug use. Secondary prevention targets high-risk groups and strives to prevent abuse and addiction. The nurse can identify high-risk groups, assess them for any drug-related problems, and offer interventions. Tertiary prevention targets the addicts and their families, and the nurse can refer to treatment, offer counseling for the addict and/or family, and assist with identifying community resources.
25. An enabler is a person who shields or prevents the addict from experiencing the consequences of the addiction. As a result, the addict does not understand the cost of the addiction and thus is "enabled" to continue to use.

38 Violence and Human Abuse

Chapter Summary

The most powerful obstacle to culture, according to Freud, is man's innate, independent, and instinctual tendency toward aggression. Other scholars have convincingly argued that aggression and violence are not innate, but rather are learned behaviors. Regardless of the cause, violence seems to be ever-present.

Violence and human abuse are not new phenomena, but they have increasingly become community health concerns. Communities around the country are voicing anger and fear about increasing crime and violence.

Violence and abuse within the family are not always as easily identifiable as street crimes. Detection of family violence and abuse can be particularly difficult because of the nature of the problem, the associated guilt, and the potential for punishment. The community health nurse is in a position to assess, evaluate, and intervene in matters of community and family violence.

To do this, the community health nurse needs to understand the dynamics of violence and human abuse. The chapter examines the causes of community violence and its effects. It also looks at various types of intrafamily violence.

Annotated Outline

I. Nature of problem: Violence and human abuse are not new phenomena, but are increasingly becoming public concerns. Between 1980 and 1984, the numbers of murders, robberies, larceny-thefts, and burglaries all showed decreases. Forcible rape and aggravated assault increased during this same period.

   Although family violence is more difficult to measure, the extent of this community health problem should not be underestimated. The roots of human abuse and violence lie both in the people directly involved, as well as in the social system in which they live.

II. Social and community factors influencing violence
   - A. Work: People are expected to be productive, contributing, and self-sufficient. However, some jobs can be repetitive, boring, and nearly lacking in stimulation, or supervisors and other forms of organizational control may discourage creativity and reward conformity. Adults often go home feeling physically and psychologically drained, setting the stage for family violence.
   - B. Education: Schools have assumed many responsibilities traditionally assigned to the family, such as sexual development and discipline. However, in large classes, isolation is often the primary method of dealing with children who do not conform to norms of expected behavior.
   - C. Media: The media often portray people as happy and fun-loving, with all the wonders money can provide. Yet for many Americans, the hope of buying many of the nonessentials seems like an unrealistic dream and provides fertile ground for the development of abusive patterns. The media also portray the world as a violent place and give sanction to violence when the good guys conquer the bad guys.
   - D. Organized religion: Religion often provides a sense of worth or power and some degree of closeness and intimacy. However, often a contradictory relationship has existed between abuse and religion. For example, many religious groups uphold the philosophy of "spare the rod and spoil the child," and others uphold victimization of people by their disapproval of divorce. The rigid guidelines resulting from religious tenets may result in feelings of guilt and low self-esteem.
   - E. Population density and diversity: A community's population, size, location, and surroundings can influence the potential for violence. It is the type of high-density area that determines the nature and amount of crime. The potential for violence tends to increase among highly heterogeneous populations.
   - F. Community facilities: In determining the potential for crime and violence in a community, consider the role of recreational and spectator sports in providing socially acceptable outlets for a variety of feelings, including aggression, anger, and frustration. Although the absence of community facilities can increase the likelihood of violence, their presence alone does not prevent violence or crime.

III. Violence against individuals or self

A. Homicide includes any violent death that is neither a suicide nor an accident; this includes deaths caused by murder, nonnegligent manslaughter, justifiable homicide (self-defense), and legal executions. Abusive-prone people are at risk for homicidal acts because of their inability to deal with stressful situations in nonviolent ways.
B. Assault: The difference between homicide and assault is the response time and quality of emergency transport and treatment facilities. The emotional trauma resulting from a violent attack often compounds the physical health problems.
C. Rape: Because research shows statistics that connect community level variables and rape rates, the appropriate level of intervention is at the community level. Interventions should be aimed at attitudes toward rape and pornography, and toward supportive, effective rape treatment programs.
D. Suicide: The third leading cause of death among persons age 15 to 24 years is suicide. Factors often associated with suicidal attempts include broken homes, frequent relocation during childhood, marital disharmony, emotional immaturity, cruelty to children, and extreme jealousy.

IV. Family violence and abuse
A. Development of abusive patterns: Several factors characterize people who become involved in family violence, including the way they were raised, the unique characteristics of family members, and the nature of the crisis. The most predictably present characteristic is previous exposure to violence. Many abusers were themselves victims of or witnesses to family violence.
B. Definition: Child abuse is the physical and emotional neglect of children. Physical abuse refers to the extreme episodes of burning, beating, branding, or kicking. Emotional abuse includes extreme debasement of a child's feelings. Many children are also sexually abused.
C. Abuse of female partners: Violence against female partners has greater prevalence than other forms of violence, a greater potential for homicide, more serious long-term consequences, and will have effects upon children in the household. Women's socialization may keep them in a battering relationship.
D. Abuse of the elderly: Violence against the elderly includes neglect as well as physical or psychological assault. The elderly are abused with regard to shelter, clothing, nutrition, physical and safety needs, and emotional needs.

V. Community health nursing interventions
A. Primary prevention: On the community level, a stance against violence should be a priority. Laws, personal security, and self-defense measures help to prevent violence. Identification of risk factors also promotes prevention.
B. Secondary prevention: Initiation and support of measures to reduce further abuse are needed. Community services available for support and assistance may need to be identified for both victims and their abusers.
C. Tertiary prevention: Therapeutic intervention involves dealing with the psychological damage caused by being abusive and having been abused. This requires a longer period of time than other types of intervention.

Additional Critical Thinking Activities

1. Read the newspaper and/or watch television news shows for five days to determine a profile of the types of violent crimes committed in your area or state. Assess the reasons given for the crime, the age and sex of persons involved, and family involvement, if indicated. Compare your findings with your text. Identify two nursing interventions, based on your findings, that could be implemented in your community at the primary, secondary, and tertiary levels. Write a report based on your assessment.
2. Spend a Saturday morning watching children's cartoons and commercials. Assess the type of violence, the type of characters represented (good or bad, male or female, ethnicity, etc.), and the types of toys promoted during this time period. Discuss the role of the media as "portraying the world as a violent place" and how this influences social and community violence. Produce a written analysis of your findings.
3. Assess your community's recreational facilities and activities to determine how well your community provides socially acceptable outlets for aggression. Attend at least one recreational or sporting event. Observe the participation of the spectators. Relate your observations to your text's contention that "spectator sports, organized by the community . . .allow members of the community to vicariously express feelings of anger and frustration." Analyze your community's ability to provide such outlets, and make two recommendations for improving your community's facilities.
4. If an agency will provide you with the names of one or more of the clients, interview them to determine their perceptions of the service they received and their level of satisfaction. What suggestions might clients offer the agency or the

community in general for becoming more responsive to the needs of victims of violence?

5. What gaps in services for victims of violence do you notice in your community? What agency or group might pick up this kind of effort?
6. Interview a clergyman, school principal, or person in a management position in a large employment site in your community to determine:
   A. His perceptions of his responsibility to reduce violence in the community.
   B. Efforts he is making to decrease or prevent violence.
   C. His perception of the nature and amount of violence as a community health problem.
   D. His suggestions for making the community a safer place to live.
7. During a home visit, analyze the home's level of protection from outsider intruders. Do the residents hold safety as a priority? Do they see violence as a potential problem for them?

Critical Analysis Questions

1. Between 1980 and 1990, which forms of violence rose?
2. Why is violence against the family difficult to accurately measure?
3. What general category of people are at greatest risk for homicide?
4. Describe three root causes of violence that exist in most communities.
5. List four types of community facilities that typically offer release of angry and hostile feelings to residents.
6. Name four ways that families can reduce their vulnerability to intrusions that could threaten their safety.
7. If you suspected that a child has been abused, what ten factors would you assess?
8. Differentiate between child neglect and physical abuse.
9. Describe emotional abuse.
10. Name five of the reasons battered women give for remaining in a violent marriage.
11. Discuss the three-phase cycle often seen in spouse abuse.
12. Describe the nursing approach considered most useful with victims of violence.
13. Describe what is included in abuse of the elderly.
14. According to this chapter, why is rape so underreported?
15. Describe a primary prevention program for rape.
16. Select one population at risk in your community for becoming victims of violence, and develop a comprehensive community health nursing plan for primary, secondary, and tertiary prevention relative to the violence to this group.
17. Victims of emotional abuse tend to hold in their feelings to avoid incurring additional scorn. Name five symptoms that result from repression of feelings.
18. What is the most common form of abuse of the elderly?
19. If you assessed elderly abuse as a problem for families with whom you are working, what would be your first action?
20. Caring for an elderly person in the home can often be taxing for caretakers. What kinds of resources are available in your community that might ease the family stress?

Answer Key

1. Forcible rape, aggravated assault, and homicide among adolescents.
2. Because of lack of accurate reporting or because of embarrassment, fear, and other emotions, families are often hesitant to report violence and abuse.
3. People who know one another are responsible for about 50% of homicides, and of these, 30% are among family members.
4. Changing social conditions, including employment decreases; multiple demands being made on people; institutions that are nonsupportive in meeting human needs; the work ethic of "hard work produces a life of comfort"; the media with its presentation of all the good things in life; organized religion, in which guilt plays a major role in the teachings of the church; the school, when children are not taught proper avenues for dealing with feelings, especially anger.
5. Recreational areas; organized and informal sports; movie theaters; tennis courts; parks; YMCAs and other groups with health clubs and organized exercise programs; spectator sports; educational, cultural, and religious institutions.
6. Keep doors and windows locked, trim shrubs around the home, keep lights on during high crime periods, organize a neighborhood watch program, install a home security system, learn self-defense measures.
7. See boxed material in Chapter 24 of text.
8. Physical neglect is the failure to provide adequate food, clothing, shelter, hygiene, or necessary medical care, whereas the idea of emotional neglect implies the omission of basic nurturing, acceptance, and caring. In contrast, physical abuse refers to one or more episodes of violence, often resulting in serious physical damage to the internal organs, bones, central nervous system, or sense organs.

9. Extreme debasement of a person's feelings so that the person feels inadequate, inept, uncared for, and worthless.
10. Hope that the husband will reform, feelings of no place to go, financial problems because of unemployment and lack of money, fear of living alone, belief that it is a sign of failure to seek a divorce, feeling the husband needs them, fear of retaliation from the husband.
11. (1) Tension-building phase, in which the victim tries to calm the abuser by being compliant, nurturing, and generally nonoffensive. (2) Battering phase, in which the woman is punished for "misbehavior." (3) Apologetic phase, in which the batterer is contrite and even attempts to convince the victim that the out-of-control episode will not occur again.
12. A listening, nonjudgmental approach that encourages the person to discuss and deal with the feelings associated with the past and to plan for the future. (This can only be used with older children and adults.)
13. Often includes actual physical mistreatment as well as neglect, rough handling, failure to take them to the bathroom, withholding medication, giving foods they cannot chew or otherwise eat, implying they are worthless or useless.
14. Fear of retaliation, public ridicule, guilt about the attack, and fear of the treatment they will receive from the police and health care providers.
15. Provides information about the dangers in going places with strangers and about avoiding high-risk locations; discusses safeguarding the home against possible entry; teaches self-defense.
16. Answer should be a synthesis of measures described throughout the chapter.
17. Hyperactivity, overeating, psychosomatic and dermatological problems, vague complaints, stuttering, truancy, general hostility, and aggression.
18. Rejection.
19. Find out if those who are seen as the rejectors realize the implications of their actions, and help them consider other ways of relating to the aging relative.
20. Home-related services include home health aides, nursing care in the home, meal delivery, home repair services, day care and respite care centers, monetary assistance, counseling, and educational programs focusing on the needs of the aged.

39 Communicable Disease Risk and Prevention

Chapter Summary

The nature and scope of communicable diseases has changed remarkably during the past century. In 1900, communicable diseases were the leading cause of death in the United States. While many of the previous deadly communicable diseases have been conquered, new ones have emerged to take their place. Thus, the problem of communicable disease is not less than in 1900, although it is much different. Infectious diseases account for 25% of all physician visits annually. The advent of AIDS, the reemergence of tuberculosis, the onset of new diseases such as Hantavirus Pulmonary Syndrome, and the increase in antibiotic sensitive strains of bacterial infections pose significant community health problems.

Annotated Outline

I. Transmission of communicable diseases
   A. The transmission of communicable diseases depends on the successful interaction of the infectious agent with the host and the environment. These three factors are referred to as the epidemiologic triad. Changes in the characteristics of any of these three factors may result in disease transmission. There are four main categories of infectious agents that can cause infection or disease: bacteria, fungi, parasites, and viruses. A human or animal host may harbor an infectious agent. Four factors influence the spread of disease: host resistance, immunity, herd immunity, and infectiousness. Whether disease develops following exposure to an infectious agent depends on many factors, including the infective dose, the infectivity of the infectious agent, and the immunity and immunocompetence of the host. Likewise, incubation period is different from communicable period. Incubation period is the time interval between invasion by an infectious agent and the first appearance of signs and symptoms of disease, while communicable period refers to the time interval during which an infectious agent may be transferred directly or indirectly from an infected person to another person. The disease spectrum also varies from a subclinical infection to a severe and fatal disease.

II. Surveillance of communicable disease: Surveillance is a system of close observation of all aspects of the occurrence and distribution of a communicable disease through systematic collection, orderly consolidation and analysis, and prompt dissemination of all relevant data.
   A. Elements of surveillance: The chapter describes the ten elements of surveillance and discusses the roles that community health nurses play at different levels of the surveillance system in collecting data, making diagnoses, reporting cases, and providing feedback information to the general public.
   B. List of reportable diseases: Each state varies in the diseases that must be reported. The Centers for Disease Control and Prevention (CDC) are excellent sources of information about reportable diseases.

III. Emerging infectious diseases: Emerging infectious diseases are those in which the incidence has actually increased in the past two decades or has the potential to increase in the near future. A variety of factors influence the emergence of these diseases. Most of the influential factors relate to consequences of activities and behavior of the human hosts, and to environmental changes, such as deforestation, urbanization, and industrialization.

IV. Prevention and control of communicable diseases: Communicable disease control programs seek to reduce the prevalence of a disease to a level at which it no longer poses a major public health problem. Elimination focuses on removing the disease from a large geographic area, such as a country or region of the world. Eradication refers to the irreversible termination of all transmission of infection by extermination of the infectious agents worldwide.
   A. Primary prevention of communicable disease seeks to reduce the incidence through health promotion and education. Secondary prevention seeks to reduce the prevalence of disease or to diminish the morbidity through early diagnosis and treatment. Tertiary prevention seeks to reduce complications and disabilities

related to disease through treatment and through mental and physical rehabilitation.

V. Vaccines—preventable diseases: Vaccines are one of the most effective methods of preventing and controlling communicable diseases. Many current diseases; e.g., polio, diphtheria, pertussis, and measles, are controlled by vaccines, but have not been eradicated. Community health nurses play a major role in immunizing people. This chapter provides information about the immunization schedule followed in the United States and discusses common diseases that respond effectively to immunizations, such as measles, rubella, or influenza.

VI. Foodborne and waterborne diseases: Food infection results from bacteria or from viral or parasitic infection of food. Food intoxication results from toxins produced by bacterial growth, chemical contaminants (heavy metals), and a variety of disease-producing substances found naturally in certain foods, such as mushrooms and some seafood. As discussed in this chapter, much foodborne illness can be prevented through effective food preparation, handling, and storage. Examples of commonly experienced foodborne diseases are salmonellosis and *Escherichia coli*.

Waterborne pathogens usually enter water supplies through animal or human fecal contamination and frequently cause enteric disease. They include viruses, bacteria, and protozoans. Hepatitis A is the most well known waterborne viral agent. The CDC defines an outbreak of waterborne disease as an incident in which two or more people experience similar illness after consuming water that epidemiologic evidence implicates as a source of the illness.

VII. Vectorborne diseases: Vectorborne diseases are transmitted by vectors, usually insects, either biologically or mechanically. The two most common in the United States are Lyme disease and Rocky Mountain spotted fever.

A. Lyme disease is transmitted by Ixodid ticks that are associated with white-tailed deer and the white-footed mouse. It is most prevalent in northeastern, north-central and the Pacific coast states, and it occurs most often in the summer. If not treated, it can have serious health consequences.

B. Rocky Mountain spotted fever occurs most often in the Southeast in Oklahoma, Kansas, and Missouri. It is transmitted via tick vector; the vector differs by region of the country. Clinical signs include sudden onset of moderate to high fever, severe headaches, chills, deep muscle pain, and malaise.

C. Vaccines are not available for any tickborne diseases except tularemia. The best preventive measures include wearing protective clothing when doing outside work and, prior to going inside, conducting a systematic assessment for ticks.

VIII. Diseases of travelers: People traveling outside the United States should consult with public health agencies or other knowledgeable sources to learn which diseases are prevalent and what precautions should be taken. Some of the common infectious diseases that can affect travelers are malaria, food and waterborne diseases, and diarrheal diseases.

IX. Zoonosis: A zoonosis is an infection transmitted under natural conditions from a vertebrate animal to a human. Means of transmission include animal bites, inhalation, ingestion, direct contact, and arthropod intermediates. Rabies is an example.

X. Parasitic diseases: Parasitic diseases are more common in developing countries than in the United States, due to the tropical climate in many of the countries and to their often inadequate prevention and control measures. Several factors at the present time are leading to an increase in parasitic infections: international travel, immigration, an increase in AIDS, and recognition of how selected parasitic diseases are transmitted. A common parasitic infection is enterobiasis (pinworm).

Community health nurses play a key role in the prevention, diagnosis, and control of parasitic infections. Diagnosis of parasitic diseases is based on history of travel, characteristic clinical signs and symptoms, and use of laboratory tests.

XI. Nosocomial infections: Nosocomial infections are acquired during hospitalization or developed within a hospital setting. They may involve patients, health care workers, visitors, or anyone who has contact with a hospital. In 1985, in response to concerns about the transmission of the HIV virus in health care settings, CDC developed a strategy of universal precautions for blood and body fluids. Tuberculosis remains a serious infectious disease; it is mainly transmitted by exposure to tubercle bacilli in airborne droplets from persons with pulmonary tuberculosis during talking, coughing, or sneezing. The common symptoms are cough, fever, hemoptysis, chest pains, fatigue, and weight loss.

Additional Critical Thinking Activities

1. Working with a partner in your class, complete a self-assessment related to prevention of communicable disease. For example, what have you done or what will you do to achieve primary prevention from possible communicable diseases that affect people of your age group? If you or your partner has had a communicable disease in the past, what secondary and tertiary prevention measures did you employ? Now that you have

read this chapter, what measures do you think you might have employed?
2. Prepare tables that compare/contrast the leading three reportable communicable diseases in your community with both state and national incidence of these diseases.
3. Looking at the list of nationally notifiable infectious diseases in the text box, find the incidence of at least ten of these diseases in your community. Contrast that incidence in your community with state and national data.
4. Using Table 39-1, complete an assessment of the factors in your own community that are most likely to promote/constrain the emergence of three specific infectious diseases. You may choose the diseases based on the patterns in your community.
5. There are ten Golden Rules for Safe Food Preparation (see text box). Review your eating patterns for the last 48 hours. Identify which of the golden rules you adhered to and which you violated. Develop a plan for altering your future behavior, related to those instances in which you failed to observe one of the golden rules.

Critical Analysis Questions

1. List and define the three components of the epidemiologic triad.
2. List the four main categories of infectious agents that may cause infection or disease.
3. Differentiate between natural immunity and acquired immunity.
4. Differentiate and give examples among primary, secondary, and tertiary prevention of communicable disease.
5. The chickenpox virus is one of the most contagious of all microbial agents. The characteristic agent that best describes this organism's ability to spread rapidly among school age children is called:
   a. pathogenicity.
   b. infectivity.
   c. dosage.
   d. virulence.
6. Which of the following is a nationally notifiable disease?
   a. influenza
   b. measles
   c. cancer
   d. congestive heart disease
7. Match the following diseases with their mode of transmission:
   1. Lyme disease
   2. E. coli
   3. Hantavirus
   4. Legionella pneumophia
   a. inhalation of aerosolized rodent urine and feces
   b. air cooling systems, water supplies
   c. bites of infective Ixodid tick
   d. ingestion of contaminated food
8. There are several opinions about whether the United States should pay for health care to illegal immigrants. Discuss the pros and cons of doing so.
9. Name nine diseases for which United States children are routinely immunized.
10. Since immunizations are important forms of primary prevention, describe at least four ways that you might provide immunizations in a way that might encourage people to participate.
11. True or False? Only the successful interaction of the infectious agent and the human host is needed for disease transmission.
12. True or False? Most of the factors causing the emergence of infectious diseases are influenced by human behavior and activities.
13. True or False? Active immunization refers to immunization through the transfer of a specific antibody from an immunized individual to a nonimmunized individual.
14. True or False? Virulence refers to the ability of an infectious agent to produce a severe pathological reaction in the host.
15. True or False? Nosocomial infections are infections that are acquired at home before being admitted in the hospital.
16. True or False? Universal precautions emphasize strict adherence to the rule that the blood and body fluids of all patients should be handled as if they contain HIV and other blood-borne pathogens.
17. True or False? Reactivation of latent tuberculosis infection is common in the elderly, in immunocompromised patients, substance abusers, underweight and undernourished persons, and in those with diabetes, silicosis, or gastrectomies.

Answer Key

1. Agent: Causative factor invading a susceptible host through an environment favorable to produce disease.
   Host: Human or animal that provides adequate living conditions for any given infectious agent.
   Environment: All that is external to the human host including physical, biological, social, and cultural factors.
2. Bacteria, fungi, parasites, viruses.
3. Natural immunity is species-determined innate resistance to an infectious agent, whereas acquired immunity is the resistance acquired by a host due to previous natural exposure to an infectious agent.

4. Primary prevention seeks to reduce the incidence of disease through health promotion and education (immunization, malaria chemoprophylaxis, universal precautions in health care workers, safe sex).
   Secondary prevention seeks to reduce the prevalence of disease or to diminish the morbidity of the disease through early diagnosis and treatment (skin testing for tuberculosis, serological screening for HIV, screening for STDs, partner notification in AIDs and STDs).
   Tertiary prevention aims to reduce complications and disabilities related to disease through treatment and through mental and physical rehabilitation (pneumonia chemoprophylaxis for people with AIDs).
5. b
6. b
7. 1. c, 2. d, 3. a, 4. b
8. Con: To provide health care is costly, and illegal immigrants generally do not have coverage for health care costs, nor can they pay themselves. To pay is to encourage them to come and to stay. Some, especially pregnant women, will come for health care and will come so that their children can be United States citizens.
   Pro: Untreated immigrants can bring infectious diseases and other illnesses into the United States and can infect innocent citizens. If they are not treated early, the condition may worsen and will be much more costly to treat when they finally seek care at an emergency room or other part of a hospital. Will the hospital turn them away?
9. Hepatitis B, diphtheria, pertussis, tetanus, polio, Hemophilus influenza type B, measles, mumps, rubella.
10. Set up immunization stations at places like schools, the worksite, churches, shopping areas, and polling places during elections.
11. False
12. True
13. False
14. True
15. False
16. True
17. True

40 HIV, Hepatitis and Sexually Transmitted Diseases

Chapter Summary

Sexually transmitted diseases (STDs) have recently become the focus of greater concern for many reasons. The rise in incidence of the incurable viral STDs, such as HIV and HBV, are well known. Other factors, like the association between genital warts and cervical cancer, and the rise in reported cases of antibiotic-resistant gonorrhea, are posing new challenges. Nearly all STDs are acquired through behaviors that can be avoided or changed. If left untreated, STDs can result in infertility, stillbirths, and congenital defects.

This chapter examines HIV, HBV, and other STDs. The implications for community health nursing practice in providing primary, secondary, and tertiary prevention are reviewed.

Annotated Outline

I. HIV infection: HIV infection and AIDS have had a political and social impact as decisions are made about controlling their spread and associated costs. However, the disease remains costly, with much of the health costs covered by Medicaid. In 1990, the Ryan White Comprehensive AIDS Resource Emergency Act was passed to provide services to persons with AIDS in communities with the largest number of AIDS cases.

A. Pathogenesis: HIV enters specific cells. Among these are cells of the nervous system, immune system, and integumentary system. It is the infection of the T4, or T helper cell, that causes the major impairment of immune system functioning and leaves the host susceptible to opportunistic diseases like cancers, bacteria, fungi, and viruses.

B. Natural history of HIV: Upon entering the body, the virus infects cells, such as the T4 cell, and becomes latent for several months or years. During this period of infection, the HIV does not cause overt signs of physical illness in the host, even though the virus may be transmitted to others. Approximately three or four weeks after inoculation, many persons experience an acute retroviral syndrome characterized by fever, rash, and lymphadenopathy. Antibodies to HIV are detected in the blood from six weeks to three months following infection, although some researchers have noted that detectable antibody levels may take up to 42 months to appear. Symptomatic illness may take an average of 11 years to develop.

C. Transmission: HIV is transmitted in specific and identifiable ways that are greatly influenced by behavior and, as such, are preventable. Generally, infection results from exposure to infected blood or other body fluids during sexual contact, through transfusions or other exposure to HIV contaminated blood or other blood products, through perinatal transmission, or through sharing injectable drug paraphernalia. HIV transmission has occurred through exposure to blood, semen, vaginal secretions, and breast milk. Although the virus has been isolated in several other fluids, including saliva, tears, cerebrospinal fluid, synovial fluid, amniotic fluid, and urine, no cases of transmission by these fluids have been documented. Having an infection with one STD may facilitate infection with another STD because of open lesions providing a portal of entry or because of decreased immune system functioning of the host.

D. Distribution and trends: Studying the distribution and trends of HIV infection and AIDS gives information about risk behaviors and groups that need education about HIV and STD preventions.

1. Gender: Of those reported to have AIDS, males outnumber females, but the proportion of increase in recent years is greater for women. The high number of male cases reflects the impact of HIV on the male homosexual, bisexual, and hemophilia populations. In 1992, for the first time, heterosexual transmission was greater than injection drug use (IDU) transmission in women.
2. Age: Forty-six percent of all reported AIDS cases are between the ages of 30 and 39 years, and nearly ninty percent are between the ages of 20 and 49 years. Because of the lengthy incubation period, infection occurs most often in the adolescent and early adult years. Of growing concern is the increasing

number of infants with AIDS, which directly parallels the increase in the number of women with AIDS. Perinatal transmission is the primary source of HIV infection in those under 13 years of age.

3. Race/Ethnicity: AIDS has disproportionately affected minorities. Although African-Americans make up 12.1% of the American population, they represent 31.8% of those reported to have AIDS. African-American women and their infants are particularly affected.
4. Geographic location: AIDS has occurred mostly in urban areas, with the highest prevalence occurring in Florida, New York, New Jersey, California, District of Columbia, and Texas. The number of cases of AIDS is expected to grow in rural areas in the future.
5. Seroprevalence: HIV seroprevalence is of great importance toward understanding recent transmission patterns, so that prevention efforts can be mobilized toward populations who are most at risk. Identifying cases of AIDS (the disease) gives only a picture of the transmission pattern from several years ago. Identifying those who are most at risk is difficult to do, but one method of learning recent transmission patterns is to screen specific groups within the population for evidence of HIV infection. These screenings, referred to as seroprevalence studies, have been conducted on military, hospital, clinic, and prison populations in an attempt to ascertain infection patterns and rates.

E. HIV testing: Testing for the HIV antibody is important for early recognition and management of the infection, because preventive care and medication may delay the onset of symptomatic AIDS. The HIV antibody test is the most commonly used test. The test does not determine if the person has AIDS, nor does it test for the virus. The most commonly used tests are the ELISA and the Western Blot, which are used in conjunction with one another. Their accuracy is over 99%. People who believe they may be infected should be tested three months after their last exposure, because it takes the body that long to develop antibodies and to give an accurate test result.

F. Perinatal HIV infection: Women who are HIV positive must consider the health risks to themselves and their infants and should be counseled to prevent pregnancy. Estimates are that 13% to 40% of women infected with HIV will pass the virus to their infants. Zidovudine therapy initiated early in the pregnancy may decrease the risk of transmission to the fetus, so current recommendations are that pregnant women be tested for this reason.

G. Pediatric AIDS differs greatly from AIDS in adults because the incubation and survival periods are shorter for children, and the physical signs and symptoms differ. In children, the signs are failure to thrive, diarrhea, developmental delays, and bacterial infections.

H. AIDS in the community: AIDS is a chronic disease and, as such, afflicts individuals who are living and functioning in the community. During episodes of illness, much of the care is provided in the home. The CHN teaches families and significant others about personal care and infection control, and can assist employers by identifying the importance of sponsoring educational programs on HIV. Policies for school attendance have been outlined by state departments of health and the Centers for Disease Control. Because HIV is not casually transmitted, students with AIDS should be allowed to continue to attend school, except when outbreaks of childhood diseases and other infectious diseases occur or when there is a risk to other students due to uncontrolled drainage of body fluids, such as drooling or incontinence. A multidisciplinary group made up of a health department representative, a teacher, a physician, a parent, and the school nurse should meet to determine the child's placement and should also be consulted as needs arise or conditions change.

I. HIV and the workplace: Policies for the workplace have been developed by unions and businesses. Workers who are HIV infected are protected by the 1974 Vocational Rehabilitation Act from discrimination based on the HIV infection alone.

J. Resources: Community-based AIDS service organizations and others, such as home health agencies and hospices, are frequently involved in the provision of support services and care.

II. Other sexually transmitted diseases: There has been an increase in the incidence of several other STDs, such as genital herpes, human papillomavirus infection (genital warts), chancroid, syphilis, and antibiotic-resistant gonorrhea.

A. Bacterial infections: With the exception of antibiotic-resistant gonorrhea, STDs caused by bacteria are curable with antibiotics.

1. Gonorrhea: Neisseria gonorrhea is a gram negative, intracellular diplococcus that infects the mucous membranes of the genitourinary tract, the rectum, and the pharynx. Signs and symptoms of gonorrhea include urethral or vaginal discharge, dysuria, or there may be no symptoms at all. Gonorrhea

is the most common of all reported communicable diseases. Antibiotic-resistant strains were first identified in 1976 when 15 cases were reported; this number had risen to 64,972 cases by 1990. Currently, penicillin and tetracycline-resistant strains have been identified. The development of pelvic inflammatory disease (PID) is a risk for women who do not seek treatment. PID can result in ectopic pregnancy and infertility.

2. Syphilis: Syphilis is caused by the spirochete, Treponema pallidum. The incidence of syphilis peaked in 1990 and is beginning to decline. The signs and symptoms of syphilis include the development of a chancre (ulcerative lesion) approximately three weeks after inoculation. If left untreated, the infection will progress to secondary syphilis, latency, and tertiary syphilis.
   a. Primary syphilis: The first sign of infection is a chancre at the site where the spirochete enters the body. The lesion begins as a macule, progresses to a papule, and later ulcerates. If left untreated, the infection will progress to secondary syphilis, latency, and tertiary syphilis.
   b. Secondary syphilis: Signs and symptoms include rash, lymphadenopathy, mucosal ulceration, sore throat, and fever.
   c. Latency: During the latent phase there are no clinical signs, but the client has historical or serological evidence of infection.
   d. Tertiary syphilis: Tertiary syphilis may include the complications of blindness, congenital damage, cardiovascular damage, or psychoses. Tertiary syphilis may occur from 2 to 30 years after initial infection.
   e. Congenital syphilis: The incidence of syphilis in pregnancy and congenital syphilis has increased at alarming rates in recent years. Syphilis is transmitted transplacentally and, if untreated, can result in premature stillbirth, blindness, deafness, facial abnormalities, crippling, or death in the newborn.
3. Chlamydia: Chlamydia infects the genitourinary tract and rectum. Symptoms may include dysuria, urinary frequency, and purulent vaginal discharge. The incidence of Chlamydia infection is unknown, but mandatory reporting has recently begun in some states. The infection is commonly asymptomatic in women. For this reason, it may be left untreated. Women infected with chlamydia are frequently also infected with gonorrhea. Untreated Chlamydia infection is the primary cause of PID.
4. Chancroid: Chancroid is caused by a bacteria, Hemophilus ducreyi, and is characterized by ulcer-type lesions that may appear similar to the chancroid that develops with syphilis. Usually one to two lesions occur, but there may be up to ten, whereas typically with syphilis, a single ulcer occurs.

B. Viral infections: Sexually-transmitted diseases that are caused by viruses have no cure. This results in life-long chronic diseases that require symptom management and measures to control the spread of infection.
   1. Hepatitis B Virus (HBV): The number of new cases of HBV increased by 37% between 1979 and 1989, and is found mostly in health care workers, persons with multiple sex partners, and foreign-born Asian Americans. HBV is a blood-borne pathogen and has the same transmission mechanisms as HIV. HBV is more hardy and can live on environmental surfaces at room temperature for up to one week. HBV vaccine is routinely given as part of the immunization schedule in infants and children. An OSHA mandate requires that health care workers and other workers exposed to blood and body fluids as part of their employment be offered the vaccine at the expense of the employer.
   2. Herpes simplex virus-2 (genital herpes) causes lesions that begin as vesicles which ulcerate and crust within one to four days. Initially, the virus infects the genitalia and surrounding skin. It then remains latent in the sacral nerve and may reactivate periodically with or without visible vesicles. Some people experience a prodrome that may range from a mild, tingling sensation 48 hours prior to eruption, to shooting pains in the legs or hips up to 5 days before eruption. Herpes is a lifelong infection, since there is no cure. Major concerns include that it has been linked to cervical cancer, spontaneous abortions, and risk of transmission to the newborn that may result in neurological damage.
   3. Genital warts: Genital warts are caused by the human Papillomavirus (HPV). Transmission occurs through direct exposure to the wart and possibly to body fluids that contain the virus. Many HPV infections are subclinical, which makes recognition and control difficult. Genital warts spontaneously disappear over time, but have been linked to the development of cervical cancer and may infect the fetus during pregnancy.

III. Community health nurse's role in preventing STDs and providing related services

A. Primary prevention: Most STDs are not curable, so the emphasis is on prevention. Activities to prevent and control STD include risk assessment, client education and counseling, partner notification, street outreach, and education of community groups.

1. Risk assessment: Performing a risk assessment provides an opportunity for the community health nurse to teach about human sexuality, assess the client's ability and desire to discuss risk behaviors, and identify the client's needs. A thorough sexual and IDU history should be conducted with individuals and their partners.

2. Intervention: Client education for preventing STDs includes the following:

a. Safer sex: Sexual abstinence is the most effective means of preventing STD, but for many people that is undesired. In these situations, information about making sexual behaviors safer must be taught. Condoms can prevent the spread of many STDs through preventing the exchange of body fluids. Some condoms contain viricidal and bactericidal lubricants, like nonoxynol-9. There is evidence that nonoxynol-9 may be an irritant to the vaginal lining, so its use should be limited to women who do not have a sensitivity to it. A female condom is available; its main advantage is that women control its use.

b. Injection drug use: During injection drug use, needles may be shared. This provides efficient transmission of bloodborne pathogens such as HIV. Bleach rinses of needle-injecting equipment may disinfect it. Drug treatment programs are ultimately needed to reduce use of addictive drugs.

c. Community outreach: Because of the illegal nature of IDU and the poverty associated with HIV, many people at risk do not seek health care. Community health nurses go into communities where those at risk live, to provide risk reduction education, counseling, and referral.

d. Community education: Community health nurses may provide educational sessions about STDs to community groups. These sessions are most effective when delivered in settings where groups regularly meet, such as churches or businesses. Topics covered include the characteristics of HIV and other STDs, how they are transmitted, the trends in occurrence, and the consequences of infection for individuals and society.

3. Evaluation: Evaluation may be based on behavior change toward safer behavior, but the best indicator is whether the incidence of the disease declines.

B. Secondary prevention: Secondary prevention includes activities that involve the early identification and treatment of STDs.

1. Testing for HIV: The community health nurse should recommend that persons who have engaged in high-risk behavior be tested. Persons who have a history of STDs, multiple sex partners, or injection drug use, or who are a homosexual or bisexual male or have sex with a prostitute should be offered the HIV antibody test. If HIV infection is discovered before the individual is symptomatic, antiretroviral therapy may be started based on the T-4 lymphocyte count. Testing also provides an opportunity for risk-reduction counseling.

a. HIV test counseling: Pretest counseling is important to assess the reasons why the client presents for the test, to teach the client that the test is for antibodies to the virus and not a diagnosis of AIDS, and to provide risk reduction education. Post-testing counseling: if the test is negative, the client should be counseled about risk-reduction activities. The possibility of a false-negative test for up to three months after infection is likely, and clients should have the test redone if there is a chance that they were recently infected. If the test is positive, counseling includes an assessment of the client's ability to cope with his illness and giving appropriate support and referrals, partner notification, and risk-reduction education. Community health nurses must be adept at interviewing, educating, and counseling skills, because of the sensitive nature of discussing sexual and other risk activities.

b. Partner notification: Partner notification or contact tracing is done by the client or by the health professional. It involves confidentially identifying and notifying exposed sexual and injection drug use partners of clients who have a reportable STD. Plans are made for the partner to seek follow-up care.

C. Tertiary prevention: Tertiary prevention involves caring for persons when the disease is present to prevent further decline. With the viral STDs, this prevention is focused on managing symptoms and psychosocial support regarding coping with the disease and developing meaningful sexual relationships despite having a chronic infection.

1. Universal precautions: Many persons with HIV return to their homes as the illness progresses and are unable to care for themselves. Universal precautions must be taught to all caregivers of the client.

IV. Clinical application: Indications for community health nursing practice are cited throughout the chapter. The case study involves counseling a pregnant woman who is infected with HIV and has a history of injection drug use.

V. Summary: This chapter describes the major STDs, their prevention, control, and treatment. The role of the community health nurse in providing primary, secondary, and tertiary preventive services is described.

Additional Critical Thinking Activities

1. Develop a teaching and counseling plan for a client who has just learned of his/her HIV infection.
2. Attend a sexually transmitted disease clinic at the health department. What specific services does the community health nurse provide?
3. Begin a file of articles from magazines and newspapers that discuss AIDS and other STDs. What types of stories related to STDs are covered?
4. Interview the individual(s) who carries out partner notification at the local health department. How do they contact a person under 18 years of age? What strategies do they use to bring the contact in for treatment? How do they locate and make contact? How do they maintain confidentiality?
5. Identify three local community agencies that provide services to those with AIDS or other STDs. List the services that each provides, their fees, and hours of service.
6. Compare the incidence of AIDS, gonorrhea, and syphilis in your state to the national average. To whom are these diseases reported within your locale?

Critical Analysis Questions

1. Which STDs are associated with cervical neoplasm?
2. Identify the STDs that may be asymptomatic, and list potential complications that may result from a lack of treatment.
3. STDs that result in ulcerative lesions are:
   a. herpes, gonorrhea.
   b. human papillomavirus, chlamydia.
   c. syphilis, gonorrhea.
   d. chancroid, syphilis.
4. The epidemic occurrence of genital herpes is significant for which of the following reasons?
   a. It is a painful disease that may recur chronically if not treated initially.
   b. There is an association between genital herpes and cancer of the cervix.
   c. Infants born to infected mothers may be severely affected.
   d. All of the above statement are true.
5. The first sign of herpes simplex virus-2 is the development of newly formed ______________ on the skin.
   a. linear burrows
   b. open ulcerations
   c. vesicles
   d. diffuse patches
6. Herpes simplex infections are contagious to other individuals by which of the following mechanisms?
   a. inhalation of airborne virus
   b. direct contact with the lesions
   c. percutaneous absorption of virus through intact skin
   d. inoculation of viruses through use of contaminated needles
7. After infection with HIV, seroconversion from a negative to a positive antibody test most commonly occurs in:
   a. 2 weeks.
   b. 6 weeks.
   c. 1 year.
   d. 3 1/2 years.
8. A 29-year-old woman seeks advice from you. She is considering taking the HIV antibody test. Which of the following are important points to discuss?
   a. to whom she will not reveal the results of the test (e.g., family, friends, current, past, and future sexual partners)
   b. how the results would change her life and behaviors, specifically sexual behavior
   c. issues of suicide, depression, guilt, and isolation, if the results are positive
   d. All of the above statements are true.
9. Early symptoms of pediatric AIDS infection include:
   a. failure to thrive, developmental delays.
   b. Kaposi's sarcoma, developmental delays.
   c. toxoplasmosis, oral candidiasis.
   d. fatigue, shortness of breath, skin rashes.
10. Pediatric AIDS differs from adult AIDS in that:
    a. the incubation period is shorter.
    b. mortality rate is lower.
    c. some of the accepted opportunistic infections for case definition are different.
    d. a and c
    e. all of the above

11. True or False? Most people infected with HIV look healthy and feel well.
12. True or False? The presence of HIV antibody in an infant is conclusive evidence of HIV infection.
13. What sexual behaviors are considered to be "safe?"
    a. dry kissing, oral sex with a condom, rimming
    b. fisting, dry kissing, touching
    c. masturbation on open skin, oral sex on a woman
    d. external water sports, fantasy, oral sex with a condom
14. The enzyme-linked immumosorbant assay (ELISA) test, which evaluates the presence of the antibody to HIV, has the following shortcomings:
    a. false-positive results, because the test is so sensitive
    b. false-negative results, because it takes a certain amount of time for the body to produce antibodies
    c. both a and b
15. True or False? The use of condoms lubricated with nonoxynol-9 should be recommended to everyone because of their viricidal properties.

Answer Key

1. Herpes simplex virus-2; human Papillomavirus (genital warts).
2. Asymptomatic STDs include HIV infection. Chlamydia and gonorrhea include PID, which can result in acute pelvic infection in women, nfertility, and ectopic pregnancy. Genital herpes can result in cervical cancer and poses a risk to the fetus in a pregnant woman. HIV infection may develop into symptomatic AIDS.
3. d
4. d
5. c
6. b
7. b
8. d
9. a
10. d
11. True
12. False
13. d
14. c
15. False

41 Community Health Nurse in Home Health and Hospice

Chapter Summary

The purpose of this chapter is to present another aspect of community health nursing—home health care. Home health care is different from other areas of health care in that it is the only health care setting in which the health care providers practice on the client's turf. Several components directly affect the nurse who is practicing in the home care setting. These elements will be discussed in the chapter to acquaint the nurse with the roles, functions, and responsibilities of practice.

Annotated Outline

I. Definition of home health care: Home health care in today's society includes an arrangement of health-related services that are provided to people in their place of residence.

Several definitions are explored, all of which integrate the components of home health care—the client, family, health care professionals (including nurses), and goals to assist the client to return to an optimum level of health and independence.

II. History of home health care: Home health care was born in the United States in the 1800s. By 1890, there were 21 visiting nursing associations, most of them employing only one nurse. In the 1940s, hospitals began to take a more serious interest in home care because of the number of chronically ill clients being hospitalized. The Montefiore Hospital Home Care Program, established in 1947, was the model for contemporary comprehensive home care services.

III. Types of home health care agencies: Home health agencies are divided into five general types, based on the administrative and organizational structures: official, private/voluntary, combination, hospital-based, and proprietary.

Regardless of the type of agency, all must meet licensure, certification, and accreditation.

A. Official agencies: Official, or public, agencies are those agencies operated by the state or local governments, such as health departments. Official agencies can offer more comprehensive types of community health services based on their objectives of health promotion and disease prevention. Community health nurses in these agencies may provide general home care, as well as providing care through clinics.

B. Voluntary/private nonprofit agencies: Voluntary agencies are supported by charities such as the United Way and other third party payers. With the advent of Medicare, the private, nonprofit agency emerged as a viable alternative. These agencies are governed by a board of directors representative of the community they serve. Voluntary charitable agencies were the first home health agencies.

C. Combination agencies: In some communities, home health agencies of the official and voluntary type have merged to provide home health care to decrease cost and prevent duplication of services.

D. Hospital-based agencies: Hospital-based agencies differ from other home health care agencies in that the already-established hospital board of directors is responsible for governing the agency. Clients of the agency have existing inpatient services available to them.

E. Proprietary agencies: Proprietary agencies are ineligible for tax exemption and can be licensed and certified for Medicare by the state licensing agency. The owner of the agency is responsible for governing.

F. Summary: Regardless of the type of home health agency, the primary goal should be to provide quality home health care to the community, based on the health needs of the people.

Competition is paramount in home health care. To survive in the competitive arena, one must continue to provide quality care and also be cost effective, without compromising accountability.

IV. Educational requirements for practice: Demonstration of professional competency is the foremost requirement for home health nurses. NLN advocates baccalaureate education as the minimal level of professional preparation for a community health nurse.

In home health care, the baccalaureate-prepared nurse usually functions in the role of a staff nurse, whereas the holder of a master's degree is best suited to be a practitioner, administrator, or educator.

V. Scope of practice
   A. Objectives in home health care: Objectives include practicing health promotion techniques, assisting clients in the prevention of illness and in the promotion of well-being, facilitating positive health behaviors for the client who has had an illness episode, and allowing the client and family to participate in setting their health care goals.
   B. Contracting: Contracting is a vital component of all nurse/client relationships. Contracting is directly related to use of the nursing process and can be either formal or informal, depending on the client's needs.
   C. Practice functions of the home health care nurse: Nursing services were the first home health services in the United States. Nursing still remains the service most frequently used. Home health care nursing involves both direct and indirect functions.

      Direct care involves "laying on of hands," teaching, and serving as a role model for the client and family to develop positive health care behaviors.

      Indirect client care is given by the nurse while serving as a consultant to other health personnel providing care, while participating in team conferences to provide for coordinated care and continuity for optimal client care, and while supervising other health personnel providing care.

VI. Integration of Standards of Community Health Nursing Practice in home health care: The home health care nurse practices in accordance with the Standards of Community Health Nursing Practice developed by the ANA and uses the nursing process as a framework for client care.
   A. The ANA Standards of Community Health Nursing Practice are reviewed, are related to the home health care nurse, and are related to the nursing process.

VII. Interdisciplinary approach to home health care: Interdisciplinary collaboration is a legally required, expected, and integral process in the home health care setting. Effective collaboration leads to continuity of care for the client. In home health settings, professionals experience stress associated with changing roles and overlapping boundaries. Successful interdisciplinary functioning requires that each health provider brings to the setting and shares his professional knowledge, skills, attitudes, and competencies.
   A. Responsibilities of the disciplines: Responsibilities and functions of the various disciplines are dictated by Medicare regulations, professional organizations, and state licensing boards.
      1. Physician: Each client in home health care must be under the current care of a physician to certify that the client does have a medical problem. A nurse can make an assessment visit without physician approval, but must have the physician's certification if a plan of care is to be developed. This plan must be reviewed by the physician at least every 60 days in collaboration with other health professionals. Physicians in the community serve in an advisory capacity for policy development.
      2. Physical therapist: Physical therapists provide maintenance and preventive or restorative treatments for clients in the home. They provide direct and indirect care to clients. The physical therapist provides direct care to enhance neuromuscular and functional abilities of the client and indirect care by consulting with staff members and by contributing to team conferences.
      3. Occupational therapist: Occupational therapists help clients to achieve their optimal level of functioning by teaching them to develop and maintain the abilities to perform activities of daily living in their homes. They also consult and attend team conferences.
      4. Speech pathologist: Speech pathologists deliver direct care services to clients to assist them to develop and maintain maximum speech and language ability.
      5. Social worker: Social workers assist clients directly by interviewing or referring clients to appropriate community resources. The social worker also provides consultation resource identification and application, crisis intervention, and equipment procurement.
      6. Homemaker home health aide: The role of the home health aide is to assist clients to reach their maximal level of independence by temporarily assisting with personal hygiene. The home health aide is directly supervised by the nurse or physical therapist. Additional functions include light housekeeping and other homemaking skills.

VIII. Accountability and quality assurance
   A. Quality control mechanisms: All home health care agencies are accountable to the clients and families, to their reimbursement sources, and to themselves for observance of professional standards.

      Quality is demonstrated through evaluations reflecting that appropriate and needed care has been given to clients in a professional manner. Documentation in agency records is the major data source for quality control.

B. Accreditation: The purpose of the accreditation process is to evaluate the administrative practices of the agency, based on the major assumption that there is a relationship between the quality of administration and the quality of services delivered to the community. Currently, accreditation is voluntary; however, it may become a requirement in the future.

C. Regulatory mechanisms: Home health regulation is mainly carried out at the state level, with state health departments certifying home health agencies according to the federal regulations set forth by the Health Care Financing Administration. Failing to meet the certifying criteria can result in loss of licensure and the closing of the agency.

IX. Financial aspects of home health care

A. Reimbursement mechanisms: Medicare and Medicaid are the principal funding sources for home health care, with private third party insurance a growing source.

1. Medicare: The use of home health services under Medicare has increased significantly since the 1972 amendments. Clients must meet specific criteria to qualify for Medicare payment for home health services. The person's physician must certify his treatment plan and his need to be confined to the home.

   Medicare emphasizes episodic care and "skilled" nursing, and does not reimburse for prevention of illness or injury.

2. Medicaid: Medicaid provides health services to low-income persons. Medicaid is administered by the states, but is state and federally funded. Medicaid covers home health services, including skilled and unskilled services such as personal care.

   Medicare and Medicaid comparisons are given.

3. Private insurance: Private third party payers may offer home health care reimbursement as a part of an individual or group insurance package. Some states have laws requiring private insurance to offer home health care.

4. Payment by individual: Persons who do not have health insurance or who need or desire home health services above and beyond Medicare reimbursement levels may pay for it themselves.

5. Nursing visit charges: The Health Care Financing Administration continuously gathers data about use of home health care services because of their interest in cost containment and quality of care. Several factors affect charges: type of service, geographical area, salaries in area, population characteristics, type of agency, and staffing patterns.

B. Cost effectiveness: Public attention is now being focused on home health care as a cost-effective alternative to institutionalization.

X. Impact of legislation on home health care services: The federal government plays a significant role in the delivery of home health services. The Social Security Act of 1935 was the first important bit of legislation to provide federal social insurance. This legislation formed the foundation for the two major health insurance programs, Medicare and Medicaid. The 1939, 1950, 1956, and 1960 amendments to the Social Security Act had an indirect effect on home health. The 1965 amendments introduced Medicare and Medicaid. The 1966, 1967, 1972, 1980, 1981, 1990, and 1993 amendments have led to progressive expansion of these two programs.

XI. Trends and issues in home health care

A. Legal and ethical issues confronting the home health nurse: The legal and ethical issues confronting the nurse include program fraud and abuse; defining skilled nursing care; determining frequency of client visits, of physician support, and of subsequent service underuse; and accountability for practice.

B. Issues in the 1990s: The major issues of the 1990s will be deregulation and restructuring of the home health care system, quality care, alternative care to hospitalization, cost, and competition.

C. National health objectives: Because nurses are working in the homes of clients, they are in a key position to promote the achievement of the national health objectives as the objectives relate to specific age groups.

D. Clinical preventive services task force: The home health nurse can use the age-specific protocols developed by this task force for assessing clients, care planning, and health education.

E. Indigent care: There is no legal right to health care in the United States. Nursing has the opportunity to ameliorate this deficit through health care reform, clinical research, public advocacy, and devising cost-reduction strategies.

F. High technology nursing: The DRG incentive for early hospital discharge has created a precipitous transfer of high-technology nursing skills from the hospital to the home care setting.

G. Pediatric home care: This area has changed tremendously over recent years as children are being treated outside the institutional environment. Pediatric home care in the future will continue to assist parents in the care of their children at home if resources and interventions continue to be appropriate.

H. Family responsibility, roles, and functions: The term *family* refers to the caretaker responsible for the client's well-being. A major issue is whether home health care services should be used as respite or relief type of care. The family primarily assists in maintaining the client at home for as long as possible and in providing a quality of care.

I. Hospice home care: People with terminal disease now are offered the opportunity to die at home, if it is their choice, with the supportive services that home care can provide. Health care providers who work with the dying often experience stress that must be identified and appropriately dealt with so that quality client care continues to be delivered.

Reimbursement for hospice care is currently provided through federal programs.

XII. Clinical application: Clinical application is the initiation of home health services.

Additional Critical Thinking Activities

1. Make a joint home visit with an experienced home health care nurse to:
   A. Evaluate the process and content of the nurse/patient interaction to determine if the visit was merely ritual or therapeutic, and describe the process of the visit.
   B. Compare actual roles and functions with the Standards of Community Health Nursing Practice.
   C. Assess level of skilled care the patient received and to determine whether it was needed and appropriate. (Was it within the four criteria described in the section on roles and functions? Answer the four questions in relation to the home visit made.)
2. Make a joint home visit with another home health care professional, and assess as in the preceding activity. Also attend a patient care conference meeting and write a summary of the process of the group.
3. Assess an elderly group of persons regarding their knowledge of Medicare relative to home health care. The sample can be obtained by contacting organizations that are primarily made up of elderly persons; for example, senior citizens' centers, church groups, or an elderly housing project. Prepare a talk regarding home health care for these people to inform them of what they are entitled to and what resources are available to them in their community.
4. Spend a day with a hospital discharge planner to assess needs of skilled or supportive services using Gikow's decision-making model.
5. Investigate the types of agencies in your community, the actual number that provide home health care, and what services they provide. (This information can be obtained through a local health systems agency.)

Critical Analysis Questions

1. Define in your own words "home health care."
2. a. List and describe the types of home health agencies.
   b. Give their similarities and differences.
3. Give reasons for the educational requirement for the home health care nurse.
4. Interpret the nursing process and the Standards of Community Health Nursing Practice into the home health care setting.
5. a. What are the basic home health care disciplines?
   b. How can they collaborate effectively?
6. Which governmental agency governs the regulation of Medicare and home health agencies?
7. What effect does HCFA have on nursing practice?
8. Why is reimbursement a special consideration for the home health care nurse?
9. True or False? Hospice care does not provide for terminally ill patients in the home because all patients wish to die in the hospital.
10. True or False? Deregulation will adversely affect home health care.

Answer Key

1. Definition should include the following aspects: home care is a component of health care; services are provided to patients and families in place of residence; purpose is to promote, maintain, and/or restore health; assistance should be given to return patient to optimal level of function; and services are coordinated and planned.
2. a. Official—public funding; operated by government agencies such as health department; home care is component; offers health education.
   Voluntary/private—third party reimbursement; has board of directors, is nonprofit.
   Combination—combination of public and private; funded with public dollars; has board of directors.
   Hospital-based—managed by hospital.
   Proprietary—profit-making.
   b. All offer basic home health services; differences are in administration and organization.
3. A baccalaureate degree prepares the practitioner for entry into professional nursing according to

professional nursing organizations. Competency and skills are important characteristics. A general baccalaureate education provides a foundation of linking theory into clinical practice.

4. See the boxed material in Chapter 41 for outline of contents.
5. a. Registered nurse, physical therapist, occupational therapist, speech therapist, social worker, and physician.
   b. Case conferences, in-service programs, and documentation in patient's record.
6. Health Care Financing Administration.
7. Provides and assures quality care is being delivered to Medicare beneficiaries.
8. Reimbursement mechanisms dictate what type of care is to be given and set standards for practice at this time; payment for service depends on skilled services and adequate documentation.
9. False
10. False

42 Community Health Clinical Nurse Specialist and Family Nurse Practitioner

Chapter Summary

The roles of community health clinical nurse specialists (CNSs) and family nurse practitioners (FNPs or NPs) are examined in this chapter. Debates on the similarities and differences in the two roles of CNS and NP have taken place over the past decade. The overlapping of functions of CNSs and NPs are becoming more evident, and future nursing education programs may prepare a blended "advanced practice nurse."

Annotated Outline

I. Historical perspective: Changes in the health care system and nursing have occurred in the past few decades because of a shift in societal demands and needs. Trends, such as an improvement in technology, self-care, cost-containment measures, accountability to the client, third-party reimbursement, and demands for humanizing technical care, have influenced the new roles of CNS and NP.
   A. The CNS role began in the early 1960s and grew out of a need to improve client care. CNSs educate patients and their families, provide social and psychological support to patients, serve as role models to nursing staff, consult with nurses and staff in other disciplines, and conduct clinical nursing research.
   B. In the United States during the 1960s, a shortage of physicians occurred, and there was an increasing tendency among physicians to specialize. The number of physicians who might have provided medical care to communities and families across the nation was thus reduced. As this trend continued, a serious gap in primary health care services developed.
   C. The NP movement was begun in 1965 at the University of Colorado by Dr. Henry Silver and Dr. Loretta Ford. They determined that the morbidity among medically deprived children could be decreased by educating community health nurses to provide well-child care to children of all ages. As a profession, nursing's priorities have traditionally been to care for and support the well, the worried well, and the ill, in both physiological support and physical care services previously provided only by physicians. Preparing nurses as primary health care providers was not only consistent with traditional nursing, but was also responsive to society's critical need for primary health care services, including health promotion and illness prevention . In 1965, as with the NP role, the physician assistant (PA) role was initiated at Duke University. This program was intended to attract ex-military corpsmen for training as medical extender.

II. Education: Educational preparation for the community health CNS includes a master's degree and is based upon a synthesis of current knowledge and research in nursing, public health, and other scientific disciplines. In contrast to the CNS, educational preparation of the NP has not always been at the graduate level. Early NP programs were continuing education certificate programs, and the baccalaureate degree was not always a requirement. The recent trend, however, has been toward graduate education for NPs.

III. Credentials: The academic degree and accreditation are important to the community health CNS and NP; however, licensure and certification affect their practice most directly. The purpose of professional certification is to confirm knowledge and expertise and provide recognition of professional achievement in defined areas of nursing. Certification is a means of assuring the public that nurses who claim competence at an advanced level have had their credentials verified.
   A. The ANA began its certification program in 1973 and has offered NP certification examinations since 1974. Since 1992, a master's or higher degree in nursing is required for all NP exams.
   B. The certification exam for clinical nurse specialists in community health nursing was first offered in October 1990. Qualifications for this examination include a master's or higher degree in nursing with a specialization in community/public health nursing practice.

IV. The advanced practice role: Although the roles of CNS and NP are merging, some common features exist.
   A. Clinician: Most differences between the roles of the community health CNS and NP are seen

in clinical practice. Although the CNS's practice includes nursing directed at individuals, families, and groups, the primary responsibility is to take a leadership role in the overall assessment, planning, development, coordination, and evaluation of innovative programs to meet identified community health needs. The CNS provides the direction for community health care indicated by identified and documented health needs and resources in a particular community, in collaboration with community health nurse generalists, other health professionals, and consumers. The NP applies advanced practice nursing knowledge and physical, psychosocial, and environmental assessment skills to manage common health and illness problems of clients of all ages and both sexes. The NP's primary "client" is the individual and family. In the direct role of clinician, the NP assesses health risks and health and illness status, as well as the response to illness of individuals and families. The NP also diagnoses actual or potential health problems; decides on treatment plans jointly with clients; intervenes to promote health, protect against disease, treat illness, manage chronic disease, and limit disability; and evaluates with the client and other primary health care team members the effectiveness, comprehensiveness, and continuity of the intervention .

B. Educator: The educator role of the community health CNS and NP includes health education within a nursing framework (as opposed to health educators who may not have a nursing background) and professional nursing education. The CNS and NP enhance wellness and contribute to health maintenance and promotion by teaching the importance of good nutrition, physical exercise, stress management, and a healthy lifestyle. They provide education about disease processes and the importance of following treatment regimens. In addition, they provide anticipatory guidance and educate clients on the use of medications, diet, birth control methods, and other therapeutic procedures.

C. Administrator: The community health CNS and NP may function in administrative roles. As health administrators, they may assume the responsibility for all administrative matters within the setting.

D. Consultant: Consultation is an integral part of practice for the community health CNSs and NPs. Consultation involves problem solving with an individual, family, or community to improve health care delivery. Steps of the consultation process include assessing the problem, determining the availability and feasibility of resources, proposing solutions, and assisting with implementation, if appropriate.

E. Researcher: Improvement in nursing practice depends on the commitment of nurses to developing and refining knowledge through research. Practicing CNSs and NPs are in ideal positions to identify researchable nursing problems. They can apply their research findings to the community health practice setting.

V. Arenas for practice: Positions for NPs and CNSs vary greatly in terms of scope of practice, degree of responsibility, power and authority, working conditions, creativity, and reward structure. These factors and their effect on practice are influenced by Nurse Practice Acts and other legislation (e.g., reimbursement and prescriptive privileges) that governs the legal practice in each state.

A. Private/joint practice/independent practice: Research indicates that the opportunities for NPs in private practice settings increased throughout the 1980s. Currently, the CNS role in private/joint practice is not seen as frequently as that of the NP. This may change as health care continues to shift from primarily acute care settings, such as hospitals, to innovative models of community-based preventive care. The independent practice option is more likely to be chosen by NPs and CNSs in states that have established legislation to facilitate this nursing practice.

B. Nursing centers: Nursing centers or clinics, a type of joint practice developed by advanced practice nurses, provide opportunities for collaborative relationships for CNSs, NPs, baccalaureate-prepared nurses, other health care professionals, and community members.

C. Block nursing: Block nursing is an innovative nursing model designed to allow the elderly to stay in their homes when they are not totally independent. The beginning of block nursing was seen in the earliest days of professional nursing, when people sought service on a fee basis from nurses who lived in their community. More recent block nursing models involve NPs and CNSs collaborating with baccalaureate-prepared nurses in the case management of individuals and families in a specific geographic area. These individuals and families receive professional nursing assessment and care from the NP, while the CNS mobilizes and coordinates community agencies and volunteers to provide needed supportive services.

D. Parish nursing: The parish nurse concept began in the late 1960s in the United States when increasing numbers of churches employed registered nurses to provide holistic, preventive health care to the members of their congregations. The parish nurse functions as health educator, counselor, group facilitator, client advocate, and liaison to community resources.

E. Ambulatory/outpatient clinics: NPs and CNSs may be employed in the primary care unit of an institution (e.g., the ambulatory center or outpatient clinic). Ambulatory/outpatient facilities are cost-effective and can improve the hospital's image in community service. Hospital clinics generally provide hospital referral, hospital follow-up care, and health maintenance and management for nonemergent problems. The population served is usually more culturally and economically diverse and represents a larger geographic area than that served by private practices.

F. Emergency departments: Persons without accessible health care, such as the medically uninsured and the homeless, frequently do not seek health care services until they become ill. Hospital emergency departments are increasingly used for nonemergent primary care. Although this is an inappropriate use of expensive health resources, it is a result of the current system, which limits access to routine and preventive health care.

G. Long-term care facilities: Many NPs and CNSs view long-term care facilities as exciting areas for practice and as a way of increasing quality of care while containing costs. Federal legislation provides reimbursement for NPs and CNSs associated with physicians to provide care to clients in Medicare-certified nursing homes and to recertify eligible clients for continued Medicare coverage.

H. Industry: Community health CNSs and NPs are increasingly useful in occupational health programs as businesses and industries seek ways to control their health care costs. The CNS in an industrial setting assesses the health needs of the organization based on claims data, cost/benefit health research, results of employee health screening, and the perceived needs of employee groups. With their advanced administrative and clinical skills, CNSs plan, implement, and evaluate company-wide health programs. NPs in occupational settings generally practice independently, with physician consultation as needed.

VI. Government

1. U.S. Public Health Service: The U.S. Public Health Service operates two services—the National Health Service Corps, which places health practitioners in federally designated areas with shortages of health manpower, and the Indian Health Service, which provides health services to Native Americans. Nurse practitioners are primarily sought by the National Health Service Corps, while nurse anesthetists and BSN graduates are primarily sought by the Indian Health Service at this time.
2. Armed Services: Currently the Army, Navy, and Air Force have programs providing educational leave and tuition to pursue advanced degrees for nurses on active duty. NPs are used in ambulatory clinics serving both active duty and retired personnel and their dependents. Certified NPs are authorized to provide CHAMPUS services and are directly reimbursed. CNSs use their skills with needs assessment and program planning/evaluation to develop programs aimed at improving the health of the aggregate identified.
3. Public Health Departments: Public health departments are increasingly employing community health nurses with master's degrees. These CNSs and NPs have administrative and clinical skills to work collaboratively with physicians and to manage and implement clinical services provided by the health departments.

J. Schools: School health nursing, discussed in Chapter 44, involves comprehensive assessment and management of care, with particular emphasis on health education to promote health behaviors in children and their families. CNSs and NPs may be employed as school health nurses by school boards or county health departments to provide specific services to schools.

K. Other arenas

1. Health maintenance organizations (HMOs): HMOs emphasize health promotion and disease prevention services to reduce health risks and avoid expensive medical care. NPs are often employed in HMOs to provide cost-effective basic health care services. Recently, HMOs have been contracting with Medicare to provide services to enrollees. NPs often deliver these services but, in this case, must work in collaboration with a physician.
2. Home health agencies: NPs and CNSs are well qualified to provide home health care that yields positive outcomes for clients and their families because of their knowledge and skills in the following areas: (1) public/community health principles, (2) family and individual counseling skills, (3) health education and strategies for adult learning, and (4) increased decision-making.
3. Correctional institutions: Inmates are a population with health needs that can be met by CNSs and NPs. Community health CNSs

are an asset within prison systems, planning and implementing coordinated health programs that include health education as well as health services. Where personnel resources are limited, CNSs provide counseling for inmates and their families to prepare prison clients for transition to the community upon their release. NPs often practice in health clinics on-site at prisons, providing both primary health care services and health education programs.

VI. Issues and concerns

A. Legal status: The legal authority of nurses in advanced practice is determined by each state's nurse practice act and, in some states, by additional rules and regulations for practice. Community health CNSs have less need than NPs for expanded practice within the traditional nursing domain. The community health CNS role involves acting as a consultant-facilitator, and guidelines for practice are more frequently defined by the nurse practice act. In the 1970s, regulations for the direct care role performed by NPs, including diagnosis and treatment, were less defined in state nursing laws than they are today, and the legal statutes of NPs were being questioned. Since 1971, when Idaho revised its nurse practice act to include the practice of NPs, states have amended their nurse practice acts or revised their definitions of nursing to reflect the new nursing roles. It was recently reported that NPs in 37 states are regulated by their state boards of nursing through specific regulations. In an additional eight states, NPs function under a broad nurse practice act, but with no specific title protection. However, in six states, NPs are still regulated by both the state board of nursing and the board of medicine.

B. Reimbursement: The third-party reimbursement system in the United States, both public and private, is complicated. As health care costs rise at an average of 10% per year, many people need a third-party payer to receive health care services. In order to practice independently or work collaboratively with physicians, NPs need to be reimbursed adequately. Because states regulate the insurance industry, availability of third-party private reimbursement depends largely on state statute. Advanced practice nurses require direct access to these third party payers. The most common mechanism through which NPs and CNSs acquire access to direct payment are mandated benefits laws and nondiscrimination provisions.

C. Institutional Privileges: Because of their direct care role, NPs in community health are more concerned than CNSs about institutional privileges. It is often difficult for NPs to obtain hospital privileges within institutions where their clients are admitted. The traditional hospital nurse is automatically responsible to and governed by the department of nursing as a condition of employment. However, if an NP is employed in a private joint practice with a physician, there is rarely a mechanism for clinical privileges to be granted by the department of nursing, because the nurse is not employed by the hospital.

D. Employment and role negotiation: For NPs and CNSs to collaboratively provide comprehensive primary health care, they must understand and develop negotiation skills. Positive working relationships with health professionals, organizations, and clients require role negotiation, particularly when few guidelines exist or a role is new and undeveloped. NPs and CNSs need to assess the internal politics of the organization as part of their role negotiation. Networking is another necessary skill. Forums, joint conferences, collaborative practice, and research provide opportunities to expand their functions.

VII. Role stress: Factors causing stress for advanced practice nurses include legal issues (as discussed previously), professional isolation, liability, collaborative practice, conflicting expectations, and professional responsibilities. NPs and CNSs should identify self-care strategies to cope with predictable stressors, some of which will be discussed below.

A. Professional isolation: Professional isolation is a source of conflict for NPs and CNSs. Because they practice across all age groups, NPs and CNSs are likely to be sought for remote practice employment sites. Rural communities unable to support a physician, for instance, may find the NP an affordable and logical alternative for primary health care services. The autonomy of practice in these sites attracts many NPs and CNSs, who may fail to consider the disadvantages of isolated practice.

B. Liability: All nurses are liable for their actions. Because more legal action is appearing in the judicial system, specifically concerning NPs and CNSs, the importance of liability and/or malpractice insurance cannot be overemphasized. Although malpractice insurance is not a prerequisite to functioning as an NP or CNS, most nurses carry their own liability insurance. It is in the best interest of NPs and CNSs to thoroughly investigate the coverage offered by different companies rather than to assume that the coverage is adequate. Practitioners who function without a physician on-site are particularly vulnerable.

C. Collaborative practice: The future of NPs and CNSs depends upon whether they make a recognizable difference in the health of families and communities and upon their ability to practice collaboratively with physicians. Collaborative practice denotes a collegial relationship with mutual trust and respect. Working out a collaborative practice takes a considerable amount of time and energy. Until such practice relationships evolve within joint practice situations, the quality health care that nursing and medicine can collaboratively provide will not be achieved. The arrangement demands the professional maturity to work together without territorial disputes, and the structure and philosophy of the organization must support joint practice as a mechanism for health care delivery.

D. Conflicting expectations: Services provided by NPs and CNSs in health promotion and maintenance are often more time-consuming and complex than just the management of clients' health problems. NPs and CNSs frequently experience conflict between their practice goals in health promotion and the need to see the number of clients required to maintain the clinic's economic goals. The problem is compounded when the clinic administrator or physician views NPs or CNSs only as medical extenders, and reimbursement to them is limited.

E. Professional responsibilities: Professional responsibilities contribute to role stress. Most states require NPs and CNSs in expanded roles to be nationally certified and to maintain certification. Recertification requires documentation of continuing education hours in primary health care topics. Because the practitioner is in a minority role in nursing, continuing education may not be locally available and may require travel and lodging expenses in addition to time away from practice. Anticipating professional responsibilities and attendant expenses in financial planning decreases these concerns. Negotiating with the employer for education leave and expenses should be part of any contract.

VIII. Trends: In the United States, there are over 100,000 advanced practice nurses, half of which are NPs and nurse midwives and half of which are CNSs. While the trend has been for physicians to be more interested in specialty medicine, nurses have leaned more toward primary health care. Numerous studies have shown that the independent judgments of NPs and physicians were similar. However, nurses were generally more likely to talk with patients about their health and medical regimens in relationship to their family environments and lifestyles, and were more likely to include health promotion and disease prevention counseling. The need for NPs and CNSs is increasing, especially in light of health care reform, social changes, and complex specialized health problems. More CNSs/NPs may appear in inpatient settings.

Additional Critical Thinking Activities

1. Explore the development of the NP and CNS roles locally.
2. Compare and contrast the local, state, and national NP and CNS movements.
3. Outline ways the CNS and NP complement other team members in a specific health care arena.
4. Investigate the CNS and NP programs within the state or region to determine the educational requirements for admission and the type of degree or certification conferred upon graduation.
5. Review a specific state's nurse practice act, as well as any rules and regulations governing expanded role practice.
6. Negotiate clinical observation experiences with a CNS or NP.
7. List settings locally where NPs and CNSs are employed.
8. Identify potential CNS or NP sites for employment.
9. Scan the classified advertisement section of a local newspaper, as well as professional journals, for number and types of positions available.
10. Examine state practice acts to determine who is legally authorized or permitted to write medication prescriptions.
11. Review state laws to determine the feasibility of partnership with other providers, of third-party reimbursement, and of insurance laws.
12. Outline job descriptions for a CNS or an NP.
13. Interview a practicing CNS or NP for his or her perception of stressors.
14. Discuss three mechanisms to combat professional isolation.

Critical Analysis Questions

1. Compare and contrast the roles of the NP, PA, and CNS.
2. How did state nurse practice acts accommodate the expanded roles of NPs and CNSs?
3. Briefly discuss the rationale behind the trend to educate NPs at the master's level.
4. Identify five role functions for both the CNS and NP.

5. Describe one of the above role functions.
6. Briefly discuss the role of the CNS and NP in the industrial or occupational health setting.
7. Describe third-party reimbursement under the Rural Health Clinic Services Act of 1977 (PL 95-210).
8. Discuss the necessity of role negotiation skills for the CNS and NP.
9. Identify eight benefits for which the CNS and NP should negotiate in contracting for employment.

Answer Key

1. See text for a description of the roles of the CNS and NP.
2. By rules and regulations passed under the authority of state boards of nursing. By revising the definition of nursing practice.
3. As NPs increased their knowledge and clinical expertise, the realization of the complex knowledge and skills necessary to provide accountable primary health care services became apparent. Such skills are effectively built on a professional nursing base.
4. Health practitioner, health educator, health administrator, health consultant, and health researcher.
5. Health practitioner: CNSs are skilled in the area of needs assessment, program planning, and program evaluation. NPs are skilled in physical assessment skills and learn to diagnose and treat a variety of common, acute, and self-limiting diseases.
   Health educator: CNSs and NPs intervene while the client is well to assist with health maintenance and promotion. During illness, they educate clients about the disease process, what can be expected, and the importance of adhering to the treatment regimen. Anticipatory guidance is provided to educate the client about the use of medications, diet, and other therapeutic procedures.
   Health administrator: CNS and NP may be in a position to assume ultimate responsibility for all administrative matters within a clinical or community agency, including supervision of clinical staff. They serve as decision makers and problem solvers and are involved in business management, policy making, finances, public relations, evaluation, and future planning.
   Health consultant: CNSs and NPs may serve as consultants to other nurses or physicians on a formal or informal basis, providing them with information to be used in improving client care. They may also consult with other health care providers or with organizations, schools, or programs educating CNSs and NPs.
   Health researcher: CNSs and NPs use research knowledge and skills to answer questions relevant to nursing practice. Identifying, defining, and investigating clinical nursing problems and reporting findings foster collegial relationships with other professions and contribute to health policy and decision making.
6. CNSs and NPs in occupational or industrial settings generally practice without direct physician supervision. Their major concern is with the health and welfare of the worker; therefore, concentration is on health maintenance, promotion, and education activities. Responsibilities include direct nursing care for on-the-job injuries and accidents, and care of nonoccupationally-related illnesses (such as follow-up of workers with hypertension and diabetes).
7. PL 95-210 applies only to NPs providing care in federally recognized, medically undeserved areas. Under the provision of the act, Medicare and Medicaid funds are made available for reimbursement of clinics operated or owned by qualified nonphysician providers. A physician is not required to see the clients or to be physically present for the clinic or provider to be reimbursed, but a physician is required to provide medical direction and to be available for consultation, emergency assistance, and client referral.
8. If the CNS or NP is going to collaboratively provide comprehensive primary health care, negotiation skills must be thoroughly developed. This is particularly true because NPs and CNSs find themselves considering pioneer positions in which few if any guidelines exist, or in which the position is new and underdeveloped.
9. Health insurance, retirement, sick leave, educational leave, holidays, vacations, personal leave, and malpractice insurance.

43 Community Health Nurse Manager and Consultant

Chapter Summary

This chapter describes the theory and skills that are relevant to community health nurse managers and consultants. While the chapter focuses on community health nurses with formal roles as managers and consultants, it also addresses the managerial and consulting aspects of all community health nurses' roles. Community health nurses are relied upon to organize clinical services and to manage resources used in service delivery. Nurse managers and consultants play pivotal roles in delivering high quality, cost-effective community nursing services. The chapter explains the major theories used in functioning as a community health nurse manager and consultant, the goals of nurse management and consultation, and the skills that underpin both roles.

Annotated Outline

I. Introduction to the community health nurse manager and consultant role

A. Purpose of the chapter: This chapter examines the roles and functions of community health nurse managers and consultants, emphasizing nursing clinical leadership, personnel management, and consultation on issues related to community health nursing services.

B. Major trends and issues affecting the community health nurse manager and consultant roles: Certain trends and issues influence the ways that community health nurse managers and consultants function. Cost containment pressures affect the ways jobs are designed and have created an emphasis on redesigning jobs through cross-training. Managed care is a macro-level trend that is a response to cost containment pressures. Capitated managed care creates incentives for health promotion and illness prevention. It may also create incentives to enroll the healthiest individuals in managed care plans, creating greater health risk for vulnerable populations. Vertically integrated organizations that include community services attempt to provide a seamless system of care for clients. Clients are demanding a greater voice in health care delivery, whether they are individuals, families, or communities. One way that organizations encourage individual and family involvement is through continuous quality improvement programs. These programs include ways to help organizations compare their service delivery with others through the use of benchmarks and report cards. Professional standards, accreditation standards, and clinical guidelines provide guidance for the ways that services are delivered.

C. Definitions: Community health leadership refers to influence exerted by community health nurses to improve client health. Community health management refers to the ways that community health nurses handle resources for the provision of clinical services. Consultation is a process of empowering clients that helps them perceive, understand, and act on events within the client's environment.

II. Management

A. Goals: The goals of community health nursing management are to achieve organizational and professional goals for client services and clinical outcomes, to empower personnel to perform their jobs effectively and efficiently, and to develop new services in response to community health needs.

B. Theories of management and leadership: Micro-level theories are based in psychology, whereas macro-level theories originate in sociology. Micro-level theories used by community health nurse managers include scientific management, neoclassical management, motivation theories, and leadership theories.

C. Intrapersonal/interpersonal management and leadership theories applied to community health nursing management: Scientific management is based on the concept of efficiency through specialization, and neoclassical management emphasizes workers' human needs and group dynamics. Motivation theories that are helpful in community health nursing management include Alderfer's ERG theory and Hackman and Oldham's Job Redesign Theory (which was based on ERG theory). Job Redesign Theory offers guidance for cross-training because it suggests that workers with high growth-need strength will be motivated by job enrichment, but not by job enlargement. Locke's Goal Setting Theory and Vroom's Expectancy Theory both indicate that workers are motivated by those outcomes they desire and by their beliefs about the likelihood of achieving those outcomes. Reinforcement theory and social learning theory argue that people are motivated by what they learn about the actual outcomes of their behavior. Contingency leadership theory says that the optimum leadership style depends on the nature of the relationships between the leaders and followers, and on the nature of the task and the situation. Path-goal leadership theory argues that leaders should facilitate others' goal achievement by removing obstacles to goal achievement. Transformational leadership incorporates both the needs of the organization and of the individual. Transformational leaders motivate others to envision new ways of doing things that are based in personal and professional values. Transformational leadership is compatible with the concept of learning organizations.

D. Organizational level theories applied to community health nursing management: Structural contingency theory predicts that the most effective organizational structure depends on the situation. In the past, many health care organizations possessed more mechanized structures. Currently, many are moving toward more organic structures, though they are often quite large. Decentralization creates more responsibilities for first-line community health nurse managers. Institutional theory explains the importance of organizational norms and values on informal organizational structure. Resource dependence theory provides helpful explanations of power dynamics as groups attempt to gain the resources they need. Systems theory helps community health nurse managers and consultants understand the distributional effects of policies on multiple groups. Roy's extension of her Adaptation Model of Nursing to nursing management further helps community health nurse managers and consultants analyze the effects of changing circumstances on organizational effectiveness.

E. The community health nurse manager role: Community health nurse managers may serve as team leaders or program directors, divisional directors, agency directors, or commissioners of health. They function as coaches, facilitators, role models, advocates, visionaries, program planners, teachers, and supervisors. They have ongoing responsibility for clients, groups, and community health, and for personnel and fiscal resources.

III. Consultation

A. Goal: The goal of consultation is to empower clients to be more effective problem-solvers. The functions of a consultant differ from those of managers because consultation is typically a temporary and voluntary relationship. Internal consultants function within the organizations by whom they are employed, while external consultants are employed temporarily on a contractual basis.

B. Theories of consultation: Purchase-of-expertise and the doctor-patient model are both content models of consultation. Purchase-of-expertise consultation involves hiring a professional helper to provide expert information or service.The client defines the need for the consultant in this model. This model is likely to be effective only when problems are simple and the client needs specific expert information. In the doctor-patient model, the consultant is employed to diagnose the problem and to prescribe solutions. The empowerment goal of consultation may not be met since the client does not help diagnose the problem. Process consultation engages the client in diagnosing the problem and developing the solution. This model emphasizes the collaborative process between consultant and consultee.

C. Process consultation: Proactive consultation is directed toward anticipating and preventing a future problem. Reactive consultation is directed toward solving an existing problem. Accurately identifying the client is critical to effective consultation. Five intervention modes are the following: acceptant, catalytic, confrontation, prescriptive, and theory-principles. Acceptant intervention emphasizes clarifying the emotional reactions to a problem. Catalytic intervention helps clients understand the problem by gathering additional data or by integrating existing data. Confrontational intervention presents clients with facts that reveal the client's underlying values and assumptions. Prescriptive intervention involves the consultant telling the client how to solve the problem. In the theory-principles intervention mode, the consultant helps clients learn how to use theories in their problem-solving. The choice of an intervention mode depends on the nature of the problem. Blake and Mouton (1983) identified four categories of problems. Power/authority problems result from questions about who has the right to make decisions. Morale/cohesion problems occur when clients feel powerless. Norms/standards problems occur when norms or standards are changed or violated. Goals/objectives problems result when goals are changed or clients are unable to meet goals.

D. The community health nurse and the use of process consultation: The consultative contract defines the expectations held by the consultant and the client. The areas that should be included in a contract are as follows: client and consultant goals, the problem, the consultant's resources, the time commitment, limitations of the contract, cost, conditions under which the contract may be broken or renegotiated, intervention modes, expected client benefits, methods of data collection, client resources, potential interventions, evaluation methods, and confidentiality. The seven phases of consultation are (1) the initial contact with the client; (2) definition of the relationship; (3) selection of a setting and an approach; (4) data collection and problem diagnosis; (5) intervention; (6) reduction of involvement and evaluation; and (7) termination. The initial contact is exploratory, while the terms of the relationship and the contract are negotiated in the next phase. At this point, the setting for the consultation is decided upon, the time schedule is set, the goals of the intervention are established, and the mode of intervention is chosen. Data gathering methods may include direct observation, individual and group interviews, questionnaires or surveys, tape recordings, analysis of existing data, and focus groups. After completing the intervention, the nurse disengages and reduces contact with the client. After the relationship is terminated, the nurse provides a written summary of findings and recommendations. Both client and consultant have complementary responsibilities throughout the process.

E. The nurse consultant role: Generalist nurse consultants work in official generalized community health agencies, while specialist nurse consultants work with community health agencies that provide programmatic approaches to service delivery. Primary care clinics, long-term care agencies, and home health agencies often prefer nurse consultants who possess both generalized and specialized knowledge. Generalist consultants may be required to function in a dual supervisor-consultant role, although the consultant must ensure effective communication to avoid conflict. Both internal and external consultants function as resource persons and facilitators.

IV. Skills required by management and consultant roles

A. Leadership skills: Leadership skills essential to both the community health nurse manager and consultant roles include abilities to articulate a vision and to influence others to achieve that vision, to empower others to achieve clinical goals,to balance attention to people and tasks, to delegate tasks and supervise others, to manage time, and to make decisions effectively. The Essential Public Health Services Work Group of the USPHS articulated the vision and mission of public health in the United States. Community health nurse managers and consultants should also use the ANA Standards for Community Health Nursing Practice and the Standards for Organized Nursing Services when developing vision, mission, and organizational goal statements. The concept of service leadership focuses leaders' attention on the needs of clients, whether clients are individuals, families, groups, or communities. Empowering others to achieve clinical goals means helping others to acquire the knowledge, skills, and authority to make effective, timely decisions. Leaders must balance attention to both people and tasks. Contingency leadership theory to help select the proper balance is based on the characteristics of the people, the task, and the situation. Leadership involves effective delegation, because delegation not only helps increase efficiency, but also and perhaps more importantly, helps develop others' talents. Delegation is becoming increasingly important and complex as community health nurses work with more individuals who are cross-trained to take on tasks for which they were not prepared in their initial educational programs. Many of these are unlicensed individuals, such as lay community health workers. Effective delegation involves determining the appropriate tasks to delegate (those which do not require professional education), appointing the appropriate person (someone who has been prepared to perform the task and is competent), and providing adequate supervision and ensuring that the task is competed safely and effectively. Direct delegation involves speaking personally to the individual to whom responsibility for the task is delegated. Indirect delegation occurs as a result of policies and procedures that transfer responsibility for a task to someone other than the person who is ultimately accountable for that task. State nurse practice acts and professional organizations provide guidance on delegation. Good leaders must be able to make effective decisions. Vroom and Yetton's theory helps select the amount of participation best for particular decisions. The Bernhard and Walsh decision model helps nurses choose from among several alternative decisions based on the goals for the decision. Leaders must possess critical thinking skills. Critical thinking incorporates values, makes assumptions explicit, and encourages creativity and innovation.

B. Interpersonal skills: Community health nurse managers and consultants need to be effective communicators, motivators, coaches, contractors, supervisors, team builders, and managers of diversity. Because community health nurse managers and consultants work with people from many different cultural and work backgrounds, good communication skills are particularly important. Communication must be culturally sensitive. Community health nurse managers and consultants need to be able to create a motivating climate and to use employee appraisal and coaching to help foster motivation and skill development. Contracting involves identifying expectations and responsibilities held by both parties. Handling criticism involves both the give and take of criticism related to job performance. Constructive criticism focuses on the behaviors necessary to meet job expectations. Supervision is an active process of coaching and ensuring that the outcomes of a delegated task are effective. Supervision may occur on-site or off-site. Off-site supervision is particularly important for community health nurse managers since so many community health workers function independently in a variety of off-site locations, including clients' homes, in schools, and in residential facilities. Interdisciplinary teams are widely used to manage client services and quality improvement activities. The workplace is becoming increasingly diverse, and managers and consultants must understand how to foster an appreciation for diversity and must create a positive and welcoming workplace environment.

C. Organizational skills: Community health nurse managers and consultants should be skillful with planning, organizing, implementing and coordinating, monitoring and evaluating, improving quality, and managing fiscal resources. Several documents are available to assist with community health planning. The Year 2000 National Health Objectives found in Healthy People 2000 should form the basis for program planning. The Model Standards for Community Health Programs provide guidelines for adapting the year 2000 objectives to local conditions. The Assessment Protocol of Excellence in Public Health gives suggestions for health departments to help them meet the year 2000 objectives. A Planned Approach to Community Health provides guidelines for ways to collaborate with the community in meeting personal and community health needs. The Five-Stage Process for Change also depicts a method of collaborating with the community on service planning. This model is based on a partnership built on trust. Organizing services involves determining the sequencing and timing of activities, and ensuring that the resources needed to implement a plan are available. Implementing plans includes ensuring that the relevant regulations have been followed and that work is both coordinated and documented. Attention should be paid to the change process during this phase. Monitoring and evaluating services should be based on professional and accreditation standards, clinical guidelines, and on relevant regulations. In addition to standards and guidelines, one other programmatic decision-making tool is the concept of screening test sensitivity and specificity. Highly sensitive tests are not likely to yield false negatives, and highly specific tests are not likely to yield false positives. Community health nurse managers and consultants must also possess skills in fiscal management. They must be able to estimate the cost of nursing services in managed care environments using community health assessment skills, epidemiologic projections, and actuarial consultation. They must also be able to develop justifiable budgets and to analyze variances from planned expenditures.

D. Political skills and power dynamics: Community health nurse managers and consultants use political skills such as skills in negotiation, conflict resolution, and managing power dynamics. Principled negotiation emphasizes collaborative problem-solving. Collaboration, confrontation, and participation in problem-solving are most likely to result in win-win conflict resolution. Power dynamics influence the extent to which managers are able to secure the resources necessary for clinical services. Perceptions of consultants' power are likely to influence their effectiveness.

V. Educational requirements: Both first-line community health nurse managers and generalist consultants should have a minimum of undergraduate nursing preparation.

Additional Critical Thinking Activities

1. Have several class members conduct interviews with community health nurse managers and community health nurse consultants to identify what they think are the most effective ways to motivate work behavior. After sharing the results with the class, ask class members to debate which approaches to encouraging work motivation they think are most effective. Does their opinion change if they are talking about motivating professionals? If so, why? (A useful resource for this phase of the discussion would be Joseph

Raelin's book, *Clash of Cultures*, in which he talks about the difficulty of trying to impose bureaucratic management styles on professionals, whose education has socialized them to be autonomous thinkers whose primary allegiance is not to the organization.) Ask them to consider the ethical implications of reinforcement as a motivating technique. Finally, ask them to consider the practical implications of trying to determine each individual's personal goals and needs, and whether community health nurse managers should focus on these needs, or on organizational needs. Encourage them to discuss how they would balance attention to people and tasks, as described in the text.

2. Ask class members to review the policy and procedure manuals from several different community health agencies, including, if possible, home health, school health, occupational health, and a nurse-managed clinic. Have them identify those policies and procedures that reflect indirect delegation. Who is accountable for the nursing care delivered through the indirect delegation provided for in the policies? Ask class members to develop strategies for providing either on-site or off-site supervision for the delegatee in those cases. Class members could break into small groups for this phase of the activity and write their strategies on newsprint. The newsprint summaries can then be taped to the walls in the classroom for the entire class to discuss.
3. Ask class members to work in small groups of three or four to develop an innovative community health program that supports at least one of the Year 2000 National Health Objectives. They should select a target population and conduct a needs assessment, comparing the data they gather with state and national data, if available. Ask students to use the Model Standards to develop a strategy for meeting one community health need that is tailored to the needs and strengths of their community. If the program involves any type of health screening, the students should determine the extent to which the screening test they plan to use is both sensitive and specific to the problem. Their program plan should include goals and objectives, an implementation plan, a budget and brief justification, and an evaluation plan.
4. Ask class members to read this scenario and discuss the questions that follow.
   Theresa Adams, RN, works for a small home health agency. She supervises the care provided by Bertha Dunn, who is the home health aide employed by the agency. Theresa has noticed that the patients do not seem to have been well-cared- for when she makes her supervisory visits. She learned that 78-year-old Mrs. Rose had lost ten pounds over the last month and had been coughing a lot during that period of time. "Don't think anything about it, dear," Mrs. Rose had said. "This is just a little cold." Theresa also noticed that several patients had not been getting their sheets changed regularly, and that Ms. McDonald's leg dressing had not been changed for a week. Theresa learned that 83-year-old Mr. Isom had run out of food stamps and had eaten only cereal and canned cake frosting for the last two days, and that Bertha had said nothing about it to anyone. The worst thing was that Mr. Stanley insisted that he was missing some money from his wallet, and that he thought Bertha had borrowed it. "What should I say to Bertha?" wondered Theresa. "It is so awkward to approach her about these things because she gets so defensive. If I mention it to the director, Bertha is likely to lose her job, and I know she needs the money."
   What other information would Theresa need to help her better understand the situation?
   What do you think Theresa should do?
   Role play a discussion between Theresa and Bertha, assuming that Theresa is trying to obtain more information from Bertha.
   Discuss the legal and ethical implications of this case. For which aspects of Bertha's care is Theresa accountable?

Critical Analysis Questions

1. Describe what is meant by a "seamless system of care" and explain how community health nurse managers could ensure that clients receive such care.
2. Differentiate between micro- and macro-level theories of management, and give examples of how community health nurse managers and consultants might use these theories.
3. Explain what contingency leadership theory suggests for choosing a leadership style with workers having different abilities and personalities.
4. Explain the difference between the content and process models of consultation. Which model would you recommend for community health nurse consultants and why?
5. Explain what variance analysis is, and describe the kinds of questions community health nurse managers and consultants might ask about the three different kinds of variances.

Questions 6-10 refer to the following situation.

Kaneesha Clark, BSN, has been contacted by a local home health agency to consult with them about the low morale in the agency. The issue that precipitated the visit was that the agency was considering instituting a policy to screen all employees for human immunodeficiency and hepatitis B viruses, and removing any individuals who were positive from the home infusion team. Staff members were angry about not being involved in the discussion and argued that such a policy was ineffective and discriminatory.

6. During Kaneesha's data gathering, she learned that staff resented having little say in many decisions that affected them. Based on this information, which intervention mode would you recommend to Kaneesha?
   a. the catalytic mode
   b. the theory-principles intervention mode
   c. the prescriptive mode
   d. the acceptant mode
7. Kaneesha is discussing the potential for delegating more decision-making authority with the staff. Which of the following should she point out is among the purposes of delegation?
   a. improving morale
   b. developing others' talents
   c. compliance with JCAHO requirements
   d. helping staff understand management's problems
8. Kaneesha understands that it may not be appropriate to involve staff in every organizational decision. According to Vroom and Yetton (1973), which of the following factors should one consider when deciding whether to involve others in making a decision?
   a. the extent to which the individual needs others' ideas and information
   b. the extent to which the individual is comfortable with group process
   c. the extent to which one espouses a participatory approach to management
   d. the extent to which others might be interested in the issue under consideration
9. Management and staff in the home health agency developed several potential solutions to the morale problems. Kaneesha decided to use the Bernhard and Walsh decision-making model to help them select the most preferred alternative. Which of the following describes this model?
   a. The model uses nominal group technique for voting on the most preferred alternative and then selecting the alternative with the most votes.
   b. The model involves developing a decision tree for identifying the most preferred outcomes of each alternative.
   c. The model involves identifying the goals of the decision and ranking each alternative based on the extent to which it will help achieve those goals.
   d. The model involves analyzing which alternative will be the easiest to implement and then adopting that alternative as the most realistic.
10. In helping the agency work through the particular issue about screening employees for human immunodeficiency and hepatitis B virus, Kaneesha focuses on the sensitivity and specificity of the screening tests available for these two viruses. Because the staff are concerned about false positives, which of these two characteristics of screening tests should Kaneesha focus on initially?
    a. screening test specificity
    b. screening test sensitivity
    c. the combined sensitivity and specificity of the screening tests
    d. neither

Answer Key

1. A seamless system of care refers to reducing service fragmentation from the client's perspective. Because many services that clients need (especially clients who are vulnerable, chronically ill, or require long term care) are provided by multiple agencies, clients often perceive the current health care system as fragmented and not responsive to their needs. Community health nurse managers can ensure that coordinating mechanisms are in place through means such as creating interagency coordinating councils, establishing referral policies and monitoring them for effectiveness, training staff to use a holistic perspective when working with clients, and assisting clients in order to meet their needs in a comprehensive way along a continuum of care.
2. Micro-level theories of management are based in psychology and explain intrapersonal processes such as work motivation. Some micro-level theories also explain interpersonal processes, such as leadership and group dynamics. Macro-level theories are based in sociology and explain organizational dynamics, such as the effects of variations in organizational structure, organizational change, power dynamics, and the effects of values and norms on organizational culture. Community health nurse managers and consultants use micro-level theories when they select strategies for motivating others or when they choose a certain leadership style for a particular situation. These theories are also used when analyzing group and team dynamics. Community health nurse managers and consultants use macro-level theories when analyzing potential changes in organizational structure and when analyzing power dynamics and organizational culture.
3. According to contingency theory, managers should focus more of their attention on supervising task accomplishment when the worker is not very familiar with the task or is not self-directed.

Blanchard, Zigmari, and Zigmari (1985) recommend that the leader coach closely supervise and follow up on the results of the work activity in this type of situation. On the other hand, the leader should function more as a facilitator and less as a supervisor with individuals who possess technical expertise, are highly motivated, and are self-directed. These individuals primarily need guidance and opportunity from the leader.

4. Schein (1969) described two content models of consultation. The purchase of expertise and the doctor-patient model are both content models because they focus on the content (or nature) of the problem. The process consultation model, on the other hand, focuses on the problem-solving process and emphasizes collaboration between the consultant and the consultee. It is usually best to employ the process model, because this model empowers consultees to solve future problems by helping them actively identify the nature of the problem and engage in its resolution. However, if problems are simple and the client needs specific, expert information, the purchase-of-service model may be appropriate. Schein (1989) argues that, while process consultation is the ideal, the three models do not need to be mutually exclusive. He recommends that consultants be willing to offer their opinions and advice at various points throughout the consultation.
5. Variance analysis occurs when one evaluates the differences between planned and actual expenditures and attempts to determine why variations from the budget occurred. Some variations from the budget are not under management's control, such as when the prevailing wage rate increases. However, many variations are under management's control, so evaluating the reasons for their occurrence may lead to changes in management behavior and ultimately to greater efficiency. The three types of variances are wage or price variance, which occurs when the price that must be paid for either labor or supplies increases; quantity variance, which occurs when either more labor time or supplies have been used than expected; and volume variance, which occurs when a greater number of services have been provided than anticipated, usually because more clients have been seen. Community health nurse managers and consultants should inquire about the type of variance that may have occurred, since this will not be apparent from the variance report itself. They should also determine whether the variance had any impact on quality of clinical services (e.g., providing fewer services than desirable may lead to a favorable variance, but lower clinical quality). Finally, they should determine whether the variance suggests that efficiency can be improved through managerial action.
6. d; The acceptant mode is best for morale/cohesion or power/authority problems because the issue generally causes feelings that block decision making.
7. b; Other purposes for delegation include increasing organizational efficiency and improving time management.
8. a; Other factors Vroom and Yetton (1973) recommend considering when choosing the degree to which others participate in making a particular decision are the extent to which those affected by the decision will be likely to support a decision they do not participate in making, and the time constraints.
9. c
10. a; Screening test specificity refers to the extent to which the test is specific to a particular health problem and is not likely to yield false positives. Screening test sensitivity refers to the extent to which the test is likely to detect all cases of a particular health problem and not yield false negatives. Ideally, screening tests will be both highly specific and highly sensitive, although that is often not the case.

44 Community Health Nurse in the Schools

Chapter Summary

It has been said that the most fragile members of society—children and youth—are the most likely to receive inconsistent health care. For children between 5 and 12 years of age, accidents, cancer (including leukemia), influenza and pneumonia, homicides, upper respiratory infections, malnutrition, and dental disease are the major problems interfering with school attendance. For adolescents, pregnancy, substance abuse, accidents, homicide, suicide, and venereal disease are the most common conditions leading to school failure.

The nutrition of school-aged children and youth has changed from that of a diet deficient in food to a diet that is excessive in empty calories and deficient in many of the body's essential nutrients.

Annotated Outline

I. Health problems of school-age children: Alcohol is still the most widely used substance among teenagers. In 1985, over one million teens became pregnant, and over 31,000 of these teens were younger than 15 years. Annually, 2.5 million teens are infected with a sexually transmitted disease. As of 1993, 629 children under 13 years were infected with AIDS. High school absenteeism is associated with low educational achievement, and poor children and adolescents are at higher risk for absenteeism than their more affluent counterparts.

The health problems of school-age children today involve social, emotional, behavioral, and technological aspects that require a wide range of services provided by skilled professionals who are flexible and able to coordinate their efforts.

II. History of school nursing: Lillian Wald is credited as the originator of school nursing when, in her work at Henry Street Settlement, she found a 12-year-old boy was excluded from school because of eczema. She and Lina Rogers conducted health inspections for five years and uncovered thousands of children who were not allowed to go to school because of health conditions. Between 1903 and 1904, 39 nurses were recruited by the New York Health Department to work with school-aged children. By 1909, municipalities throughout the United States were employing school nurses. After World War I, school nurses shifted their priorities from case-finding of communicable diseases to include primary prevention such as vision and hearing screening. By the 1920s, the role of the school nurse had expanded to include that of health educator and counselor. During World War II, school nurses gave up their more labor-intensive roles of health educator and counselors and focused on consultation, coordination, and serving as a liaison between school, home, and the community. Today the role of school nurse includes policy-making activities to assure a more organized school health program.

III. Components of the school health program: The three components are health services, health education, and environmental measures.

A. Health services: School services typically include health screenings, basic care of minor complaints, administration of medications, surveillance of immunization status, case finding for early identification of health problems, nursing care to children with special health needs, and, in some school districts, primary health care and health promotion activities.

1. Screening: Basic screening tests determine whether children can hear, see, speak, and communicate. They also assess whether physiological development and anthropometric measurements are appropriate for their age. The nurse's responsibility is to determine, with the family and team members, the appropriate resources for additional workup for children with symptoms.
2. Case finding: School nurses are trained to identify children who have undetected health problems and whose problems did not surface in screening programs.
3. Immunizations: Polio, measles, mumps, rubella, and diphtheria/tetanus vaccines are required for school entry. Each school has a procedure for guaranteeing that children are immunized.
4. Basic care for minor complaints: Each school building should have first-aid supplies and essential equipment, and a health room should be available. Increasingly,

nurses involve teachers in first-aid responsibilities.

5. Administration of medication: A large number of children in schools need to take medication, and the role of the nurse is guided by a set of basic requirements.
6. Counseling: The school nurse as counselor provides information, listens objectively, and is supportive, caring, and trustworthy.
7. Case management: The majority of the registered nurses in the schools function in the consultant/coordinator role and have extensive involvement in case management.
8. Primary health care and health promotion: School nurses are especially well prepared to conduct school-wide health promotion and preventive health care campaigns.
9. Students with special needs: The number of students with disabilities, handicaps, and chronic health conditions enrolled in regular schools has increased considerably since the enactment of the Education for All Handicapped Children legislation in 1975. Most of the students eligible for services under Public Law 94-142 have specific learning disabilities and are generally in good health. In 1986, the Education for All Handicapped Children Act was amended by PL 99-457, which changed the limit for mandated health and education services to include disabled children three to five years of age.

B. Health education: Health education efforts must relate to the values and beliefs of students and their families. This component should include instruction that fosters wellness.

C. Environmental health: This refers to the physical and psychosocial factors, such as infectious agent control and the physical and social environment of children. School safety is important.

IV. Roles and functions of school nurses

A. Specialists: Both school nurse practitioners (SNPs) and clinical nurse specialists (CNSs) care for disabled or chronically ill children, including those who are mentally ill. SNPs are registered nurses with advanced preparation in primary health care. The newest role is community health nurse specialist for school-age children.

B. Credentials: In addition to RN licensure, many nurses elect to become certified as a school nurse, school nurse practitioner, or community health nurse through a national certifying organization such as the American Nurses Credentialing Center.

V. Management of the school health program: There are four essential steps to the management of a school health program. These are planning, organizing, directing, and controlling the quality of the program through proper evaluation.

A. Planning: School nurses rely on pivot management; that is, creating the school health team by using the personnel already in the system, such as teachers, students, parents, administrators, and other health workers employed by the schools. A needs assessment is the starting point for program development. Plans must include who will provide the services and who is the target audience. Schools must have clear written policies and procedures to guide their work.

B. Organizing: It is useful to develop the health programs under a single department, office, or division so that needs can be met and duplication can be avoided.

C. Directing: As the health needs of students become more complex and the level of care delivered in schools increases, there will be an increased need for school nurses.

D. Controlling: Efforts to evaluate school health programs are still in the developmental stages. Nurses can rely on school health practice standards and school health standards provided by some states.

VI. Innovations in school health

A. School-based health centers: Schools are good sites for health surveillance and primary care because virtually all children can be reached on a regular basis through their schools. School nurse practitioners with appropriate physician back-up can provide a comprehensive and affordable set of primary health care services.

B. Family resource/service centers: Many states are looking at organized centers to provide families a one-stop shopping arrangement including child and adolescent health care services, education, and employment opportunities for parents.

C. Employee health: Some school health programs meet health care needs of teaching staff and other school employees, such as medical services and employee wellness programs.

Additional Critical Thinking Activities

1. Find out from the community health nursing staff in community health agencies and from school nurses hired by the local board of education how school health is administered in your community. Compare your findings with your readings.
2. Talk with school nurses in your community and discuss:
   A. Nursing roles.
   B. Nursing functions.
   C. Issues and concerns.

Compare your answers from the interview to your reading.
3. Debate with your classmates the roles and functions of school nurses.
4. Select three articles that focus on the school nurse to determine a historical perspective of changes within the role. Utilize professional nursing journals for your research. Use the following guidelines as you conduct your study.
   A. Select one article from the 1950s, one article from the 1970s, and one article from the present decade.
   B. Review the article for the following points:
      (1) Role of the nurse
      (2) Responsibilities of the nurse
      (3) Common health problems
      (4) Educational preparation
      (5) Certification
      (6) Stresses within the role
   C. Compare and contrast the articles as to the above points.
   D. Prepare a summary of your findings in a written analysis.

Critical Analysis Questions

1. Identify four major health problems of school-age children.
2. List three major health problems of school-age adolescents.
3. Name the founder of school nursing.
4. List the components of the school health program.
5. List and briefly describe the roles and functions of the school nurse.
6. Discuss the role of the school nurse practitioner.
7. List the four essential management functions that are used in school health.

Answer Key

1. Accidents, cancers (including leukemia), influenza and pneumonia, homicides, upper respiratory infections, malnutrition, dental disease.
2. Substance abuse, accidents, suicide, homicide, venereal disease.
3. Lillian Wald.
4. Health services, including the administration of medications; verification of immunization status; case finding; dealing with students with special needs; primary health care and health promotion and basic care for minor complaints; health education, including environmental health.
5. (See text for description.) Case management, counseling, serving as a school health specialist.
6. School nurse practitioners are registered nurses with advanced practice skills in primary care who can serve as the primary care provider for students who have no personal physician. They also work as part of the school health interdisciplinary team to make and implement school health policies.
7. Planning, organizing, directing, and controlling.

45 The Community Health Nurse in Occupational Health

Chapter Summary

This chapter deals with the community health nurse's role with workers. In the past decade, there have been major changes in the nature of work, the workplace, the global economy, and the health care system. Since the interaction between the workplace and the health of the worker will continue to develop, it is clear that the scope of occupational health nursing will grow. This chapter describes the community health nurse's role with the working population and discusses work-related health and safety concerns and the principles for preventing and controlling adverse work-related interactions.

Annotated Outline

I. The evolution of nursing roles in occupational settings: Nursing care for workers began in 1888 and grew rapidly during the early 1900s when workers began to allege that having accidents was not just part of the job. The field of industrial nursing began in the first half of the twentieth century, and both the interest in the health of workers and the role of occupational health nursing has grown, especially in the last two decades.

II. Workers as a population aggregate: There are more than 100 million workers over 16 years of age in the United States, and they work in 6.3 million different work sites.

   A. Characteristics of the workforce: The workforce is changing as more women, more older people, and more people with chronic illnesses are being employed.

   B. Characteristics of work: The nature of work is changing with the greatest proportion of workers being in the service industries, in professions, and doing clerical work, in contrast to manufacturing and agriculture. Of the new jobs created between 1984 and 1994, 73% were in professional administration, sales, technical, and precision crafts.

   C. Work-health interactions: In 1993, 2.2 million workers reported that they lost time from work due to work-related illnesses and injuries. In recent years, the number and severity of work-related injuries have increased.

III. Application of the epidemiological model: In the workplace, the host is any susceptible human being; agents are biological, chemical, ergonomic, physical, or psychosocial occupational hazards. The environment includes all external conditions that influence the interaction of the host and the agents.

   A. Host: The worker is the host in the occupational setting. Certain factors such as age, gender, chronic illness, work practices, immunological status, ethnicity, and lifestyle habits correlate with greater risk.

   B. Agents: The five categories of work-related hazards are described below.

      1. Biological: These agents involve living organisms whose excretions or parts are capable of causing human disease, often by an infectious process. Examples are hepatitis B and tuberculosis, with high risk groups being health care workers or dry cleaners who work with solvents.

      2. Chemical: Only several hundred of the two million known chemicals have been carefully studied for their affect on humans. Because of the frequent and multiple sources of exposure to chemicals, most people have a low level of chemical build-up in their tissues. The reproductive health effects of chemicals is the most crucial concern.

      3. Ergonomic: These agents involve the transfer of mechanical energy from the work to the person by such means as vibration, repetitive motion, poor workstation fit to the worker, or by lifting heavy loads.

      4. Physical: These agents affect health when they transfer physical energy from the workplace to the worker, such as through extreme temperatures, noise, radiation, or lighting.

      5. Psychosocial: These agents involve conditions that pose a threat to the psychosocial and/or social well-being of individuals and groups of people. Their effects are evidenced in stress and burnout.

   C. Environment: Both physical and psychosocial aspects of the environment affect the agent/host interaction. For example, physical qualities such as heat, ventilation, and humidity affect the interaction, as do such things as feelings of worth to the organization and acceptance by both coworkers and supervisors.

IV. Organizational and societal efforts to promote worker health and safety: These effects are becoming increasingly important as the cost of worker illnesses and injuries affect workers and their families, as well as their employers and their insurers.

A. On-site occupational health and safety programs: Typically, these programs are provided by a team of occupational health and safety workers, with the largest single group being occupational health nurses. The nurse collaborates with a physician via telephone or by on-site discussion. The range and scope of the team depends on the size of the workforce and the diversity of services needed. In recent years, there has been a significant growth in employee health promotion programs and employee assistance programs. The latter help employees learn strategies for coping with a range of stressors occurring both on the job and in their personal lives.

B. Legislation: The government has worked to improve the regulations governing occupational health and safety. The Occupational Safety and Health Act established two agencies to carry out the purposes of the act, assuring "safe and healthful working conditions for working men and women." These agencies are the Occupational Safety and Health Administration (OSHA) and the National Institute for Occupational Safety and Health (NIOSH).

V. Disaster planning and management: The legislation of the Superfund Amendment and Reauthorization Act requires written disaster plans that are shared with key resources in the community. The potential for disaster within the workplace must be identified, and this is best achieved by completing an exhaustive chemical inventory.

VI. Nursing interventions with working populations: An occupational health history should be incorporated into all routine nursing assessments. It is important to recognize the possibility of a relationship between health and occupational factors.

A. Assessment of individuals and families: Occupational health histories should include a list of current and past jobs the person has held, questions about exposure to specific agents and relationships between the symptoms and activities at work, and job titles or history of exposures and other factors that may enhance the client's susceptibility to occupational agents. Questions about the client's occupational history can be woven into existing assessment tools.

B. Assessment of the workplace: Not only are individual clients assessed, but the workplace itself should be assessed. This assessment is known as the "plant survey." The purposes of the plant survey are to learn about the work processes and materials, the requirements of various jobs, the presence of actual or potential hazards, and the work practices of employees. Plant surveys begin with an understanding of the type of work that occurs in the workplace and also include characteristics of the employee group.

VII. Clinical application: The clinical application demonstrates the use of the epidemiological triad in a company that replaced its computer equipment with new machinery that had adverse effects on worker health.

Additional Critical Thinking Activities

1. Develop a presentation to a community group on the role and scope of practice of the occupational health nurse. Use an actual company in your town. You may wish to interview the occupational nurse or, if there is no nurse on-site, interview a manager in human resources to identify what health care needs might be handled by an occupational health nurse. Make an on-site visit and talk with workers to identify possible host, agent, and environment interactions.
2. Identify the hazards for student nurses with the occurrence of occupational health disruptions. Identify all possible factors that might influence health, then take one factor and do an in-depth analysis of potential health effects. Describe how the health disruption might be prevented, and list all possible interventions.
3. Identify a person with a job-related health disruption, such as carpal tunnel syndrome. Look for past and present types of employment, and identify the likely causative factors. Develop a care plan to alleviate the symptoms or to enable the person to cope more effectively.
4. Make a site visit to an industry in your town. Identify the possible occupational health hazards according to the five types of agents (biological, chemical, ergonomic, physical, and psychosocial). Develop plans of action to avoid the hazard(s) leading to health disruptions.

Critical Analysis Questions

1. Name the three categories of workers that are increasing due to economic, policy, and lifespan changes.
2. Describe how work has changed over the past 50 years.
3. List the five major types of agents that affect occupational health.
4. List at least five types of work-related diseases/conditions and the category of worker most likely to be affected.
5. List three components of the environment that can affect health.
6. Which of the following age groups has the greatest risk of experiencing a work-related accident?
   a. females aged 18 to 30 years
   b. males aged 18 to 30 years
   c. females aged 31 to 40 years
   d. males aged 31 to 40 years
7. List four types of professionals who are likely to be members of the occupational health team.
8. List four commonly used types of protective equipment for guarding against physical agents in the workplace.
9. List the two agencies established by the Occupational Safety and Health Act of 1970.
10. Describe an employee assistance program.
11. Discuss workmen's compensation.
12. Describe the goals of a disaster plan.

Answer Key

1. Women, older people, individuals with chronic illnesses.
2. Has moved from agricultural and manufacturing to service, professional, technical, and clerical.
3. Biological, chemical, ergonomic, physical, and psychosocial.
4. See Table 45-1 for more examples

Asbestosis	Demolition workers
Asthma	Animal handlers, bakers
Dermatitis	Embalmers
Silicosis	Foundry workers
Lead poisoning	Battery maker

5. Heat, odor, ventilation, light, interpersonal relationships, organizational culture.
6. b
7. Nurse, physician, industrial hygienist, safety professional.
8. Hearing guards, eye guards, protective clothes, and devices for monitoring against exposure to radiation.
9. Occupational Safety and Health Administration (OSHA); National Institute for Occupational Safety and Health (NIOSH).
10. Addresses personal problems of workers, such as marital tensions, substance abuse, financial difficulties, interpersonal problems.
11. State laws that govern the financial compensation paid to workers who sustain work-related injuries.
12. To prevent or minimize injuries and deaths of workers and residents of an area, to minimize property damage, to effectively triage, and to foster the assumption of necessary business activities.

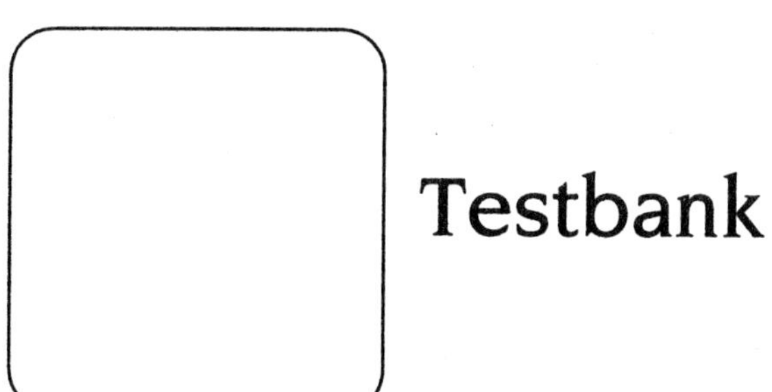

Testbank

Chapter 1

1. A community health program developed to improve the care of the people in rural Appalachian Kentucky was known as the:
   a. American Red Cross.
   b. Shattuck Report.
   c. Henry Street Settlement House.
   d. Frontier Nursing Service.

2. The person noted for contributions to the establishment of visiting nursing services is:
   a. Edwin Chadwick.
   b. Pearl McIver.
   c. Mary Nutting.
   d. William Rathbone.

3. Which of the following was *not* a recommendation of the Shattuck Report?
   a. establishment of state health departments and local health boards
   b. environmental sanitation
   c. proposals on smoke and alcohol control
   d. provision of supplemental food for low income persons

4. Which of the following has not been a central issue in the 1990s debate about health-care reform?
   a. access to care
   b. cost
   c. public health aims
   d. quality

5. Establishment of the Henry Street Settlement and rural health nursing services through the Red Cross are two accomplishments attributed to:
   a. Mary Breckenridge.
   b. Florence Nightingale.
   c. William Rathbone.
   d. Lillian Wald.

6. Which of the following is noted for concern about the environment and improving conditions for sick and injured soldiers?
   a. Edwin Chadwick
   b. Florence Nightingale
   c. William Rathbone
   d. Lillian Wald

7. Which nursing organization was formed to strengthen the union of nursing organizations and to promote ethical standards?
   a. American Nurses Association
   b. District Nursing Association
   c. International Council of Nursing
   d. National League for Nursing

8. A major provision of the Social Security Act of 1935 was the establishment of:
   a. the Frontier Nursing Service to provide nursing service to rural communities.
   b. state and local community health services and training of personnel.
   c. district nursing to provide home health care to sick people.
   d. community-based settlement houses.

9. An accomplishment for which the Frontier Nursing Service was noted is:
   a. improvement of the care of sick and injured soldiers.
   b. establishment of a fee-for-service program for workers at Metropolitan Life Insurance Company.
   c. reduction of infant and maternal mortality regardless of environmental conditions.
   d. increasing funding for communicable disease treatment.

10. Factors affecting community health nursing after World War II include all of the following *except*:
    a. higher quality of care expected by veterans.
    b. increased community health content in nursing curricula.
    c. increased funding targeted to specific health problems such as venereal disease and mental illness.
    d. a more prosperous economy, prohibition, and increasing use of the automobile.

Chapter 2

1. The core functions of public health include all of the following *except*:
   a. assessment.
   b. prevention.
   c. assurance.
   d. policy development.

2. Which of the following statements about public health is accurate?
   a. Prevention of early deaths can be more effectively accomplished by medical treatment than by public health approaches.
   b. Expenditures and resources for public health have increased in recent years.
   c. Historically, gains in the health of populations have been related largely to changes in safety, sanitation, and personal behavior.
   d. Reform of the medical insurance system is the single change needed to improve the health of Americans.

3. An *aggregate* is best defined as:
   a. a high-risk population group.
   b. a school or institutional setting.
   c. a collection of individuals who share at least one characteristic.
   d. a geographic location within a community.

4. Which of the following is the feature that is *least* useful in distinguishing public health nursing from other nursing specialties?
   a. use of political processes to affect public policy as an intervention strategy
   b. concern for the connection between health status and environment
   c. practice that occurs in noninstitutional settings
   d. emphasis on health promotion, health maintenance, and disease prevention

5. Barriers to specialization in public health nursing include all of the following *except*:
   a. the belief by nurses that direct care is the only role for a nurse.
   b. structures and roles that limit practice.
   c. limited knowledge of public health science and population-oriented methods.
   d. lack of skill in preventive health strategies.

6. Monitoring of the population's health status is part of the core public health function referred to as:
   a. assessment.
   b. prevention.
   c. assurance.
   d. policy development.

7. Making sure that essential community-wide health services are available is referred to as:
   a. assessment.
   b. prevention.
   c. assurance.
   d. policy development.

8. The minimum educational preparation for public health nursing specialists is:
   a. baccalaureate degree.
   b. baccalaureate degree with population-focused preparation.
   c. master's degree with population-focused preparation.
   d. doctoral degree.

9. Which of the following statements is true with regard to a population focus in public health nursing?
   a. Attention is given to the highest risk populations.
   b. Direct caregiving is limited to preventive measures such as administration of immunizations.
   c. Attention is given to persons both inside and outside the health care system.
   d. Only populations outside institutional settings are considered.

10. A strong need exists to prepare public health nurses for positions in:
    a. direct caregiving.
    b. education.
    c. institutional settings.
    d. health care policy development.

Chapter 3

1. Which of the following is not a major concern plaguing the U.S. health care system?
   a. access to care
   b. cost
   c. quality
   d. advances in technology

2. Which of the following is not a role of the state health department?
   a. protection of the food and drug supply
   b. establishment of health codes
   c. ongoing assessment of health needs
   d. regulation of the insurance industry

3. Cost shifting involves making up for lost revenue from uninsured clients by:
   a. charging more for services to those who are able to pay.
   b. denying insurance coverage to those who are sick or at risk for getting sick.
   c. decreasing funding to clinics, causing many uninsured people to seek care at the emergency room.
   d. basing the cost of health insurance on the level of income earned.

4. Which of the following statements about future population trends in the United States is erroneous?
   a. Immigration will constitute about half of the population growth in the United States.
   b. The birth rate is expected to continue to rise.
   c. Growth in the number of people aged 50 years or older is expected to increase substantially.
   d. Hispanics will become the largest minority group.

5. Health care cost containment measures include:
   a. decreasing the number of primary care physicians.
   b. increasing the number of advanced practice nurses.
   c. downsizing community-based services.
   d. increasing physician specialization.

6. A personal health care system that provides for first-contact, continuous, comprehensive, and coordinated care with intervention directed primarily at an individual's pathophysiological process is referred to as:
   a. primary care.
   b. primary health care.
   c. primary prevention.
   d. secondary prevention.

7. Which of the following statements about primary health care is *not* true?
   a. Care is community-focused.
   b. Emphasis is on curative care.
   c. A wide variety of health care team members provide care.
   d. Individual, family, and community self-reliance is encouraged.

8. Which of the following terms refers to early diagnosis and treatment, including screening activities?
   a. primary care
   b. primary prevention
   c. secondary prevention
   d. tertiary prevention

9. Which of the following is *not* a component of the community-oriented primary care (COPC) model?
   a. Health care delivery focuses entirely on public health to the exclusion of primary care.
   b. Active participation of people who live in the community is emphasized.
   c. Consensus building among diverse community leaders is important in addressing health needs.
   d. Allocation of more money into community care is assumed to ultimately save money and improve outcomes.

10. Which of the following statements about the public health system is false?
    a. It is mandated through national, state, or local laws.
    b. State health departments play an insignificant role in health care financing.
    c. The U.S. Public Health Service provides health care to medically underserved populations.
    d. Services offered by local health departments vary greatly.

Chapter 4

1. Which of the following statements concerning the global burden of disease is accurate?
   a. It is an indicator that combines losses from both premature death and disability.
   b. It is a less adequate description of the outlook of health in the world than are mortality statistics.
   c. It does not measure the impact of communicable diseases.
   d. It accurately measures the impact of familial dysfunction and violence.

2. The major factors contributing to high infant mortality rates in lesser developed countries are:
   a. nutritional deficiencies.
   b. diarrheal and respiratory diseases.
   c. malaria and tuberculosis.
   d. alcohol and drug abuse.

3. A world health problem with high mortality that has received little attention to date is:
   a. diarrheal disease.
   b. tuberculosis.
   c. malnutrition.
   d. maternal mortality.

4. Which of the following statements about nutrition and world health is inaccurate?
   a. Stunting is related to inadequate protein intake.
   b. Iron deficiency results in increased appetite and exaggerated sensation of hunger.
   c. As a result of menstruation and child bearing, women are most susceptible to iron deficiency.
   d. Malnutrition can increase susceptibility to communicable disease and illness.

5. The intergovernmental organization which focuses its efforts on assisting countries in Latin America is the:
   a. Pan American Health Organization.
   b. World Bank.
   c. World Health Organization.
   d. United Nations Children's Fund.

6. Effects of the removal of political and economic barriers between countries include all of the following except:
   a. stimulation of economic growth and development.
   b. increased risk of exposure to diseases and environmental health hazards.
   c. spread of diseases such as AIDS and tuberculosis.
   d. decreased movement of population groups.

7. Health problems in need of control in developed countries include:
   a. hepatitis.
   b. malaria.
   c. polio.
   d. smallpox.

8. Of the following countries, which is referred to as a lesser developed country?
   a. France
   b. Japan
   c. Indonesia
   d. Sweden

9. According to a resolution adopted at the Alma Ata conference, the major key to attaining Health for All by the Year 2000 is:
   a. technological development.
   b. stable economy.
   c. primary health care.
   d. health commodification.

10. Nurses who work in international communities need to recognize that:
    a. health is directly related to economic development.
    b. availability of technology automatically improves care.
    c. the promotion of pharmaceuticals for all people is essential regardless of local traditions.
    d. all of the above

11. Worldwide, the largest cause of death from a single agent is:
    a. acquired immune deficiency syndrome.
    b. malaria.
    c. hepatitis.
    d. tuberculosis.

12. Which of the following statements concerning short-course chemotherapy (SCC) programs for TB control is false?
    a. The cost per client is lower than in longer programs.
    b. More clients complete the program.
    c. A combination of drugs is used.
    d. Clients are hospitalized.

13. Which of the following is *not* an incentive for a lesser developed country to engage in a bilateral arrangement with a more economically advanced country?
    a. economic enhancement
    b. national defense
    c. protection of private investments
    d. opportunities to conduct medical research

14. Which of the following statements reflects the relationship of economic development to health care throughout the world?
    a. Resources may be diverted from health and education to military and technology needs.
    b. Importation of drugs and other health care products depends on a network of foreign exchange that is influenced by economic and political factors.
    c. Improvement in the overall health status of a country contributes to its economic growth.
    d. All of the above are true.

15. Most deaths to women around the world are related to:
    a. diarrheal and respiratory infections.
    b. malnutrition.
    c. pregnancy and childbirth.
    d. tuberculosis.

Chapter 5

1. The measure used to compare the costs of health care in the United States with other countries such as Canada is the:
   a. consumer price index.
   (b) gross domestic product.
   c. gross national product.
   d. price inflation factor.

2. The economic theory used by community health nurses who work with aggregates would be:
   a. microeconomic theory because they are concerned with factors that determine prices and affect resource allocation.
   b. microeconomic theory because of the positive effect of competitiveness on health care costs.
   c. macroeconomic theory because they are concerned with the supply, demand, and costs of services available to their clients.
   (d) macroeconomic theory because they are concerned with policy to support programs to improve the health of the community.

3. Which of the four developmental stages in the U.S. health care delivery system showed a shift away from infectious diseases?
   a. the first stage (1800 to 1900)
   b. the second stage (1900 to 1945)
   (c) the third stage (1945 to 1984)
   d. the fourth stage (1985 to the present)

4. Which of the following statements about the current supply and demand of health care products is *not* accurate?
   a. More primary care physicians and fewer specialty physicians are needed.
   (b) The demand for nurses is increasing.
   c. Hospitals are using nonlicensed assistive personnel to replace nurses.
   d. More nurses are employed by community-based settings.

5. Which of the following is *not* a valid assumption regarding the reasons for price inflation?
   a. development of new health care technology
   b. duplication of services
   c. increased wages for health care personnel
   (d) decreased availability of insurance and types of coverage

6. The age group with the least health care expenditures has been those:
   (a) under 19 years.
   b. 20 to 44 years.
   c. 45 to 64 years.
   d. 65 years and over.

7. Which of the following factors has contributed most to the growth in health care expenditures?
   a. changes in population demography
   b. intensity of services
   (c) price inflation
   d. medical research costs

8. Which of the following is *not* a demographic change contributing to increased expenditures for health care?
   (a) decreased ability of elderly persons to pay for services
   b. increased number of elderly women who are heavier users of health services than men
   c. decline in family social support
   d. increased use of complex medical and surgical services

9. Which of the following statements is accurate in describing how the baby boom generation becoming middle-aged will affect health care costs?
   a. Costs will decrease because they are a healthier group than the elderly.
   b. Costs will decrease because they are less oriented to preventive care.
   (c) Costs will increase because the numbers of middle-aged persons requiring long-term care will increase.
   d. Costs will increase because they are more likely to have acute health problems than chronic conditions.

10. Currently, the source of health care financing contributing the highest percentage is:
    a. the consumer.
    b. public health funding.
    (c) third-party payment.
    d. out-of-pocket payment.

11. Which of the following statements about the Medicare program is accurate?
    (a) Part A provides coverage for hospitalization.
    b. Part A requires payment of a monthly premium for coverage.
    c. Part B provides payment for home health services and extended care facilities.
    d. Part B is available without cost to all elderly people who have paid social security taxes.

12. Which of the following statements about the Medicaid program is inaccurate?
    a. The program provides financial assistance to pay for medical services for families with dependent children, the blind, the elderly, and the aged poor.
    b. The state has complete authority to decide what services are provided to participants below poverty-level incomes.
    c. The program is jointly sponsored and financed by the federal and state governments.
    d. The medically indigent are required by law to pay a monthly premium.

13. A major contributor to costs in the Medicaid program in the past has been:
    a. nursing home care.
    b. family planning and EPSDT.
    c. physician services.
    d. home care.

14. Which of the following represents an attempt to regulate and change physician fee structure by shifting physician reimbursement from surgical procedures and technologies to prevention and promotion?
    a. resource-based relative value scale
    b. "unbundling" of hospital services
    c. health care rationing
    d. diagnostic related groups

15. The pay-or-play system of financing introduced by the Health Security Act was proposed to:
    a. provide universal access to care.
    b. reduce the costs to businesses in providing insurance to employees.
    c. create a single-payer system.
    d. decrease the length of stay in hospitals.

16. The following statements relate to poverty and health care financing. Which statement is incorrect?
    a. Health care access may be denied to those who are poor and unable to qualify for public programs.
    b. The need for long-term care may result in poverty.
    c. The typical uninsured person is a retired elderly adult.
    d. Those in poverty are more likely to experience ill health.

17. Health care reform is likely to result in a two-tiered system. Which of the following is *not* expected to be a component of the two-tiered system?
    a. a free market system in the second tier for purchasing additional health care
    b. decreased equity in access to care
    c. care in the second tier limited by individuals' ability and willingness to pay
    d. costs and use of services controlled by government and corporations in the first tier and by the consumer in the second level

Chapter 6

1. The "right to health" means that:
   a. the government is obligated to initiate services to maintain or to improve health.
   b. people have the right not to have their health interfered with by the actions of others.
   c. specific health care services such as immunizations and family planning are the right of all people.
   d. services to achieve complete physical, mental, and social well-being must be available for all people.

2. Advance directives are based on the principle of:
   a. autonomy
   b. beneficence.
   c. justice.
   d. utility.

3. The Patient Self-Determination Act requires all health care institutions receiving Medicare or Medicaid funds to provide information to clients regarding:
   a. explanations of financial charges.
   b. confidentiality of medical records.
   c. availability of services according to place of residence.
   d. the right to refuse medical and surgical care.

4. Withholding information from clients about the seriousness of their condition involves violation of the duty of:
   a. accountability.
   b. advocacy.
   c. confidentiality.
   d. veracity.

5. The nurse speaking in support of the best interest of a vulnerable client population reflects the duty of:
   a. advocacy.
   b. caring.
   c. confidentiality.
   d. veracity.

6. The moral obligation to prevent harm to clients is based on the principle of:
   a. autonomy.
   b. beneficence.
   c. justice.
   d. paternalism

7. When the community health nurse makes a decision about allocation of resources in order to provide the greatest good to the greatest number of people, the decision is based on which of the following?
   a. entitlement theory
   b. egalitarian theory
   c. maximin theory
   d. utilitarian theory

8. Promoting freedom of choice for clients in decision making supports the principle of:
   a. autonomy.
   b. beneficence.
   c. justice.
   d. paternalism.

9. In most nursing situations, the professional ethic generally places least emphasis on observance of the principle of:
   a. autonomy.
   b. beneficence.
   c. justice.
   d. self-determination.

10. The Code for Nurses with Interpretive Statements prescribes rules for professional behavior that are considered:
    a. moral principles.
    b. morally obligatory and legally required.
    c. statements of professional etiquette.
    d. a guide for conduct between professional groups.

11. The duty to observe confidentiality may be overridden when:
    a. it conflicts with other duties toward the client.
    b. the client expresses intent to harm self or others.
    c. it conflicts with duties toward society in general.
    d. all of the above

12. The obligation to provide an explanation to someone for actions performed in the role of the nurse is:
    a. accountability.
    b. autonomy.
    c. caring.
    d. self-determination.

13. In which of the following situations would paternalism be justified?
    a. when the nurse's recommendation will have greater benefit than the client's choice would
    b. when withholding information may prevent grief
    c. when necessary to prevent life-threatening physical harm
    d. when the community disagrees with the individual's decision

14. The essential elements of informed consent are:
    a. confidentiality, freedom from coercion, and veracity.
    b. information, comprehension, and voluntariness.
    c. self-determination, privacy, and understanding.
    d. information, accountability, and advocacy.

15. Community health nursing guided by the public health ethic is most strongly based on:
    a. beneficence and utility.
    b. paternalism and entitlement.
    c. autonomy and egalitarianism.
    d. confidentiality and maximin theory.

16. The theory of justice which emphasizes improving the position of the least advantaged members of the community is:
    a. entitlement theory.
    b. utilitarian theory.
    c. maximin theory.
    d. egalitarian theory.

17. The theory of justice which takes the position that all citizens have claim to an equal amount of resources is:
    a. entitlement theory.
    b. utilitarian theory.
    c. maximin theory.
    d. egalitarian theory.

Chapter 7

1. When nurses support the use of those aspects of the client's culture that promote healthy behaviors, they are using:
   a. cultural accommodation.
   b. cultural brokering.
   c. cultural preservation.
   d. cultural repatterning.

2. To meet a client's needs, it is sometimes necessary to integrate into the client's care a culturally relevant practice that lacks scientific utility. This is known as:
   a. cultural accommodation.
   b. cultural brokering.
   c. cultural preservation.
   d. cultural repatterning.

3. Assisting clients in making changes in culture behaviors when those behaviors are harmful to the client's well-being is called:
   a. cultural accommodation.
   b. cultural brokering.
   c. cultural preservation.
   d. cultural repatterning.

4. When the nurse advocates and intervenes between the health care system and the client's cultural beliefs on behalf of the client, the nurse's action is called:
   a. cultural accommodation.
   b. cultural brokering.
   c. cultural preservation.
   d. cultural repatterning.

5. The process of forcefully promoting one's own values while ignoring a client's differing values is known as:
   a. ethnocentrism.
   b. cultural conflict.
   c. cultural imposition.
   d. cultural shock.

6. The belief that your cultural group determines the standards for judging the behavior of all other groups is known as:
   a. ethnocentrism.
   b. cultural imposition.
   c. racism.
   d. prejudice.

7. The belief that people born into a particular cultural group are inferior in one or more ways is known as:
   a. ethnocentrism.
   b. cultural imposition.
   c. racism.
   d. stereotyping.

8. Assuming that groups of people have certain beliefs and behaviors without recognizing individual differences within groups is known as:
   a. ethnocentrism.
   b. cultural imposition.
   c. racism.
   d. stereotyping.

9. When communicating with a client, the nurse modifies the physical distance between herself and the client. This is an example of:
   a. cultural accommodation.
   b. cultural awareness.
   c. cultural knowledge.
   d. cultural skill.

10. Which of the following statements regarding working with clients of different cultures is accurate?
    a. Individuals of the same cultural group have the same values, beliefs, and customs.
    b. There is no significant difference between racial and ethnic identity.
    c. Care that is not focused on the client's values may increase cost and interfere with positive outcomes.
    d. Stereotypes that are positive facilitate cultural competence in providing care.

11. Which cultural characteristics are associated with Hispanic clients?
    a. the importance of family involvement in decision making
    b. the belief that touching another's hair is offensive
    c. speaking in a low voice and expecting that the listener will be attentive
    d. use of acupuncture and acupressure for healing

12. Which characteristic is associated with the Asian American culture?
    a. importance of direct eye contact when communicating
    b. shaking hands with people of the opposite sex
    c. female-dominated households
    d. emphasis on harmony and avoidance of conflict

13. The key to a successful cultural assessment lies in:
    a. the nurses awareness of their own culture.
    b. focusing first on dietary patterns.
    c. relying on the translator to influence the client.
    d. asking comprehensive questions even if the client becomes offended.

Chapter 8

1. All of the following are potential sources of exposure to radon *except*:
   a. cracks in basement walls and floors.
   b. dermal contact.
   c. inhalation of air.
   d. ingestion of water.

2. Exposure to which of the following substances may be the number one environmental health problem in the United States?
   a. asbestos
   b. lead
   c. pesticides
   d. radon

3. Young children may be at greater risk for exposure to hazardous substances than adults because:
   a. they are attracted to physical hazards by curiosity.
   b. they absorb and store some toxic substances more easily.
   c. they spend more time in the home.
   d. all of the above

4. An intervention targeted specifically to prevent lead poisoning in black children would be education to:
   a. reduce play on wooden playground equipment.
   b. keep children out of basements with cracked walls or floors.
   c. avoid folk remedies.
   d. increase dietary calcium.

5. One of the most common agents identified in water-borne illness is:
   a. giardia.
   b. hepatitis.
   c. malaria.
   d. salmonella.

6. Which of the following statements about dose response to environmental exposures is accurate?
   a. The threshold dose for all chemicals has been determined through animal studies.
   b. Exposures below the threshold dose result in adverse health effects.
   c. For most exposures, the type and severity of adverse health effects are dependent on dose.
   d. Low doses of substances produce allergic reactions after sensitization.

7. Which of the following statements about quantitative risk assessment is accurate?
   a. Risk assessment is mandated by law.
   b. Environmental rules and regulations are shaped by risk assessment.
   c. Risk assessment is used primarily to facilitate treatment of individuals with exposure to a hazard.
   d. all of the above

8. When environmental issues exist within a community, a key source of environmental information is:
   a. occupational health nurses.
   b. regulatory environmental agencies.
   c. local community activists.
   d. poison control centers.

9. An excellent resource to assist a community health nurse in identifying exposure pathways and providing information about available screening and treatment programs is:
   a. the local health department.
   b. an occupational health and safety agency.
   c. a poison control center.
   d. community action groups.

10. Initial assessment of environmental health can be effectively completed by:
    a. interviewing community residents.
    b. gathering information from governmental agencies.
    c. conducting a windshield survey.
    d. all of the above

11. In completing an environmental exposure history:
    a. a negative response to all questions rules out toxic exposure.
    b. a positive response to any question indicates the need for further questioning.
    c. the two factors most important in determining how much exposure a client has experienced are the source of contamination and route of exposure.
    d. all of the above

12. Occupational exposure to lead should be suspected in those who are:
    a. cigarette smokers.
    b. agricultural workers.
    c. dry cleaners.
    d. remodeling old homes.

13. Factors that may place the client at higher risk from toxic substance exposure include all of the following *except*:
    a. liver disease.
    b. pregnancy or lactation.
    c. chronic obstructive pulmonary disease.
    d. stress.

14. Which statement about testing for exposure levels is accurate?
    a. Because toxic substances remain in the body for a long time, testing any time following exposure will confirm the exposure.
    b. A positive test for a biomarker of exposure may only confirm what is already known—that an exposure has occurred.
    c. Detectable levels of a hazardous substance indicate that adverse health effects will result from the exposure.
    d. Testing is an easy, cost-effective way to measure exposure.

Chapter 9

1. The law that has had the most significant impact on the development of public health policy, public health nursing, and social welfare policy in the United States is the:
   a. Health Security Act.
   b. Occupational Safety and Health Act.
   c. Sheppard-Towner Act.
   d. Social Security Act.

2. Which of the following statements concerning the impact of governmental funding on the roles of community health nurses is correct?
   a. The designation of money for specific needs has led to more narrowly focused roles.
   b. The roles of nurse practitioners emerged primarily because of governmental funding.
   c. Community health nurses are often employed to implement programs for special populations.
   d. Block grant funding usually results in a shift toward more specialized roles.

3. The branch of the federal government that includes regulatory units such as the Department of Health and Human Services is the:
   a. executive branch.
   b. legislative branch.
   c. judicial branch.

4. The branch of the government involved in interpreting the states' rights to grant abortions is the:
   a. executive branch.
   b. legislative branch.
   c. judicial branch.

5. When Congress decides that states will administer a program rather than the federal government, money is given to states as block grants. One effect of block grants is:
   a. reduction of federal expenditures.
   b. increased federal restriction regarding the specific type of program implemented.
   c. decreased ability of the state to spend the money for programs designated by the state.
   d. guaranteed continuation of programs with demonstrated effectiveness.

6. Which of the following is *not* a health care function of federal, state, and local governments?
   a. direct services to certain individuals and groups
   b. financing of services
   c. collection and analysis of data
   d. regulating nursing practice

7. Health services to prisoners are:
   a. provided at the federal level within the Department of Defense.
   b. exempt from professional malpractice claims.
   c. required at an adequate level for all incarcerated individuals.
   d. not mandated after sentencing.

8. The term that refers to legal definition and customary practice of a particular profession is:
   a. precedent.
   b. scope of practice.
   c. sovereign immunity.
   d. self-regulation.

9. For a nurse to be found guilty of malpractice, which of the following must be proven?
   a. The nurse owed a duty to the client.
   b. Injuries provided the basis for a monetary claim through the legal system.
   c. Failure of the nurse to act in the situation in a reasonable manner led to the injuries.
   d. all of the above

10. When a nurse is employed and functioning within the scope of that employment, the employer is responsible for the nurse's negligent actions. This is referred to as:
    a. respondent superior.
    b. sovereign immunity.
    c. institutional negligence.
    d. professional immunity.

Chapter 10

1. In differentiating between a conceptual model and a theory, which of the following statements is correct?
   a. A theory is highly abstract.
   b. A theory includes operational definitions.
   c. A conceptual model is concrete and specific.
   d. A conceptual model can be directly tested.

2. A set of relational statements that present a systematic view and are used to describe, explain, and predict phenomena is a:
   a. concept.
   b. construct.
   c. model.
   d. theory.

3. The term *world view* refers to:
   a. philosophical assumptions about the nature of person-environment interactions.
   b. an individual's unique set of beliefs guiding the categorization of ideas and perception of situations.
   c. a conceptual model which determines what is considered relevant in viewing people and their environment.
   d. all of the above

4. In public health, the term *assurance activities* refers to thc:
   a. evaluation of the potential health risk factors and disease indicators in a community.
   b. monitoring of acess to and effectiveness of health services.
   c. establishment of partnerships with other agencies to develop a policy to address a problem.
   d. provision of primary care services for all clients in the community.

5. In comparison to the ANA definition of community health nursing, the APHA definition places greater emphasis on:
   a. identification of high risk groups.
   b. health promotion.
   c. nursing.
   d. public health.

6. Contemporary conceptual models of nursing may be compared in terms of four essential components. These include definitions of:
   a. person, environment, health, and nursing.
   b. person, development, environment, and health.
   c. theoretical framework, person, health, and nursing.
   d. theoretical framework, person, environment, and health.

7. According to the Neuman Systems Model, the goal of nursing is to:
   a. promote self-care of individuals, families, and communities.
   b. restore, maintain, or attain behavioral system balance at the highest level possible.
   c. help people interact with their environment in ways that lead to health.
   d. keep the client stable through assessment of stressors and appropriate intervention.

8. According to the Neuman Systems Model, nursing intervention is implemented through:
   a. promotion of adaptation.
   b. primary, secondary, and tertiary prevention.
   c. facilitation of effective behavior.
   d. repatterning of behavior.

9. Properties of systems include all of the following *except*:
   a. wholeness.
   b. openness.
   c. organization.
   d. randomness.

10. The following theorists have developed models which are applicable to nursing. Of these, whose model is best suited to community health nursing?
    a. Roy
    b. Rogers
    c. King
    d. Neuman

11. What level of intervention is most appropriate for a community experiencing chronic dysfunction as a result of losing a major source of employment?
    a. primary prevention
    b. secondary prevention
    c. tertiary prevention
    d. health promotion

12. An example of an intercommunity stressor affecting a community would be:
    a. power lines adjacent to an elementary school.
    b. bussing of students.
    c. decreased state funding for services.
    d. high teen pregnancy rate.

13. The Omaha System is best described as a classification system that consists of:
    a. the nursing diagnoses that have been used most frequently in acute care.
    b. a list of NANDA nursing diagnoses used in home care.
    c. nursing interventions generated by home care agencies.
    d. a nursing diagnoses/problem classification scheme, intervention categories, and a problem rating scale for outcomes.

Chapter 11

1. The method which attempts to identify the determinants of disease in individuals is referred to as:
   a. descriptive epidemiology.
   b. analytic epidemiology.
   c. an intervention study.
   d. an ecological study.

2. In public health, the three levels of prevention are tied to specific stages in the:
   a. epidemiologic triangle.
   b. web of causation.
   c. natural history of disease.
   d. surveillance process.

3. In the epidemiologic triangle, lifestyle factors such as diet would be considered an example of a(n):
   a. agent factor.
   b. host factor.
   c. environmental factor.
   d. causality factor.

4. Vocational rehabilitation of a person with a neuromuscular disease is an example of:
   a. primary prevention.
   b. secondary prevention.
   c. tertiary prevention.
   d. health promotion.

5. Screening for hearing defects is an example of:
   a. primary prevention.
   b. secondary prevention.
   c. tertiary prevention.
   d. health promotion.

6. Instructing new mothers regarding the proper use of infant seats is an example of:
   a. primary prevention.
   b. secondary prevention.
   c. tertiary prevention.
   d. health promotion.

7. The rate that best indicates the proportion of people exposed to an agent who develop the disease is:
   a. attack rate.
   b. incidence.
   c. prevalence.
   d. susceptibility.

8. The prevalence rate is:
   a. an estimate of the risk of developing a disease.
   b. a measure of existing disease in a population at a particular time.
   c. useful in determining factors related to disease etiology.
   d. a reflection of the susceptibility to disease.

9. The rate most useful when comparing mortality of one population group with another group is the:
   a. crude mortality rate.
   b. cause-specific mortality rate.
   c. age-adjusted mortality rate.
   d. infant mortality rate.

10. You are told that a screening test has high specificity. This means that the test:
    a. provides precise and consistent readings.
    b. accurately identifies those with the condition or trait.
    c. accurately identifies those without the trait.
    d. has a high level of false positives.

11. You are cautioned to look for confounding in a study of alcohol consumption in teenagers. Confounding is a systematic error caused by:
    a. the way subjects are selected to enter a study.
    b. misclassification of subjects in the study.
    c. the presence of an additional factor (not accounted for) that relates to the study factors.
    d. the information that subjects choose to supply about themselves.

12. In the process of ascertaining causality, factors are said to have specificity of association if:
    a. the factors possess a high strength of association.
    b. the disease can occur only in the presence of a particular agent.
    c. the risk factor precedes the onset of the disease.
    d. the relationship among factors is consistent in findings with numerous study designs and populations.

13. The measure most commonly used around the world as an indicator of overall health and availability of health services is the:
    a. crude death rate.
    b. case fatality rate.
    c. morbidity rate.
    d. infant mortality rate.

14. In planning a successful screening program, the community health nurse recognizes the need to:
    a. screen only those who are symptomatic.
    b. interpret screening tests as diagnostic for the condition.
    c. have a large supply of materials and personnel available regardless of the expense.
    d. use valid and reliable screening tests.

Chapter 12

1. Preliminary testing of the data collection methods and data analysis plan performed with clients during the design stage is known as:
   a. deliberate sampling.
   b. random sampling.
   c. pilot testing.
   d. dissemination.

2. The stage in the research process which involves comparing findings with previous research results is:
   a. action.
   b. assessment.
   c. implementation.
   d. evaluation.

3. Collection of data from participants occurs in the research process stage of:
   a. assessment.
   b. planning.
   c. implementation.
   d. evaluation.

4. Review of the study by the human subjects review committee occurs during the research process stage of:
   a. action.
   b. assessment.
   c. implementation.
   d. planning.

5. The primary purpose of institutional human subjects review committees is to:
   a. protect research participants from physical or mental harm.
   b. identify the limitations of a research study.
   c. provide information about the project's findings to funding agencies.
   d. critique the research design.

6. Which of the following is a primary consideration when doing research in the community?
   a. Qualitative methods are characterized by deductive reasoning and objectivity.
   b. The research method used will depend on the question being studied.
   c. Research should focus only on population-based problems.
   d. The conceptual framework selected needs to address environmental concerns.

7. In the research process, an uncontrollable element that limits the certainty of the research findings is called a(n):
   a. assumption.
   b. proposition.
   c. limitation.
   d. replication.

8. Communication and utilization of findings is referred to as:
   a. limitation.
   b. replication.
   c. dissemination.
   d. publication.

9. Research findings should be reported to:
   a. clinical professionals.
   b. policy makers.
   c. community members.
   d. all of the above

10. When a change occurs in a research plan, the researcher is responsible for:
    a. communicating the change to policy makers.
    b. developing an educational guide for clients.
    c. reporting the change to the human subjects review committee.
    d. discontinuing the study immediately.

Chapter 13

1. The theory that emphasizes planning educational experiences based on the individual's readiness to learn at a particular stage is:
   a. behavioral theory.
   b. social learning theory.
   c. cognitive theory.
   d. developmental theory.

2. In planning learning experiences for Andrea, who has cognitive limitations, which theory would be most appropriate to the situation?
   a. behavioral theory
   b. social learning theory
   c. cognitive theory
   d. critical theory

3. An educational program is planned that emphasizes encouraging self-expression and helping learners to grow and develop according to their natural inclinations. The theory upon which this approach is based is:
   a. affective theory.
   b. developmental theory.
   c. humanist theory.
   d. social learning theory.

4. The behavioral approach is useful when the educator:
   a. wants to change clients' beliefs about the desirability and attainability of an outcome.
   b. seeks to change learners' behavior by changing their thought patterns.
   c. has control over the feedback system.
   d. believes that learners should be encouraged to examine their emotions and engage in self-expression.

5. Which of the following models would be most appropriate for the community health nurse to use when designing an educational program to help communities change their behavior?
   a. the health belief model
   b. the health promotion model
   c. the PRECEDE-PROCEED model
   d. the social factors model

6. The PRECEDE-PROCEED model is a model that:
   a. was developed to explain the determinants of health-promoting behavior.
   b. emphasizes the implementation phase of health education programs.
   c. is most useful in working with individuals and families when modification of sociocultural factors is desired.
   d. involves the client in a problem-solving approach to provide education for an identified area of need.

7. Which of the following statements about the domains of learning is inaccurate?
   a. Each domain is a hierarchy of steps with each level of learning building on the previous one.
   b. In the cognitive domain, teaching above the client's level of understanding is encouraged in order to provide challenge.
   c. Qualities in the affective domain, such as values and attitudes, are difficult to change.
   d. Before psychomotor learning can occur, the learner must have the necessary ability and opportunities to practice.

8. In applying guidelines for effective teaching, the community health nurse would take all of the following approaches *except*:
   a. to communicate using medical jargon and technical terms to clarify the message.
   b. to establish an appropriate learning climate through the tone and appearance of media messages announcing the program.
   c. to select audiovisual aids to enhance learning.
   d. to use participatory learning for the cognitive and affective domains, as well as the psychomotor domain.

9. Which of the following statements about affective learning is correct?
   a. Affective qualities are readily changed through health education.
   b. Affective changes are easily measured.
   c. Assessment of ability to learn is not necessary for teaching in the affective domain.
   d. Praise and group support are often useful in reinforcing affective changes.

10. During the educational process, feedback should be:
    a. constructive and helpful to the learner.
    b. clear and behaviorally focused.
    c. used for modifications in the educational program.
    d. all of the above

Chapter 14

1. Which of the following statements regarding the self-care movement is inaccurate?
   a. The biomedical emphasis on treatment and cure tends to overshadow self-care.
   b. Some self-care advocates believe that medicine has been given too much credit for improvements in health.
   c. A political climate that challenges the authority of health care professionals interferes with the advancement of self-care.
   d. Emphasis on self-care or individual responsibility for health behavior may result in "victim blaming."

2. According to Leavell and Clark, primary prevention consists of two components. The two components are:
   a. health promotion and disease prevention.
   b. health promotion and specific protection.
   c. early diagnosis and prompt treatment.
   d. health maintenance and multilevel prevention.

3. An example of specific protection would be:
   a. well-child evaluation.
   b. health education.
   c. immunizations.
   d. good nutrition.

4. The term defined as "behavior directed toward keeping a current state of health" is:
   a. *health promotion.*
   b. *health promotion behavior.*
   c. *health maintenance behavior.*
   d. *health protective behavior.*

5. Which of the following statements best describes health risk appraisal and risk reduction?
   a. Data about health risks is collected and analyzed; then a health risk profile is generated.
   b. The goal is prevention or early detection of disease.
   c. The health insurance industry recognizes the potential of risk reduction for cost containment.
   d. An epidemiological approach is used to identify risks at the individual level.

6. The Guide to Clinical Preventive Services is a guide for:
   a. group risk appraisal and risk reduction.
   b. use by primary care clinicians in delivering health care services to individuals.
   c. conducting a community wellness inventory.
   d. improving environmental living conditions and sanitation.

7. One advantage of health-risk appraisal instruments is that:
   a. they are suitable for all age groups.
   b. they accurately reflect an individual's ability to initiate changes in life style.
   c. they emphasize environmental factors.
   d. they provide support to nurses in counseling and educating individuals in self-care behaviors.

8. Which of the following community studies was not a multilevel intervention program?
   a. the Framingham Heart Study
   b. the Stanford Heart Disease Prevention Program
   c. the North Karelia Study
   d. the Minnesota Heart Health Program

9. Which of the following community-based risk reduction interventions resulted in equally favorable health risk changes for all groups (both control and treatment)?
   a. the Framingham Heart Study
   b. the Stanford Heart Disease Prevention Program
   c. the Pawtucket Study
   d. the Minnesota Heart Health Program

10. The Framingham Heart Study was successful in:
    a. providing information on the effectiveness of risk reduction interventions.
    b. documenting the relationship between social variables and heart disease.
    c. identifying factors contributing to the development of coronary heart disease and high blood pressure.
    d. demonstrating the impact of mass media in modifying high-risk behavior.

11. Milio's propositions for improving health behavior emphasize:
    a. recognizing the importance of social context and resources in influencing individual health-related decisions.
    b. developing a passive partnership with the community.
    c. addressing health maintenance behavior as well as disease prevention.
    d. using the disease prevention strategy of risk reduction to help groups maximize their self-care activities.

12. In comparison with wellness inventories, health hazard appraisals are more likely to:
   a. advocate health enhancement.
   b. address health-promoting aspects of lifestyle.
   c. focus on assessment of health behaviors with clearly documented relationships to specific diseases.
   d. emphasize empowerment of individuals to achieve health.

Chapter 15

1. The community is considered the client when:
   a. the location of the practice is in the community and the focus of the practice is on the individual.
   b. the nursing focus is on the collective good of the population.
   c. families are cared for in the home setting.
   d. all of the above

2. Change for the benefit of the community as client, such as with lifestyle-induced health problems, often involves change at which level?
   a. individual level
   b. family level
   c. societal level
   d. all of the above

3. Which of the following is an indicator of community health status?
   a. educational levels
   b. health facilities
   c. suicide rate
   d. conflict containment

4. Which of the following is an indicator of community health structure?
   a. infant mortality rate
   b. effective communication
   c. crime rate
   d. emergency room utilization

5. Which of the following is an indicator of community health process?
   a. participation
   b. live birth rate
   c. racial distribution
   d. socioeconomic levels

6. Which of the following statements about the relationship between community structure and health status is accurate?
   a. There is a direct causal relationship between the provision of health care and improved health.
   b. Health service utilization patterns provide an accurate measure of quality op care.
   c. Health status is not directly related to socioeconomic level.
   d. Age is inversely related to health status.

7. Which of the following is not an essential condition of community competence?
   a. commitment
   b. effective communication
   c. local ecology
   d. participation

8. Program planning is a nursing intervention strategy focused on which of the following community dimensions?
   a. health status
   b. environment
   c. process
   d. structure

9. Primary prevention is usually the most appropriate strategy focused on:
   a. health status.
   b. environment.
   c. process.
   d. structure.

10. The main elements of a partnership are:
    a. informed, flexible, and negotiated distribution of power.
    b. rights, responsibilities, and consensus.
    c. commitment, participation, and articulation.
    d. collaboration, advocacy, and utility.

11. The process of developing data that do not already exist through interaction with community members is called:
    a. data collection.
    b. data gathering.
    c. data generation.
    d. data interpretation.

12. The method of community data collection that involves directed conversation with selected community members is known as:
    a. informant interview.
    b. participant observation.
    c. secondary analysis.
    d. windshield survey.

13. Which of the following is *not* a typical characteristic of lay advisors?
    a. conforming to community norms
    b. being influential in approving ideas
    c. being involved in formal social groups
    d. seeking advice from others

14. In evaluating a community intervention program the nurse determines whether:
    a. objectives were met.
    b. interventions used were effective.
    c. costs in money and time were commensurate with benefits.
    d. all of the above

15. The best source of information for the nurse about personal safety in the community is:
    a. other nurses or social workers.
    b. community members.
    c. direct observation.
    d. crime reports.

16. Which of the following examples best illustrates a partnership for health?
    a. assisting a school counselor and school nurse to determine the students' health education needs
    b. helping a group of citizens concerned about potential environmental hazards collect relevant health data
    c. telling a neighborhood council that smoking is the major health problem in their community
    d. developing a volunteer program for teaching parenting skills

Chapter 16

1. The percentage of U.S. residents living in rural settings is about:
   a. 5%.
   b. 15%.
   c. 25%.
   d. 40%.

2. In general, the group with the highest proportion of its population residing in rural areas is:
   a. African-Americans.
   b. Asian-Pacific Islanders.
   c. Caucasians.
   d. Native Americans.

3. Which of the following statements about rural populations in comparison with urban populations is correct?
   a. Rural communities have a higher-than-average number of residents between 6 and 17 years of age.
   b. Rural areas have a lower proportion of residents over 65 years of age.
   c. Adults in rural areas are less likely to be, or to have been, married.
   d. Adults in rural areas have more years of formal education.

4. Which of the following are factors contributing to the risk of rural residents being uninsured or underinsured?
   a. a high number of working poor
   b. a large number of self-employed workers
   c. employment in part-time or seasonal occupations
   d. all of the above

5. Compared with urban Americans, rural residents:
   a. are more likely to engage in preventive health behavior.
   b. are less likely to be exposed to occupational and environmental hazards.
   c. have higher rates of chronic illness.
   d. rate their overall health status more favorably.

6. In comparison with urban adults, rural adults:
   a. seek medical care more often.
   b. have poorer overall health status.
   c. are less likely to identify a usual source of medical care.
   d. are usually seen by a specialist rather than a general practitioner.

7. Which of the following statements concerning mental health and rural residents is inaccurate?
   a. Depression and stress are associated with the high rate of poverty.
   b. Domestic violence and substance abuse are more likely to be reported in rural areas than in urban areas.
   c. The incidence of accidents and suicides, particularly among male adolescents and young men, is escalating.
   d. Rural residents delay seeking care for emotional problems until a crisis or emergency exists.

8. Which of the following statements about occupational health risks in rural environments is inaccurate?
   a. High-risk industries include agriculture, mining, and forestry.
   b. Safety standards are enforceable on most farms and ranches.
   c. Agriculture-related accidents are a major cause of deaths and injuries, especially among women and children.
   d. Workmen's compensation insurance is provided for most farmers and ranchers.

9. Which of the following is *not* a characteristic of nursing practice in rural environments?
   a. greater independence
   b. diversity in clinical experiences
   c. professional isolation
   d. anonymity is the community

10. The rural residents described by the researcher from the University of Montana judged their health by their ability to:
    a. work and to be productive.
    b. maintain social ties.
    c. perform activities of daily living.
    d. avoid hospitalization.

11. Which of the following is *not* a component of the community-oriented primary care model?
    a. professional-community partnerships
    b. incorporation of business principles
    c. replacement of informal support services by formal services
    d. grass-root involvement

Chapter 17

1. The Healthy Cities movement began in:
   a. Canada.
   b. Germany.
   c. the United States.
   d. Russia.

2. The strategic framework provided by the Ottawa Charter for Health Promotion includes five elements. The highest priority for health promotion action is:
   a. creating supportive environments.
   b. developing personal skills.
   c. building healthy public policy.
   d. reorienting health services.

3. The model of community practice that aims to increase the problem-solving ability of the community as well as to correct the imbalance of power of disadvantaged groups is the:
   a. locality development model.
   b. social planning model.
   c. social action model.
   d. citizen participation model.

4. An example of a model of community practice that emphasizes cooperation and building a sense of community is the:
   a. locality development model.
   b. social planning model.
   c. social action model.
   d. citizen participation model.

5. An example of a model using a top-down approach to community practice is the:
   a. locality development model.
   b. social planning model.
   c. social action model.
   d. citizen participation model.

6. The higher levels of citizen participation include:
   a. partnership.
   b. information.
   c. manipulation
   d. all of the above

7. Healthy Cities emphasizes:
   a. a top-down approach with rational-empirical problem solving.
   b. a top-down approach with community practice planned by experts.
   c. a bottom-up approach with manipulation, therapy, and informing.
   d. a bottom-up approach with multisectoral planning and action for health.

8. Each of the following conditions facilitate the Healthy Cities movement *except*:
   a. political support.
   b. broad-based representation on the Healthy City Committee.
   c. larger cities.
   d. positive media response.

9. The role of the community health nurse in Healthy Cities includes all of the following *except*:
   a. orienting community leaders to the process and benefits of becoming a Healthy City.
   b. assuming leadership for the community.
   c. serving as a resource to the community assessment team.
   d. providing data-based information to policy makers.

10. Which of the following is *not* an accurate statement about Healthy Cities initiatives?
    a. They address a broad range of health problems at the local level.
    b. They focus on using community members and mobilizing local resources to improve the health of the community.
    c. They most frequently use the locality development and social planning models.
    d. They currently involve only European cities.

11. They CITYNET-Healthy Cities process encourages health professionals to:
    a. recognize that community problems are complex and cannot be easily recognized.
    b. focus on quantity rather than quality of life issues.
    c. provide therapy and treatment for the community.
    d. foster the use of advanced technology.

Chapter 18

1. Which of the following statements concerning community nursing centers is inaccurate?
   a. The need for a community nursing center is determined through an assessment of community needs.
   b. The purposes of the center are determined by the need of the community and the needs of the institution developing the center.
   c. The collaborating physician is responsible for the management of the center and its services.
   d. Primary health care can only be provided if advanced practice nurses are in the center.

2. Which of the following are *not* considered advanced practice nurses?
   a. nurse executives
   b. clinical nurse specialists
   c. nurse midwives
   d. nurse practitioners

3. Which level of services is provided by nursing centers?
   a. primary prevention
   b. secondary prevention
   c. tertiary prevention
   d. all of these

4. Which of the following groups is *not* a typical population served by nursing centers?
   a. culturally diverse clients
   b. university students and their families
   c. mentally ill persons
   d. individuals seeking treatment for major illnesses

5. Which of the following is an example of secondary prevention services that may be provided by nursing centers?
   a. immunizations
   b. blood pressure screening
   c. family planning
   d. enterostomal services

6. Which of the following services of nursing centers is an example of primary prevention?
   a. parenting classes
   b. weight control program
   c. developmental screening
   d. HIV services

7. Which of the following statements about funding of nursing centers is incorrect?
   a. In fee-for-service systems, frequently the fees have been set lower than the actual cost of delivering services.
   b. The financial component of the business plan should include a description of long-term financing.
   c. Third-party payment reimburses nurses at the same rate as physicians when the same service is provided.
   d. Funds from charities may contribute to the financial support of a center.

8. The scope of practice for nurses in nursing centers is determined by:
   a. state nurse practice acts.
   b. prescriptive authority.
   c. the collaborating physician.
   d. the nurse executive.

9. Which of the following statements concerning legislative prescriptive authority is accurate?
   a. In many states, advanced practice nurses have complete and independent authority to prescribe medication, including controlled substances.
   b. Advanced practice nurses in most states have the authority to prescribe medication with some level of physician supervision or collaboration.
   c. Advanced practice nurses have authority to dispense medication in those states in which they have authority to prescribe controlled substances.
   d. The risk of liability is decreased for advanced practice nurses without legislative prescriptive authority who use physician cosigned prescriptions.

10. Direct reimbursement for nursing services means that payment is:
    a. based on sliding scale fees.
    b. received directly from a grant-funding source.
    c. collected from clients at the time of service.
    d. made to the center rather than to a physician provider who then pays the center.

Chapter 19

1. The case manager role of providing a formal communication link among all parties concerning the plan of care management is the role of:
   a. facilitator.
   b. liaison.
   c. coordinator.
   d. negotiator.

2. The case manager role of using effective collaboration and team strategies to make arrangements for services is the role of:
   a. broker.
   b. negotiator.
   c. liaison.
   d. facilitator.

3. The role of the case manager as coordinator is to:
   a. provide information to all parties on the state of the member and situations affecting client.
   b. educate client and providers about the case management process so that informed decisions can be made.
   c. support all parties to work toward mutual goals.
   d. arrange, regulate, and balance needed health services for clients.

4. A *critical path* is best defined as:
   a. one of the five "rights" of case management.
   b. a competency required for practicing case management.
   c. a case management tool used to achieve a measurable outcome for a specific client case.
   d. an effective approach to conflict resolution.

5. In measuring outcomes, *intermediate criteria* are defined as:
   a. measurable ends to be achieved based on the problems presented by the client's condition.
   b. incremental incidents that serve to monitor progress.
   c. landmarks of an episode of health or illness care from initial encounter to transfer of accountability.
   d. the difference between what is expected from and what is occurring with the client.

6. Variance in outcomes related to broken equipment, staffing mix, or lost documentation is referred to as:
   a. provider variance.
   b. operational variance.
   c. unmet clinical quality indicators.
   d. client variance.

7. Variance data are useful in:
   a. empowering clients to assume responsibility for monitoring and adhering to a plan of care.
   b. negotiating a plan of action.
   c. reducing the risk of liability
   d. understanding why expected client outcomes have not been met.

8. Which of the following is not a condition that is typically case-managed?
   a. spinal cord injury
   b. chronic illness
   c. well-child care
   d. terminal illness

9. The ethical principle which can be influenced when care in a managed system is provided by less experienced providers is:
   a. autonomy.
   b. beneficence.
   c. confidentiality.
   d. justice.

10. Risk management strategies to reduce the provider's exposure to liability include all of the following *except*:
    a. communicating effectively with clients.
    b. providing clear documentation.
    c. carefully selecting referral sources.
    d. limiting benefits for experimental treatment.

11. Which of the following is *not* an activity of the advocacy role?
    a. lobbying for health policy
    b. serving as a mediator to assist parties to understand each other and reach agreement on an action
    c. deciding upon the plan of action for the client
    d. prioritizing the client's rights by promoting autonomy and self-determination

12. Collaborating, a behavior used in managing conflict, occurs when an individual:
    a. attempts to work with others toward solutions that satisfy both parties.
    b. pursues neither his or her concerns nor another's concerns.
    c. neglects personal concerns to satisfy the concerns of another.
    d. attempts to find a mutually acceptable solution that partially satisfies both parties.

Chapter 20

1. Which of the following statements about disaster is accurate?
   a. People with the most financial resources suffer the most from disaster.
   b. Urbanization and overcrowding have contributed to the occurrence of disasters.
   c. The number of natural disasters is steadily increasing.
   d. In order for an event to be considered a disaster, injury or death must result.

2. Disaster management requires attention to which stage of a disaster?
   a. the preparedness stage
   b. the response stage
   c. the recovery stage
   d. all of the above

3. Which of the following is *not* a description of an effective plan for disaster preparedness?
   a. complex
   b. flexible
   c. realistic
   d. implementable

4. An example of community preparedness for a disaster is:
   a. assembling an emergency supply kit.
   b. understanding the workplace disaster plan.
   c. taking a disaster training course.
   d. developing an evacuation plan to remove individuals from areas of danger.

5. Which of the following is *not* an essential attribute of the community health nurse in delivering disaster care?
   a. creativity and willingness to improvise
   b. "high-tech" skills
   c. knowledge of vulnerable populations and resources to assist them
   d. stamina and emotional stability

6. The level of disaster is determined by the:
   a. number of casualties.
   b. type or cause of the disaster.
   c. amount of resources needed.
   d. location of the area affected.

7. A one-family house fire is an example of which level of disaster?
   a. level I
   b. level II
   c. level III
   d. level IV

8. When a federal emergency is declared by the president, the agency responsible for managing all ongoing health and medical services is the:
   a. Centers for Disease Control.
   b. American Red Cross.
   c. U.S. Public Health Service.
   d. Federal Emergency Management Agency.

9. Which of the following is *not* an emergency support function of the American Red Cross?
   a. providing individual and family assistance to meet emergency needs such as food and clothing
   b. handling inquiries from concerned family members outside the area
   c. repairing public buildings and sewage and water systems
   d. coordinating relief activities with other agencies in business, labor, and government

10. Reactions to disaster vary according to:
    a. age.
    b. cultural background.
    c. adaptability to crisis.
    d. all of the above

11. A nurse working in a shelter for disaster victims would recognize which of the following as a typical reaction to stress?
    a. bedwetting in children
    b. anger and blaming
    c. headaches
    d. all of the above

12. A common reaction of elderly persons experiencing disaster may be:
    a. anger.
    b. fear of loss of independence.
    c. violence.
    d. regression.

13. The triage process in disaster involves:
    a. separating the casualties and allocating treatment based on the victim's potential for survival.
    b. assignment of tasks to the appropriate disaster response personnel.
    c. determining the level of disaster and agency involvement.
    d. participating in mock disaster drills through realistic scenarios.

14. Which of the following statements concerning disaster assessment is inaccurate?
    a. Lack of information can contribute to the misuse of resources.
    b. Different assessment priorities exist for sudden impact and gradual onset disasters.
    c. Ongoing surveillance is less important than initdal assessment.
    d. Assessments help to match available resources to a community's emergency needs.

15. Nurses working in shelters need to be prepared to deal with all of the following problems. Which of these is especially predominant in shelter situations?
    a. stress
    b. communicable disease
    c. chronic illness
    d. injuries requiring first aid

16. Symptoms of early stress and burnout in disaster workers include all of the following *except*:
    a. inability to concentrate.
    b. minor tremors.
    c. increased energy.
    d. nausea.

Chapter 21

1. The most critical step in planning a health program is:
   a. assessing need.
   b. considering alternative solutions or options.
   c. detailing the costs, resources, and activities needed to select from the proposed alternatives.
   d. weighing each alternative.

2. To promote acceptance of an effective planning process requires involvement of:
   a. clients.
   b. health providers.
   c. administrators.
   d. all of the above

3. The method used to assess consumer and participant response to health programs is:
   a. cost studies.
   b. case register.
   c. surveys and interviews.
   d. tracer method.

4. A widely used method for evaluation of health care programs that focuses on assessment of structure, process, and outcome is known as:
   a. case register.
   b. Donabedian's model.
   c. Critical Path Method.
   d. tracer method.

5. Plans for program evaluation should be developed:
   a. prior to plans for implementation.
   b. after program planning but before implementation.
   c. at the same time as plans for implementation.
   d. when the program is near completion.

6. A popular program planning method that focuses on program activities, sequencing of activities for best use of time and resources, and estimated time for program completion is:
   a. case register.
   b. Donabedian's model.
   c. Critical Path Method.
   d. tracer method.

7. A type of study to help determine the actual cost of a program is a:
   a. cost accounting study.
   b. cost benefit study.
   c. cost effectiveness study.
   d. cost efficiency study.

8. A study designed to examine the actual cost of performing program services and to focus on productivity versus cost is a:
   a. cost accounting study.
   b. cost benefit study.
   c. cost effectiveness study.
   d. cost efficiency study.

9. A study designed to measure the quality of a program as it relates to cost is a:
   a. cost accounting study.
   b. cost benefit study.
   c. cost effectiveness study.
   d. cost efficiency study.

10. A study used to assess the desirability of a program by examining costs and benefits is a:
    a. cost accounting study.
    b. cost benefit study.
    c. cost effectiveness study.
    d. cost efficiency study.

11. The community health index is a source of evaluation that includes:
    a. clinical records.
    b. incidence and prevalence data.
    c. an attitude scale.
    d. a description of available health resources.

12. Formative evaluation of a program is conducted to:
    a. assess program outcomes.
    b. determine the results of the program.
    c. assess whether planned activities are completed.
    d. identify key informants.

Chapter 22

1. Which of the following is *not* one of Donabedian's three major methods for evaluating quality care?
   a. outcome
   b. structure
   c. satisfaction
   d. process

2. The tracer method is most useful in evaluating health care:
   a. of individual clients.
   b. delivered by an individual provider.
   c. in problems with well-defined characteristics and treatment.
   d. using health status indicators.

3. The sentinel method of quality evaluation is based on:
   a. epidemiological principles.
   b. client satisfaction surveys.
   c. Donabedian's model.
   d. mandated review criteria.

4. Currently the most important component of an evaluation program for health care is:
   a. outcome.
   b. process.
   c. structure.
   d. peer review.

5. From the Total Quality Management (Continuous Quality Improvement) focus on delivering quality health care, *quality* is defined as:
   a. risk reduction.
   b. customer satisfaction.
   c. increased efficiency.
   d. improved functional status.

6. An example of a voluntary approach to quality control used primarily for institutions is:
   a. accreditation.
   b. licensure.
   c. certification.
   d. credentialing.

7. Continuous Quality Improvement focuses on:
   a. the structure of delivering health care.
   b. assigning personal blame for less-than-perfect outcomes.
   c. the contribution of systems to the outcomes of the organization.
   d. problem detection rather than problem prevention.

8. One reason for using a concurrent audit rather than a retrospective audit is that it:
   a. is less costly that the retrospective audit.
   b. represents the total picture of care the client receives.
   c. provides more accurate data for planning corrective action.
   d. identifies problems at the time care is given.

9. Of the following types of utilization review, which provides an assessment of the appropriateness of the cost of care?
   a. prospective review
   b. concurrent review
   c. retrospective review
   d. all of the above

10. A major objective of Professional Review Organizations (PROs) is to reduce:
    a. the liability of the agency by reviewing patterns of risk.
    b. inappropriate admissions and unnecessary procedures.
    c. the use of alternative care options such as home care.
    d. the practice of professionals without appropriate credentials.

Chapter 23

1. Which of the following statements regarding groups is inaccurate?
   a. All groups have a clearly stated purpose.
   b. Group purpose and member interaction are key elements of all groups.
   c. Groups are an effective way to initiate changes in individuals, families, and communities.
   d. Group activities are good indictors of the group's purposes.

2. Which of the following traits in group members is most likely to increase group cohesion?
   a. differences among group members' attitudes and values
   b. ability to tolerate conflict
   c. problem-solving skills
   d. diverse goals

3. High group cohesion is related to:
   a. decreased productivity and decreased member satisfaction.
   b. decreased productivity and increased member satisfaction.
   c. increased productivity and decreased member satisfaction.
   d. increased productivity and increased member satisfaction.

4. The term that refers to anything a group member does that deliberately contributes to the group's purpose is:
   a. productivity.
   b. maintenance function.
   c. task function.
   d. task norm.

5. The ability of a group member to help other members in the group to feel accepted is best described as a:
   a. maintenance norm.
   b. maintenance function.
   c. task norm.
   d. task function.

6. When using a group approach, it is important for the nurse to recognize the effects that differences may have on groups. Which of the following statements regarding differences in group members is true?
   a. Differences between the nurse and group members are to be expected and are unlikely to interfere with group cohesion.
   b. For some people, being different from the general population and similar to other group members is a compelling force for group membership.
   c. Members' perceptions of differences can increase group cohesion by creating competition.
   d. The less alike group members are, the stronger a group's attraction is.

7. Nurses may facilitate group cohesion by:
   a. assisting group members to better understand the experiences of others.
   b. identifying common ideas and reactions to issues.
   c. helping members refine differences in ways that make those dissimilarities compatible.
   d. all of the above

8. Which of the following is not a function of group norms?
   a. to influence members' perceptions of reality
   b. to ensure movement toward the group's purpose
   c. to challenge conformity in behavior and attitudes
   d. to maintain the group by affirming and supporting members

9. Behaviors that support group members' psychological and social well-being are most directly influenced by:
   a. group culture.
   b. maintenance norms.
   c. reality norms.
   d. task norms.

10. When individuals look to others in the group to reinforce or correct their ideas regarding a situation, they are being influenced by:
    a. group culture.
    b. maintenance norms.
    c. reality norms.
    d. task norms.

11. The commitment of the group members to return to the central goals is known as the:
    a. group culture.
    b. maintenance norm.
    c. reality norm.
    d. task norm.

12. Which of the following styles of group leadership generally results in increased productivity, cohesion, and satisfying interactions among members?
    a. democratic
    b. authoritarian
    c. paternal
    d. patriarchal

13. The leadership style that is most effective when members have limited skills or limited time is:
    a. democratic leadership.
    b. shared leadership.
    c. cooperative decision-making.
    d. patriarchal leadership.

14. A paternal leadership style:
    a. is authoritarian.
    b. supports members' involvement.
    c. is highly cohesive.
    d. limits power seekers.

15. The group member who focuses movement toward the main work of the group fulfills the role of:
    a. gatekeeper.
    b. leader.
    c. maintenance specialist.
    d. task specialist.

16. The person who facilitates or blocks communication between outsiders and group members is serving the role of:
    a. gatekeeper.
    b. maintenance specialist.
    c. peacemaker.
    d. task specialist.

17. Which of the following responses support conflict resolution?
    a. avoidance
    b. use of power to force an outcome
    c. exclusion of a member
    d. compromise

Chapter 24

1. A conceptual framework useful for understanding a family's expectations about how each member will behave is known as:
   a. developmental theory.
   b. interactional theory.
   c. role theory.
   d. systems theory.

2. A framework that focuses on the family as a unit of interacting personalities and examines the processes by which family members relate to one another is the:
   a. interactional framework.
   b. developmental framework.
   c. systems framework.
   d. structural framework.

3. The theory that focuses on common tasks of family life and provides a longitudinal view of the family life cycle is the:
   a. systems theory.
   b. structural-functional theory.
   c. interactional theory.
   d. developmental theory.

4. The approach which views the family as a whole with boundaries that are affected by the environment is the:
   a. developmental theory.
   b. structural-functional theory.
   c. role theory.
   d. systems theory.

5. The theory that provides the nurse with guidelines for using anticipatory guidance to prepare the family in coping with predictable changes is the:
   a. developmental theory.
   b. role theory.
   c. structural-functional theory.
   d. systems theory.

6. In assessing family structure, it is important for the nurse to recognize that:
   a. an individual may experience many different family structures over a lifetime.
   b. the variations in family structure are becoming less common.
   c. the traditional nuclear family is the only appropriate family structure.
   d. although there is great variation among different family structures, there is little variation within particular family structures.

7. Family demographics indicate:
   a. a decline in the number of marriages.
   b. a decline in young single adults remaining in or returning to their parent's home.
   c. a higher rate of remarriage for women than men.
   d. an increase in the divorce rate.

8. Which of the following statements about the demographics of the elderly population is inaccurate?
   a. There are more elderly women than men.
   b. More elderly men live alone compared with women.
   c. There are more widows than widowers.
   d. More women than men live below the poverty level.

9. Based on demographics, which of the following groups would the community health nurse recognize as a potentially at-risk population?
   a. unmarried mothers
   b. children in single-parent families
   c. elderly women
   d. all of the above

10. Role sharing refers to:
    a. the equal division of responsibilities by adult couples.
    b. siblings serving as a buffer between the parents and another sibling.
    c. two individuals in the same position enacting their roles in exactly the same way.
    d. traditional societal expectations regarding division of household and child-care activities.

11. Of the following family patterns, which is presently least common in the United States?
    a. the adoptive family
    b. the single-parent family
    c. the nuclear family
    d. the remarried family

12. Of the following family patterns, which is most likely to experience task overload?
    a. the single-parent family
    b. the adoptive family
    c. the foster family
    d. the nuclear family

13. Which of the following family patterns may experience challenges related to lack of role models for parenting?
    a. the single-parent family
    b. the nuclear family
    c. the adoptive family
    d. the divorced family

14. In the remarried family most of the concerns related to the stepfamily center around:
    a. economic security.
    b. the stepparent-stepchild relationship.
    c. maintenance of cultural norms for the stepfamily.
    d. handling legal issues.

15. Which of the following statements concerning vulnerable families is false?
    a. The family members may possess deep-seated assumptions about the relationship between themselves and society.
    b. The vulnerable family is subject to more abrupt loss of membership.
    c. The family should be viewed across a two-generational time frame that includes immediate family members.
    d. The shortened duration of the family life frequently results in blurring of life stages of the family.

Chapter 25

1. The model of health that focuses on the family's abilities and resources to accomplish developmental tasks is the:
   a. adaptive model.
   b. clinical model.
   c. eudaimonistic model.
   d. role-performance model.

2. The model of health which is concerned with reassessment of family values and goals and with ways to meet them is the:
   a. adaptive model.
   b. clinical model.
   c. eudaimonistic model.
   d. role-performance model.

3. Which of the following categories of health risks is most likely to be a threat to family health?
   a. a biologic risk
   b. an economic risk
   c. a life event
   d. a combination of risks from two or more categories

4. Which of the following is an example of a nonnormative life event?
   a. adoption of a child
   b. loss of a job
   c. marriage of a child
   d. retirement from work

5. Which of the following family factors is associated with a decreased risk for alcohol abuse in adolescents?
   a. family closeness
   b. clearly set and enforced rules
   c. modeling of behavior
   d. all of the above

6. The genogram is an effective technique for assessing a family's:
   a. biologic risks.
   b. economic risks.
   c. lifestyle risks.
   d. social risks.

7. An ecomap provides information useful in assessing a family's:
   a. biologic risks.
   b. economic risks.
   c. lifestyle risks.
   d. social risks.

8. Which of the following statements best describes the impact of life events on family health risk?
   a. Normative events require very little changes in family structures and roles.
   b. Positive events are unlikely to place stress on a family.
   c. Both normative and nonnormative events pose potential risks to the health of families.
   d. Negative life events require change and place stress on a family.

Chapter 26

1. Which of the following has *not* been a barrier to practicing family nursing?
   a. lack of comprehensive family assessment models
   b. limited settings in which family nursing can be practiced
   c. insurance reimbursement and coverage based on individuals
   d. medical model and disease-centered views of health care

2. According to the definition of family used in this chapter, the best way for the nurse to determine who the members of the family are is to:
   a. find out who resides in the home.
   b. determine who is related by blood or legal ties.
   c. ask the family whom they consider to be family members.
   d. assess the quality of relationships, including all nuclear and extended family members.

3. Use of the term *dysfunctional* to classify families:
   a. interferes with development of a constructive plan for family change and intervention.
   b. provides guidance for creating an intervention plan.
   c. distinguishes "good" families from "bad" families who are in need of intervention.
   d. identifies specific family behaviors for intervention.

4. The traits ascribed to healthy families are based primarily on:
   a. economic stability.
   b. attachment and relationships.
   c. absence of stress.
   d. physical health of family members.

5. Which of the following approaches to family nursing care views the family as an interactional system in which the whole is more than the sum of its parts?
   a. family as the context
   b. family as the client
   c. family as a system
   d. family as a component of society

6. Which of the following approaches emphasizes focusing on each and every member as they affect the whole family?
   a. family as the context
   b. family as the client
   c. family as a system
   d. family as a component of society

7. Which of the following is a disadvantage of conducting the family interview in the home?
   a. It may reinforce a cultural gap between the family and the nurse.
   b. It emphasizes that the problem is the responsibility of the whole family and not one family member.
   c. It requires skilled communication ability on the part of the nurse to conduct an interview in the personal space of the family.
   d. It increases the likelihood of family members feeling relaxed and demonstrating typical family interactions.

8. The Friedman Family Assessment Model is based on:
   a. the structural-functional framework and developmental and systems theory.
   b. Betty Neuman's Health Care Systems Model.
   c. identifying family strengths and stressors.
   d. the assumption that a set of internal resistance factors within each family system functions to stabilize the family.

9. The Family Assessment Intervention Model is based on:
   a. a macroscopic approach that views families as a subsystem of society.
   b. the assumption that individual's norms and values are learned primarily in the family through socialization.
   c. specific dimensions of family health related to family stability and functioning.
   d. a system of diagnostic taxonomies that focus on family problems.

10. A useful tool for describing the connections of the family members with agencies in the community is the:
    a. ecomap.
    b. Family Systems Stressor Strength Inventory.
    c. genogram.
    d. Neuman's Systems Model.

11. Which of the following areas is important to observe in the family genogram?
    a. sibling subsystems
    b. life events
    c. patterns of repetition
    d. all of the above

Chapter 27

1. According to Erikson's stages of ego development, resolution of the psychosocial conflict of autonomy versus shame and doubt results in a sense of:
   a. self-control.
   b. competence.
   c. independence.
   d. loyalty.

2. Parents can foster resolution of the psychosocial conflict of trust versus mistrust during infancy by:
   a. allowing the infant to assimilate the environment.
   b. disciplining the infant.
   c. consistently meeting the infant's needs.
   d. limiting the infant's interaction with strangers.

3. In assessing the psychosocial development of an eight-year-old, the nurse would expect a sense of:
   a. self-control.
   b. self or direction.
   c. competence.
   d. independence.

4. During which stage of cognitive development is the child very literal in the understanding of words?
   a. sensorimotor stage
   b. preoperational stage
   c. concrete operations stage
   d. formal operations stage

5. At what age is the child likely to be able to work with abstract ideas?
   a. 6 years
   b. 8 years
   c. 10 years
   d. 12 years

6. The process of integrating new experiences into existing thought patterns is know as:
   a. accommodation.
   b. assimilation.
   c. intuition.
   d. symbolism.

7. The cognitive operations of object permanence, causality, and symbolism are characteristics of the:
   a. sensorimotor stage.
   b. preoperational stage.
   c. concrete operations stage.
   d. formal operations stage.

8. The stage during which idealism may interfere with reality is the:
   a. sensorimotor stage.
   b. preoperational stage.
   c. concrete operations stage.
   d. formal operations stage.

9. Which of the following statements about immunizations is inaccurate?
   a. The recommended age for starting immunizations is generally 2 months.
   b. Minor acute illnesses are contraindications to giving immunizations.
   c. Providers are required to advise parents of risks, benefits, and possible side effects of immunizations.
   d. If an immunization schedule is interrupted once an initial immunization series has been started, it does not need to be restarted.

10. The placental transfer of maternal antibodies is known as:
    a. primary immune response.
    b. secondary immune response.
    c. natural passive immunity.
    d. active immunity.

11. Of the following, the best method of assessing a child's nutritional adequacy is through:
    a. a 24-hour dietary recall.
    b. activity patterns.
    c. developmental screening.
    d. physical growth patterns.

12. Which of the following statements about breast fed infants is inaccurate?
    a. They have a lower incidence of allergies.
    b. They require iron supplementation.
    c. Fluoride supplementation is not recommended for those whose mothers have a fluoridated water supply.
    d. Breast milk is the preferred method of infant feeding.

13. Which of the following statements about the introduction of solid foods is correct?
    a. Cereal may help babies sleep longer.
    b. High intake of solid foods may result in diarrhea.
    c. Early introduction of solids results in decreased possibility of food allergies.
    d. Cereal fortified with iron is an appropriate starter food because of the ease of digestion.

14. The fat content in the diet should be restricted to less than 30% beginning at:
    a. 1 year of age.
    b. 2 years of age.
    c. 6 years of age.
    d. 11 years of age.

15. Which of the following statements regarding adolescent nutritional needs is accurate?
    a. Adolescent girls have an increased need for protein and calories.
    b. Adolescent boys have an increased need for calories but a decreased need for protein.
    c. Adolescent girls have an increased need for protein but a decreased need for calories.
    d. Both boys and girls have increased needs for protein and calories.

16. The highest injury rate of all groups of children occurs in:
    a. infants.
    b. toddlers and preschoolers.
    c. school-age children.
    d. adolescents.

17. The leading cause of death for infants less than 1 year old is:
    a. aspiration.
    b. burns.
    c. poisoning.
    d. sudden infant death syndrome.

18. Which of the following factors may reduce the risk of sudden infant death syndrome?
    a. decreasing parental cigarette smoking
    b. positioning infants in a supine position
    c. improving access to prenatal and postnatal health services
    d. all of the above

19. Interventions to discourage smoking should focus on:
    a. the parents.
    b. the child or adolescent.
    c. public policy.
    d. all of the above

20. The homeless child syndrome includes increased risk of all of the following *except*:
    a. attention deficit disorder.
    b. environmental dangers.
    c. health problems.
    d. stress.

Chapter 28

1. In comparison with men, women are:
   a. more likely to be employed.
   b. more likely to be employed in lower-paying service jobs.
   c. less likely to depend on assistance programs such as Medicaid and Medicare.
   d. likely to earn the same salaries when performing the same work.

2. In contrast to classic developmental theories, research with women's developmental theory concludes that female identity is found through:
   a. relationships with others.
   b. autonomy.
   c. creativity.
   d. independence.

3. In comparison with men, women:
   a. are hospitalized less frequently.
   b. have higher rates of visual and hearing problems.
   c. report lower rates of work or school days lost.
   d. have a higher number of chronic conditions.

4. Which of the following statements about women and heart disease is inaccurate?
   a. Smoking cessation greatly reduces the risk for heart disease.
   b. Coronary artery disease occurs later in women than in men.
   c. Women who require cardiac surgery have higher operative mortality rates than do men.
   d. Hormone replacement therapy in postmenopausal women increases the risk of death from heart disease.

5. Which of the following is the leading cause of cancer deaths among women?
   a. breast cancer
   b. colorectal cancer
   c. lung cancer
   d. ovarian cancer

6. Barriers to smoking cessation include all of the following *except*:
   a. stress.
   b. poverty.
   c. social support.
   d. desire to maintain an acceptable body weight.

7. The most important strategy to increase survival in breast cancer is:
   a. smoking cessation.
   b. early detection.
   c. weight reduction.
   d. dietary fat reduction.

8. The Papanicolau (Pap) test is a poor screening test for:
   a. cervical cancer.
   b. endometrial cancer.
   c. ovarian cancer.
   d. none of the above.

9. The main risk factor for HIV in women is:
   a. hemophilia.
   b. heterosexual contact with a bisexual partners.
   c. injection drug use.
   d. heterosexual contact with injection drug users.

10. Which of the following statements about HIV infection in women is inaccurate?
    a. Women with HIV are prone to cervical neoplasia.
    b. Vaginal infections, especially candida albicans, are frequently the AIDS-defining markers.
    c. Women generally have more coexisting conditions than men.
    d. Postmenopausal women comprise the largest at-risk group for becoming infected with HIV.

11. Which of the following statements about eating disorders is correct?
    a. Individuals with anorexia frequently complain of weight loss.
    b. Purging is associated with anorexia.
    c. Most women with bulimia are within a normal weight range.
    d. Bulimia is considered more dangerous medically than anorexia.

12. Risk factors for osteoporosis include all of the following *except*:
    a. inadequate calcium intake.
    b. weight-bearing exercises.
    c. excessive alcohol use.
    d. smoking.

13. Which of the following may contribute to urinary incontinence?
    a. inadequate hydration
    b. obesity
    c. constipation
    d. all of the above

14. Which of the following is recommended to prevent or minimize urinary incontinence?
    a. Kegel exercises
    b. low-fiber diet
    c. citrus juices
    d. fluid restriction

15. Which of the following is an effect of hormone replacement therapy?
    a. reduced risk of heart disease
    b. vaginal dryness
    c. weight loss
    d. negative moods

16. Health care interventions for lesbian women should focus on all of the following *except*:
    a. screening for depression.
    b. decreasing the risk for vaginal infections.
    c. encouraging regular or gynecologic exams.
    d. treatment of substance abuse.

Chapter 29

1. Which of the following statements about men's health is inaccurate?
   a. Males have a lower infant mortality rate.
   b. Men have a shorter life span than do women.
   c. Rates of suicide and accidents are higher for men than for women.
   d. Men tend to avoid seeking medical help as long a possible.

2. The focus of the middle adulthood stage of development is:
   a. developing close relationships with others.
   b. establishing personal identity.
   c. contributing to the next generation.
   d. developing a citizenship role.

3. The state of morality in which the individual is guided by rules dictating right or wrong is known as:
   a. preconventional morality.
   b. conventional morality.
   c. hierarchical principles.
   d. universal principles.

4. The stage of morality in which the individual is concerned with comprehensive ethical principles apart from his or her own needs or the group's needs is known as:
   a. preconventional morality.
   b. conventional morality.
   c. hierarchical principles.
   d. universal principles.

5. Life expectancy for American men is:
   a. longer than for American women.
   b. similar to that of men in other developed countries.
   c. lower than in most other developed countries.
   d. higher than in most other developed countries.

6. In comparison with women, men:
   a. engage in more risk-taking behaviors.
   b. drink more alcohol.
   c. are exposed to more industrial carcinogens.
   d. all of the above

7. Death rates in men greatly exceed those for women for all of the following causes *except*:
   a. HIV.
   b. accidents.
   c. cerebrovascular disease.
   d. suicide.

8. The most common cancer among U.S. men is:
   a. lung cancer.
   b. prostate cancer.
   c. skin cancer.
   d. testicular cancer.

9. Which of the following statements about benign prostatic hyperplasia (BPH) is inaccurate?
   a. The major risk factor for BPH is age.
   b. BPH is usually asymptomatic.
   c. BPH is a precursor to prostate cancer.
   d. BPH may be treated with medication or surgery.

10. Which of the following groups is not at increased risk for suicide?
    a. married men
    b. unemployed men
    c. elderly men
    d. terminally ill men

11. The most predictive indicator of violence is:
    a. impulsive behavior.
    b. psychiatric disorders.
    c. alcohol or drug abuse.
    d. history of aggressive behavior and family violence.

12. Which of the following statements about alcohol is accurate?
    a. Alcohol consumption is a major drug problem.
    b. Patterns of alcohol usage established in the teen years often persist into adulthood.
    c. Alcohol is the major cause of all motor vehicle accidents among teenage drivers.
    d. all of the above

Chapter 30

1. Return migration occurs when elders:
   a. return to their hometown after retirement.
   b. relocate in urban areas.
   c. move to the Sunbelt states during the winter.
   d. select smaller homes to reduce their cost of living.

2. Which of the following statements about demographics and elders is inaccurate?
   a. The elder population is much less educated than is the younger population.
   b. The states in the Midwest and in the Great Plains have the highest proportion of elderly residents.
   c. Most impaired elders are living in institutions.
   d. Elders, especially women, are vulnerable to economic insecurity.

3. Which of the following statements about ageism is true?
   a. Ageism can result in social isolation.
   b. Ageism refers to prejudice about older people.
   c. Ageism is a form of stereotyping.
   d. all of the above

4. The psychosocial theory that views elders with great esteem as a result of their knowledge and experience is known as the:
   a. activity theory.
   b. continuity theory.
   c. exchange theory.
   d. humanistic theory.

5. The theory that involves satisfactory relationships as a sign of maturity and loss of relationships as a threat to security is the:
   a. continuity theory.
   b. exchange theory.
   c. humanistic theory.
   d. interpersonal theory.

6. The process of integrating past experiences in an attempt to find meaning in life is known as:
   a. continuity.
   b. generativity.
   c. life review.
   d. maturity.

7. The most common acute conditions experienced by elders are:
   a. ear conditions.
   b. musculoskeletal conditions.
   c. respiratory tract infections.
   d. urinary tract infections.

8. The most feared condition among the aging population is:
   a. dementia.
   b. immobility.
   c. falls.
   d. incontinence.

9. Which of the following is an example of a primary prevention strategy for elders?
   a. immunization for influenza
   b. blood pressure screening
   c. substance abuse counseling
   d. teaching Kegel's exercises to reduce incontinence

10. The goal of comprehensive assessment of elders and individualized management plans by community health nurses is to:
    a. optimize functional levels.
    b. enable elders to remain in their homes.
    c. improve quality of life.
    d. all of the above

11. When obtaining an elder's past health history, it is important to realize that:
    a. details about symptoms are not important.
    b. most elders are not able to give an accurate health history.
    c. symptoms are often exaggerated.
    d. impaired hearing and vision may interfere with communication.

12. Which of the following symptoms may indicate alcohol abuse in an elderly person?
    a. new urinary incontinence or decreased appetite
    b. anxiety or agitation
    c. palpitations and drowsiness
    d. dizziness and weight loss

13. Caregiving for elders is provided primarily by:
    a. community service agencies.
    b. female relatives.
    c. friends.
    d. health care professionals.

14. Which of the following is *not* an example of an appropriate intervention to prevent or reduce elder abuse?
    a. assessing door and window locks for security
    b. cautioning elders about letting strangers into their homes
    c. warning elders to keep cash in their homes in order to avoid unnecessary trips to the bank
    d. reporting suspected abuse

15. The term which denotes a slow, progressive loss of cognitive function and memory without loss of alertness is:
    a. confusion.
    b. delirium.
    c. dementia.
    d. depression.

16. An acute onset of changes in attention, cognition, behavior, and sleep occurs in:
    a. Alzheimer's disease.
    b. delirium.
    c. dementia.
    d. depression.

17. The major focus of care in nursing homes is on:
    a. custodial care.
    b. maximization of functional status.
    c. psychological care.
    d. rehabilitative services.

Chapter 31

1. Developmental disability refers to:
   a. physical impairment with a functional limitation that occurs at any age.
   b. short- or long-term physical impairment with functional limitations.
   c. multiple functional limitations of extended duration.
   d. chronic mental impairment that interferes with economic sufficiency.

2. Being physically compromised may result from:
   a. injuries.
   b. developmental disabilities.
   c. chronic diseases.
   d. all of the above.

3. In assessing physically compromised adolescents, it is important for the nurse to recognize that:
   a. regressive behavior is a common occurrence during adolescence.
   b. adolescents are at increased risk for further physical problems.
   c. denial is more likely to occur.
   d. safety issues are exaggerated during this period.

4. Which of the following statements concerning chronic illness and adults is inaccurate?
   a. Adults often experience social and emotional problems as well as physical.
   b. Children living in homes with a disabled adult are more likely to have serious behavioral problems and accidental injuries.
   c. Caregivers are most likely to be spouses or daughters of the affected individual.
   d. Strain on marital relationships seldom occurs in families with physically compromised adults.

5. Which of the following approaches is most likely to be effective in reducing barriers affecting physically compromised people in the community?
   a. focusing media efforts on the rights of the disabled
   b. supporting federal laws that affect the disabled
   c. using the medical model to define disabilities
   d. providing separate activities for those with and without disabilities

6. Which of the following statements about the relationship between poverty and disabilities is accurate?
   a. Disability may result in loss of income and poverty.
   b. People with low incomes are at greater risk for disabling conditions and for rapid progression of disease processes.
   c. Physically compromised adults often experience unemployment and lack of health insurance benefits.
   d. all of the above

7. People living in rural areas have:
   a. lower risk for disability than do urbanites.
   b. fewer resources for dealing with disabilities.
   c. a lower percentage of children living in poverty.
   d. less risk for injuries and chronic illness.

8. Which of the following statements about occupation and disability is inaccurate?
   a. Work-related injuries are greatly overreported.
   b. Chronic diseases can be exacerbated by worksite hazards.
   c. Worksite conditions may be associated with disabilities in workers' children as well as in workers themselves.
   d. Although laws require certain employers to make accommodations in the workplace for the physically compromised, implementation of the law is inconsistent.

9. Factors influencing the abuse of those who are physically compromised include:
   a. history of abuse in the family.
   b. stress and fatigue of caregivers.
   c. the disabled person's level of functioning.
   d. all of the above.

10. Of the following types of disabilities, which group may be especially at risk of abuse?
    a. those with physical disabilities
    b. those with mental disabilities
    c. the communicatively handicapped
    d. the mentally retarded

11. Which of the following statements best describes the health promotion needs of physically compromised clients?
    a. Health promotion problems and intervention are similar regardless of age or disabling condition.
    b. Establishment of health-promoting behavior has little or no impact on the condition.
    c. Physically compromised clients need information and counseling to ensure primary prevention of other health problems.
    d. Health promotion and disease prevention needs of children usually are well met because of increased contact with health care professionals.

Chapter 32

1. Vulnerable population groups are those who in comparison with the population as a whole:
   a. are more sensitive to risk factors and have worse health outcomes.
   b. have a single risk factor but experience worse health outcomes.
   c. have multiple risk factors but equal health outcomes.
   d. have worse outcomes with better access to health care.

2. The differential vulnerability hypothesis refers to:
   a. the resistance of certain groups to risk factors.
   b. the possession of—and increased susceptibility to—multiple, cumulative risk factors in vulnerable groups.
   c. the variability in the effects of stressors according to socioeconomic status.
   d. the increased sensitivity of the very young and the very old to risk factors.

3. In vulnerable groups, health status is strongly related to:
   a. age.
   b. economic level.
   c. race.
   d. stressors.

4. Which of the following problems is more likely in homeless people than in poor people with housing?
   a. dental problems
   b. injuries
   c. hypothermia
   d. all of the above

5. As a group, pregnant adolescents experience an increased risk for:
   a. economic problems.
   b. mental illness.
   c. substance abuse.
   d. tuberculosis.

6. Which of the following problems often accompanies substance abuse?
   a. communicable disease
   b. financial strain
   c. reluctance to seek health care
   d. all of the above

7. Which of the following is *not* a factor that increases the risk of communicable disease?
   a. development of drug-resistant strains of bacteria
   b. increased herd immunity
   c. living in a homeless shelter
   d. working in a drug treatment center

8. In public policy, the term *distribution effects* refers to:
   a. the impact of providing funds for building health facilities.
   b. the planning of health services to provide equal access.
   c. the unintended and unanticipated effects of a law on other groups.
   d. the movement of the mentally ill from institutions into the community.

9. According to the health field concept, the control and responsibility for health status lies with:
   a. individuals.
   b. families.
   c. society.
   d. individuals and society.

10. The dimension of vulnerability that results from blaming individuals for their own poverty and relieves society of responsibility for environmental and health service delivery issues is known as:
    a. disadvantaged status.
    b. disenfranchisement.
    c. powerlessness.
    d. victimization.

11. A feeling of separation from mainstream society and lack of social support is described as:
    a. disadvantaged status.
    b. disenfranchisement.
    c. powerlessness.
    d. victimization.

12. In assessing members of vulnerable population groups, the nurse's priority is to:
    a. address health care concerns before listening to clients' socioeconomic concerns.
    b. cover all questions on a comprehensive assessment form.
    c. provide financial or legal advice if needed by the client.
    d. focus on collecting the data needed to help the individual or family on that day.

Chapter 33

1. Federal poverty guidelines are used primarily:
   a. to determine financial eligibility for government assistance programs.
   b. for statistical purposes.
   c. to identify those with inadequate resources for basic needs.
   d. to provide guidelines for reform of social programs.

2. In comparison to nonpoor teens, poor teenagers are more likely to:
   a. have below-average academic skills.
   b. drop out of school.
   c. have children.
   d. all of the above

3. Which of the following statements about children and poverty is inaccurate?
   a. Children are less likely to live in poverty than are elderly persons.
   b. Children in single-family homes are more likely to be poor than those in two-parent homes.
   c. Younger children are more vulnerable to the effects of poverty than are older children.
   d. Poor children are at increased risk for chronic disease and injuries.

4. During the last 20 years, the rate of poverty in the elderly population has:
   a. increased.
   b. decreased.
   c. stayed the same.

5. Poor neighborhoods are more likely to have all of the following *except*:
   a. a greater proportion of minority groups.
   b. exposure to environmental hazards.
   c. more available health care.
   d. higher rates of crime and substance abuse.

6. The fastest growing segment of homeless people in the U.S. is:
   a. elderly people.
   b. families with children.
   c. teenage runaways.
   d. mentally ill people.

7. Which of the following statements about the homeless and mental illness is inaccurate?
   a. Deinstitutionalization of the chronically mentally ill has led to a growing number of homeless persons.
   b. Some homeless persons develop acute mental illness as a result of being homeless.
   c. About 90% of the homeless have major mental illnesses.
   d. The prevalence of alcohol and substance abuse compounds the effects of mental illness.

8. Which of the following statements regarding the impact of homelessness on health is inaccurate?
   a. Peripheral vascular disease and hypertension are exacerbated by the lifestyle of the homeless.
   b. The incidence and virulence of infections are decreasing among the homeless.
   c. Trauma is a significant cause of death and disability.
   d. Crowded living conditions result in an increased risk for exposure to infections.

9. Which of the following situations is likely to compound the effects of exposure in the homeless?
   a. diabetes
   b. nutritional deficits
   c. trauma
   d. all of the above

10. Which of the following is *not* an appropriate community health nursing intervention in caring for the poor?
    a. creating a trusting environment
    b. making assumptions about clients
    c. focusing on prevention
    d. advocating for accessible services

Chapter 34

1. Which of the following is an inappropriate approach for the community health nurse to use in working with adolescent clients?
   a. protecting the adolescent's right to privacy
   b. using neutral words in eliciting symptoms
   c. insisting that teens use appropriate terminology when expressing their concerns
   d. paying attention both to what the teen verbalizes and fails to verbalize

2. Obstacles to contraceptive services for adolescents include all of the following *except*:
   a. federal regulation requiring parental consent.
   b. lack of transportation.
   c. lack of money to pay for services.
   d. needing permission to leave school for an appointment.

3. For an adolescent female seeking an abortion,
   a. parental consent must be given to the abortion provider.
   b. parents must be notified by the abortion provider before the abortion is performed.
   c. the adolescent's right to privacy and ability to give consent varies by state.
   d. federal protection of the adolescent's right to privacy makes consent unnecessary.

4. Which of the following statements regarding U.S. teens and pregnancy is accurate?
   a. Birth rates are highest among teens in the northern states.
   b. Pregnancy rates among teens have decreased steadily.
   c. The United States has the highest rate of teen pregnancy in the developed world.
   d. Birth rates are highest for Hispanic teens.

5. Adolescents who terminate their pregnancies by abortion are more likely to:
   a. be black than white.
   b. come from a family of higher socioeconomic status.
   c. be unsuccessful in school.
   d. all of the above

6. Many teenagers who give birth:
   a. are poor.
   b. have limited educational achievements.
   c. did not plan to become pregnant.
   d. all of the above

7. Failure by teens to use birth control may be related to:
   a. lack of knowledge about a woman's fertile period.
   b. embarrassment in discussing birth control.
   c. difficulty finding facilities that offer confidential and affordable birth control.
   d. all of the above.

8. Which of the following factors increases a young woman's risk for early sexual experiences and pregnancy?
   a. history of sexual abuse
   b. parents who have high demands for their children and who offer warmth and understanding
   c. parents who communicate openly with their teens about birth control and sexuality
   d. all of the above

9. The nutritional needs of the pregnant adolescent are based primarily on:
   a. chronological age.
   b. gynecological age.
   c. prepregnancy diet history.
   d. blood protein levels.

10. The weight gain recommendations for the pregnant adolescent are based on the teen's:
    a. chronological age.
    b. gynecological age.
    c. prepregnancy weight.
    d. blood protein level.

11. The risk of low birth weight or prematurity is greater:
    a. for younger teens.
    b. for the first birth to a teen.
    c. with excessive weight gain in the mother.
    d. with low fat intake.

12. Which of the following is a risk factor for a second teen pregnancy?
    a. remaining in school
    b. reporting an unplanned first pregnancy
    c. being from a small family
    d. having a disadvantaged background

13. Which of the following statements about schooling and teen pregnancy is inaccurate?
    a. Federal legislation prohibits schools from excluding students because they are pregnant.
    b. Home instruction is provided for any young woman who requests it.
    c. Locating and affording child care is a major challenge for young parents.
    d. A closely spaced second pregnancy is less likely in young women who return to school soon after the birth.

Chapter 35

1. Migrant health centers are criticized for:
   a. inadequate number of bilingual staff.
   b. inconvenient hours.
   c. lack of dental, mental health, and pharmacy services.
   d. all of the above.

2. In comparison to the total population, migrant farm workers experience a(n):
   a. lower infant mortality rate.
   b. longer life expectancy.
   c. increased risk for hepatitis.
   d. lower rate of parasitic disease.

3. For which of the following health problems do migrant workers and their families most frequently seek care?
   a. dental problems
   b. communicable diseases
   c. gastrointestinal problems
   d. stress

4. Which of the following work conditions does *not* typically apply to migrant farm workers?
   a. lack of enforcement of safety regulations
   b. long work hours
   c. compensation for sick days
   d. exposure to chemicals

5. A common immediate effect of exposure to pesticides is:
   a. skin rashes.
   b. musculoskeletal problems.
   c. gastroenteritis.
   d. infertility.

6. Chronic exposure to pesticides may lead to:
   a. cancer.
   b. deafness.
   c. skin rashes.
   d. respiratory failure.

7. Child care for children of migrant farm workers is usually provided by:
   a. the migrant health centers.
   b. women or other children either at the camp or in the fields.
   c. the crew leaders on the farm being planted or harvested.
   d. government-funded day care centers.

8. For migrant farm workers, the final decision of whether or not to secure health care services is most often made by:
   a. the male head of the family.
   b. the wife/mother.
   c. the person needing services.
   d. the crew leader.

9. When farm workers seek health care, their expectation is that:
   a. they will be given time off work for recovery.
   b. they will be cared for in the hospital for as long as needed.
   c. they will recover and return to work rapidly.
   d. medication will be the best solution for all problems.

10. Which of the following are concerns of migrant women?
   a. sexual harassment and rape
   b. child care
   c. oppression by their families and communities
   d. all of the above

Chapter 36

1. A major objective of the National Institute for Mental Health is the:
   a. expansion of psychiatric units in general hospitals.
   b. development of education and research programs for community mental health treatment approaches.
   c. legislation and advocacy for the rights of people with mental disorders.
   d. deinstitutionalization of patients.

2. A significant problem related to deinstitutionalization of the mentally ill is:
   a. insufficient community mental health services.
   b. independent living settings with excessive supervision.
   c. overcrowding of nursing homes.
   d. increased cost of care.

3. Issues addressed by the Americans with Disabilities Act include:
   a. employment of people with mental impairment.
   b. public accommodations for the physically handicapped.
   c. public services, programs, and activities for people with mental and physical disabilities.
   d. all of the above.

4. Environmental factors that increase the risk for mental disorders in children include all of the following *except*:
   a. crowded living conditions.
   b. consistent caregivers.
   c. violence.
   d. separation from parents.

5. Most current mental health programs for adults focus on:
   a. stress reduction.
   b. monitoring and treatment of mental health problems.
   c. lifestyle management.
   d. prevention of domestic violence.

6. Conditions that threaten the mental health of caregivers of persons with severe mental disorders include all of the following *except*:
   a. guilt.
   b. stress.
   c. social support.
   d. chronic strain.

7. Which of the following contribute to depression in older adults?
   a. chronic illness
   b. terminal illness
   c. life changes in roles and social support
   d. all of the above

8. Low income and minority groups are at increased risk for mental health problems as a result of all of the following *except*:
   a. lack of access to mental health services.
   b. genetic predisposition.
   c. exposure to violence.
   d. displacement.

9. According to the Vulnerability-Stress-Coping-Competence Model, protective factors are exercised by:
   a. the ill individual.
   b. families.
   c. professional treatment programs.
   d. all of the above.

10. An important component of relapse management is:
    a. using a holistic view of the system.
    b. identifying triggers.
    c. understanding the individual's personality.
    d. providing crisis intervention.

Chapter 37

1. Which of the following factors contributes to the substance abuse problem?
   a. increased knowledge about the use of drugs
   b. social acceptability of certain drugs
   c. recognition of substance abuse as a health problem rather than a criminal justice problem
   d. control of the content and strength of illegal drugs

2. Which of the following is *not* a typical result of prohibition?
   a. Lack of quality control results in death.
   b. Violent crime and corruption among law officials increases.
   c. Stronger drugs are pushed because of their greater profits.
   d. Drug users seek health care more readily to avoid being arrested.

3. The "harm reduction" model is an approach that focuses on:
   a. education.
   b. law enforcement.
   c. scare tactics.
   d. rehabilitation.

4. Which of the following statements concerning drug addiction is inaccurate?
   a. Anyone who regularly uses a drug that alters the CNS may develop a drug addiction.
   b. All people who regularly use drugs develop addictions.
   c. Some people may be genetically predisposed to addiction.
   d. Using drugs to treat severe stress over time may result in addiction.

5. The term that refers to the expectations a person has about the drug being used is:
   a. *reinforcement.*
   b. *set.*
   c. *setting.*
   d. *tolerance.*

6. The ability of a substance to compel users to take it repeatedly (and instead of other substances) is known as:
   a. reinforcement.
   b. set.
   c. setting.
   d. intoxication.

7. *Dependence* is a term that refers to:
   a. the presence and severity of withdrawal symptoms.
   b. the difficulty in ending use of a substance.
   c. the level of intoxication associated with addiction.
   d. the amount of substance needed to satisfy cravings.

8. Which of the following factors is associated with decreased blood alcohol concentration?
   a. increased concentration of alcohol in the drink
   b. drinking without consuming food.
   c. female gender
   d. icreased body weight

9. Which of the following statements about barbiturates is accurate?
   a. Barbiturates increase heart rate and respirations.
   b. Barbiturates are more toxic to the body's organ systems than alcohol.
   c. A synergistic effect occurs when barbiturates are combined with alcohol, increasing the risk of overdose.
   d. Physical tolerance develops faster than tolerance to the effects on mood.

10. The use of benzodiazepines is noted for increased risk of:
    a. accidental overdose.
    b. life threatening withdrawal symptoms.
    c. cross-tolerance.
    d. respiratory stimulation.

11. Which of the following is a depressant?
    a. alcohol
    b. cocaine
    c. nicotine
    d. phencyclidine (PCP)

12. A history of blackouts is associated with the use of:
    a. alcohol.
    b. cocaine.
    c. marijuana.
    d. opiates.

13. The major adverse physical effect of marijuana use is:
    a. constipation.
    b. cardiac dysrhythmia.
    c. abdominal pain.
    d. respiratory tract damage.

14. Interventions to help increase resiliency in youths from high-risk environments include all of the following *except*:
    a. providing realistic appraisals and feedback.
    b. promoting competitive solutions to problems.
    c. encouraging education and skills training.
    d. stressing multicultural competence.

15. Urinalysis for drug testing can be used to determine:
    a. whether or not a certain drug has been used in the recent past.
    b. the degree of intoxication.
    c. the extent of performance impairment.
    d. all of the above.

16. In assessing for addiction, the nurse should be aware that a primary symptom of addiction is:
    a. anger.
    b. apathy.
    c. denial.
    d. violence.

17. Substance abuse among adolescents is influenced most by:
    a. parental role modeling.
    b. positive media messages.
    c. socioeconomic level.
    d. peer pressure.

18. The most successful smoking cessation method is:
    a. acupuncture.
    b. nicotine patches.
    c. self-help strategies.
    d. smoking cessation classes.

19. Brief intervention therapy involves providing substance abusers with all of the following *except*:
    a. feedback about the risks of drug use.
    b. clear advice to change risky behavior.
    c. choices for behavioral change.
    d. specific concerns regarding the client's ability to change.

20. Medical supervision is required during detoxification from:
    a. barbiturates.
    b. marijuana.
    c. opiates.
    d. stimulants.

Chapter 38

1. Which of the following statements about the influence of social and community factors is false?
   a. Unemployment is associated with violence inside and outside the home.
   b. Schools have the potential for teaching nonviolence but often are places where violence occurs.
   c. High population diversity decreases the potential for violence.
   d. Frequent violent television viewing by children has been associated with aggressive behavior.

2. Homicides are least likely to be perpetrated by a:
   a. friend.
   b. acquaintance.
   c. family member.
   d. stranger.

3. Suicide is more frequent among:
   a. females than males.
   b. blacks than whites.
   c. educated than educationally disadvantaged.
   d. poor than affluent.

4. The greatest risk factor for suicide in adult women is:
   a. divorce.
   b. unemployment.
   c. spouse abuse.
   d. terminal illness.

5. Behavior of potential abusers typically reflects all of the following *except*:
   a. an overly critical personality.
   b. apathy.
   c. unrealistic expectations.
   d. a low tolerance for frustration.

6. The factor that is most predictive of abusive behavior is:
   a. a perceived or actual crisis.
   b. social isolation.
   c. previous exposure to violence.
   d. marital strain.

7. Which of the following statements accurately reflects the situation when child abuse is present?
   a. The children are in greater need of intervention than are their parents.
   b. The most powerful child is likely to be the victim because the parent's sense of control is threatened.
   c. The abusive parents are overly sensitive to their children's needs.
   d. The family needs intervention for ineffective family functioning.

8. When abusive parents who have had a child removed by the courts are expecting another child, the pregnancy should be regarded as likely to be:
   a. a normal response to the grief of losing a child.
   b. a sign of continued poor judgment.
   c. a pathological reaction.
   d. an attempt to receive additional attention from the nurse.

9. Which of the following is *not* an indicator of actual or potential abuse?
   a. the tendency of parents to yell at or demean the child
   b. the presence of injuries not mentioned in the history
   c. extreme effort by the child to avoid or ignore the parent
   d. poor hygiene

10. A characteristic more likely to be seen in sexually abusive parents than in physically abusive parents is:
    a. fewer problems and a more positive view of the child.
    b. rigidity.
    c. loneliness.
    d. unhappiness.

11. Assessment for abuse is indicated in an adolescent who:
    a. displays inappropriate sexual activity.
    b. is truant.
    c. runs away from home.
    d. all of the above

12. Injuries characteristic of abuse are typically located on the:
    a. front of the body.
    b. back of the body.
    c. proximal parts of the body.
    d. distal parts of the body.

13. Which of the following responses to battering is most likely to increase over time?
    a. self-blaming by the woman
    b. remorse of the man
    c. severity of the abuse
    d. emotional strength of the woman

14. After ending an abusive relationship, the normal response is:
    a. anger.
    b. apathy.
    c. grief.
    d. guilt.

15. The most important risk factor for physical battering during pregnancy is being:
    a. abused before pregnancy.
    b. an adolescent.
    c. white.
    d. a substance abuser.

16. Therapeutic intervention with abused women by health care professionals includes all of the following *except*:
    a. assessment of all women for signs and symptoms of abuse.
    b. helping the woman develop a safety plan for herself and her children.
    c. assuring the abused woman that she is not to blame for the abuse.
    d. encouraging the woman to end the abusive relationship whether or not she is ready.

Chapter 39

1. The ability of an agent to produce a severe pathological reaction is known as:
   a. antigenicity.
   b. invasiveness.
   c. toxicity.
   d. virulence.

2. The ability of an agent to enter and multiply in the host is known as:
   a. antigenicity.
   b. infectivity.
   c. invasiveness.
   d. virulence.

3. The ability of an agent to produce a poisonous reaction is known as:
   a. antigenicity.
   b. invasiveness.
   c. toxicity.
   d. virulence.

4. Immunity is a characteristic of the:
   a. agent factor.
   b. host factor.
   c. environmental factor.
   d. epidemiologic triad.

5. The transference of antibodies from mother to infant is known as:
   a. active immunity.
   b. passive immunity.
   c. natural immunity.
   d. horizontal transmission.

6. A constant presence of a disease within a population is referred to as:
   a. epidemic.
   b. pandemic.
   c. endemic.
   d. herd immunity.

7. The term used to describe the occurrence of one case of smallpox in a population in which it was considered to be previously eliminated is:
   a. *endemic.*
   b. *epidemic.*
   c. *pandemic.*
   d. *infectivity.*

8. The role of the community health nurse in surveillance includes:
   a. investigating sources and contacts in outbreaks of diseases.
   b. collecting and reporting data pertaining to notifiable diseases.
   c. providing morbidity and mortality statistics to those who request it.
   d. all of the above.

9. Requirements for disease reporting in the United States are mandated by:
   a. the Centers for Disease Control.
   b. federal laws.
   c. state laws and regulations.
   d. county health departments.

10. Adoption of universal precautions by health care workers is an example of:
    a. primary prevention.
    b. secondary prevention.
    c. tertiary prevention.
    d. specific protection.

Chapter 40

1. Which part of the immunologic system suffers the greatest damage as a result of HIV infection?
   a. dendritic cells
   b. CD4 lymphocytes
   c. macrophages
   d. monocytes

2. Which of the following statements about the natural history of HIV is inaccurate?
   a. An HIV infected person may be seemingly well and symptom-free for years.
   b. The HIV virus may be transmitted during the asymptomatic period.
   c. HIV antibodies in the bloodstream serve a protective function.
   d. HIV antibodies usually appear from 6 weeks to 3 months after infection.

3. HIV transmission can occur through:
   a. exposure to blood.
   b. insect bites.
   c. sharing of school supplies.
   d. all of the above.

4. Which of the following statements about the trends of HIV infection is accurate?
   a. The number of heterosexual women with AIDS is increasing at a faster rate than in homosexual men.
   b. The rate of infection in white women is higher than in black or Hispanic women.
   c. AIDS is more prevalent in rural residents than in urban residents.
   d. The number of pediatric cases of AIDS is remaining stable.

5. Negative results of the ELISA test indicate:
   a. absence of HIV infection.
   b. absence of AIDS.
   c. the need to use the Western Blot test to verify the results.
   d. either absence of HIV infection or that the infection is in the window period.

6. In comparison with HIV infection in adults, HIV infection in infants and children:
   a. has the same signs and symptoms.
   b. has a shorter incubation period.
   c. has a longer survival period.
   d. is detected by using the same tests.

7. Which of the following statements about hepatitis B (HBV) is inaccurate?
   a. Like HIV, HBV is spread through blood and body fluids.
   b. HBV is prevalent in immigrants, health care workers, and persons with multiple sex partners.
   c. HBV has lower infectivity than HIV.
   d. Strategies for prevention include immunization and prevention of exposure.

8. Appropriate measures to prevent sexually transmitted diseases (STDs) include all of the following *except*:
   a. prophylactic antibiotics.
   b. condom use.
   c. mutually monogamous relationships.
   d. sexual abstinence.

9. Which of the following is likely to increase the risk of sexually transmitted disease?
   a. alcohol use
   b. presence of another sexually transmitted disease
   c. oral contraception use
   d. all of the above

10. Which of the following statements about herpes is true?
    a. The virus cannot be spread during the asymptomatic period.
    b. Herpes is easily cured with antibiotics.
    c. Neonatal infection may result in neurologic damage and death.
    d. The typical lesions are warts located in the genital area.

11. Infection with human papillomavirus is associated with:
    a. neurological damage.
    b. cervical cancer.
    c. blindness.
    d. stillbirths and miscarriages.

12. Which of the following statements about contract tracing is inaccurate?
    a. Clients are required to notify their partners.
    b. The community health nurse contacts health providers to verify examination of exposed partners.
    c. Contract tracing is carried out by the health department in conjunction with reportable disease requirements.
    d. Confidentiality is maintained in identifying and notifying partners.

Chapter 41

1. Which type of home health care agency is operated by the state or local government?
   a. official
   b. voluntary
   c. proprietary
   d. combination

2. Official agencies are financed primarily by:
   a. charities.
   b. individual clients.
   c. third-party payers.
   d. tax funds.

3. Voluntary home health agencies are:
   a. governmental organizations.
   b. exempt from federal income tax.
   c. profit-making agencies.
   d. governed by the owner of the agency.

4. Proprietary agencies are:
   a. exempt from federal income taxes.
   b. governed by a board of directors.
   c. profit-making agencies.
   d. reimbursed primarily by tax funds.

5. The most important aspect of the process of contracting is:
   a. the establishment of a formal written agreement.
   b. the client's participation in the process.
   c. setting of goals by the nurse for the client.
   d. compliance of the client and nurse with the contract.

6. Which of the following is *not* a direct care function of the home health care nurse?
   a. advising a hospital nurse regarding the client's usual method of care
   b. administration of medications
   c. assessing a wound
   d. teaching the client's family how to change a dressing

7. Medicare places emphasis on:
   a. chronic care.
   b. distributive care.
   c. episodic care.
   d. primary prevention.

8. Distributive care refers to:
   a. acute care.
   b. curative care.
   c. restorative care.
   d. health maintenance and disease prevention.

9. Which of the following is a component of home health care nursing?
   a. intermittent visits
   b. custodial care
   c. daily or hourly rate charges
   d. reimbursement payment to the nurse

10. Which of the following statements concerning discharge planning for the home care client is inaccurate?
    a. Discharge planning is not needed because the client and family are providing self-care.
    b. Discharge planning should begin with the initial contact with the client.
    c. Discharge planning may involve moving toward a long-term care facility.
    d. Discharge planning includes appropriate referral to other community resources as needed.

11. Home health regulation is carried out mainly by the:
    a. Joint Commission for the Accreditation of Health Care Organizations.
    b. Community Health Accreditation Program.
    c. state health departments.
    d. Health Care Financing Administration.

12. Qualifications for Medicaid reimbursement for home health care include:
    a. having homebound status.
    b. having physician certification.
    c. being either disabled or at least 65 years of age.
    d. all of the above.

13. Medicare requirements for home health coverage include:
    a. skilled service.
    b. homebound status.
    c. intermittent service.
    d. all of the above.

14. The primary objective of hospice care is:
    a. to enhance the quality of remaining life.
    b. to reduce the cost of terminal care.
    c. to keep clients at home.
    d. to provide care for terminally ill clients expected to live longer than 6 months.

Chapter 42

1. The nurse practitioner movement began at the University of Colorado with nurses providing:
   a. maternity care.
   b. well-child care.
   c. nursing home care.
   d. diabetes care.

2. Professional certification exams for advanced practice nurses are offered by the:
   a. American Nurses Association.
   b. National League for Nursing.
   c. state boards of nursing.
   d. universities offering graduate degree programs.

3. In which role are the most differences seen between the community health clinical nurse specialist and the nurse practitioner?
   a. administrator
   b. clinician
   c. consultant
   d. educator

4. An innovative nursing model designed to allow elderly clients to stay in their homes is:
   a. block nursing.
   b. joint practice.
   c. nursing centers.
   d. parish nursing.

5. One of the best ways for an interested clinical nurse specialist to establish an independent practice is to:
   a. act as a legal expert.
   b. learn complex assessment skills.
   c. market a service package.
   d. serve as a liaison for community programs.

6. Which of the following is a major focus of community health clinical nurse specialists, but not of the nurse practitioners?
   a. collaboration with other health disciplines
   b. providing anticipatory guidance and counseling
   c. planning population-focused programs
   d. assessing health deviations and risks

7. The scope of practice of the nurse practitioner is defined by:
   a. reimbursement policies.
   b. certification requirements.
   c. the nurse's educational preparation.
   d. the state's nurse practice act.

8. Which of the following is *not* a requirement for certification as a community health clinical nurse specialist?
   a. a minimum of 1,400 hours of clinical practice in the specialty
   b. a practice requirement of an average of 36 hours per week
   c. a master's degree with specialization in community health nursing
   d. documentation of continuing education in the specialty

9. The primary role of the nurse practitioner in emergency departments is usually to:
   a. triage clients.
   b. manage nonemergent client problems.
   c. assess medically uninsured clients.
   d. provide health education about preventive health care.

10. The major stressor for the family nurse practitioner or clinical specialist is likely to be:
    a. autonomy of practice.
    b. professional isolation.
    c. long work hours.
    d. collaboration.

Chapter 43

1. Which of the following statements describes managed care organizations?
   a. They actively recruit vulnerable populations.
   b. Payment for services is integrated with delivery of services.
   c. Reimbursement is usually based on fee-for-service.
   d. Hospitals are the preferred setting for service delivery.

2. When a manager pays attention to group dynamics and fosters cooperation in order to increase productivity, the approach is based on:
   a. neoclassical management.
   b. scientific management.
   c. expectancy theory.
   d. reinforcement theory.

3. Which of the following job design elements is most likely to be higher when workers are cross-trained or multiskilled?
   a. autonomy
   b. task identity
   c. job enlargement
   d. job enrichment

4. Application of which of the following theories is described by some as a way of manipulation?
   a. expectancy theory
   b. goal-setting theory
   c. Job Redesign Theory
   d. reinforcement theory

5. The theory that states that the most effective leadership style is dependent upon characteristics of the relationship between leaders and followers, the task, and the situation is:
   a. contingency theory.
   b. path-goal theory.
   c. social learning theory.
   d. transformational leadership.

6. The theory which focuses on how values and norms affect organizational activity is:
   a. structural contingency theory.
   b. institutional theory.
   c. resource dependence theory.
   d. systems theory.

7. The theory that emphasizes the interdependence of organizational players is:
   a. structural contingency theory.
   b. institutional theory.
   c. resource dependence theory.
   d. systems theory.

8. The model of consultation that is likely to be effective when problems are simple and the client needs specific expert information is the:
   a. doctor-patient model.
   b. process model.
   c. purchase of expertise model.
   d. content model.

9. The consultation model that emphasizes collaboration between the consultant and the consultee is the:
   a. content model.
   b. doctor-patient model.
   c. process model.
   d. purchase of expertise model.

10. The intervention mode in which the consultant encourages the client to share feelings and to move to more objective problem solving is the:
    a. acceptant mode.
    b. catalytic mode.
    c. confrontation mode.
    d. prescriptive mode.

11. The best intervention mode for goals/objectives problems is the:
    a. acceptant mode.
    b. catalytic mode.
    c. prescriptive mode.
    d. theory-principles mode.

12. The intervention mode that is most useful when the problem is straightforward and the client needs immediate answers to solve the problem is the:
    a. acceptant mode.
    b. catalytic mode.
    c. prescriptive mode.
    d. theory-principles mode.

13. The goal of consultation is to:
    a. solve the problem for the client.
    b. increase the client's problem-solving skills.
    c. identify the client's problem.
    d. eliminate and prevent the client's problem.

14. Which of the following is *not* characteristic of principled negotiation?
    a. bargaining based on the characteristics of the issue
    b. collaborative problem solving
    c. rigid adherence to a single position
    d. development of mutually agreeable ways of achieving goals

Chapter 44

1. The main cause of absence from school because of illness is:
   a. acute respiratory diseases.
   b. malnutrition.
   c. accidental injuries.
   d. digestive system problems.

2. The most widely abused substance among teenagers is:
   a. cocaine.
   b. alcohol.
   c. marijuana.
   d. heroin.

3. Currently the most prominent role of the school nurse is that of:
   a. health manager.
   b. school nurse practitioner.
   c. school teacher.
   d. health consultant.

4. Observation of certain students with risk factors such as absenteeism to determine whether further assessment is needed is a process known as:
   a. case finding.
   b. case management.
   c. surveillance.
   d. screening.

5. Determining the immunization status of a group of students is a process known as:
   a. case finding.
   b. case management.
   c. surveillance.
   d. screening.

6. Which of the following statements does *not* accurately reflect requirements for administration of medications in schools?
   a. Medications may be given only by licensed nursing personnel.
   b. Medications are given only with parents' written permission.
   c. Medications must be stored in a clean, locked container.
   d. Prescription medications must be in an individual pharmacy-labeled container.

7. A health care plan is a required component of the individualized education plan (IEP) for:
   a. students whose health status interferes with their ability to learn.
   b. students with chronic illnesses.
   c. disabled children 3 to 5 years of age.
   d. all students with special needs.

8. HealthPACT is a health education program that focuses on:
   a. preventing drug abuse.
   b. communicating effectively with health professionals.
   c. improving personal lifestyles.
   d. reducing cardiovascular risk.

9. The counseling role of the school nurse is best described as:
   a. providing information to students.
   b. directing students to available resources.
   c. helping students to arrive at workable decisions.
   d. listening and obtaining information from students.

10. Which of the following statements about school nurse practitioners (SNPs) is inaccurate?
   a. SNPs send fewer students home from school than do regular school nurses.
   b. SNPs resolve over 90% of the health problems they see.
   c. SNPs cost substantially more than using other community health facilities.
   d. Parents are more likely to act on the advice of SNPs.

Chapter 45

1. The principles of occupational health and safety are applicable to nursing in:
   a. businesses.
   b. industry.
   c. general nursing practice.
   d. all practice settings.

2. The majority of occupational health nurses work as nurse:
   a. administrators.
   b. clinicians/practitioners.
   c. consultants.
   d. educators.

3. Certification in occupational health nursing is provided by the:
   a. American Board for Occupational Health Nurses.
   b. Center for Occupational and Environmental Health.
   c. National Institute for Occupational Safety and Health.
   d. Occupational Safety and Health Administration.

4. Which of the following individuals are potentially at risk from work-related health hazards?
   a. currently employed workers
   b. family members and neighbors of workers
   c. retired or unemployed workers
   d. all of the above

5. Trends in the American workforce include all of the following *except*:
   a. an increasing number of women.
   b. increasing mismatches between skills of workers and types of employment.
   c. less education and mobility in the workforce.
   d. an increasing number of those with chronic illness.

6. Which of the following statements accurately describes the occurrence of work-related injuries over the past few years?
   a. The incidence and severity of injuries have decreased.
   b. The incidence of injuries has decreased, but severity has increased.
   c. The incidence of injuries has increased, but severity has decreased.
   d. The incidence and severity of injuries have increased.

7. Which of the following groups of workers is at greatest risk for experiencing work-related injuries?
   a. women of childbearing age
   b. young adult men with less than 6 months' job experience
   c. older men with diminished sensory abilities
   d. older women with chronic illnesses

8. Which of the following is *not* a factor associated with hypersusceptibility to occupational hazard exposure?
   a. dark skin
   b. malnutrition
   c. chronic obstructive pulmonary disease
   d. hypertension

9. Which of the following occupational groups is associated with increased risk of exposure to biological agents?
   a. dye workers
   b. dry cleaners
   c. agricultural workers
   d. drug manufacturers

10. Which of the following statements about chemical agents is accurate?
    a. Chemicals are not ordinarily found in the body tissues of the general population.
    b. Most chemicals have been studied to determine the effects of exposure on humans.
    c. Chronic exposure to low-level doses of workplace chemicals below standards constitutes a potential health risk.
    d. Human effects of chemical exposure are associated with single agents rather than with the interaction of agents.

11. Which of the following statements regarding workplace reproductive hazards is accurate?
    a. Women of childbearing age are excluded from jobs with potential reproductive hazards.
    b. Toxicity to common agents such as mercury has been demonstrated only in males.
    c. Workers must be informed about the potential reproductive health effects.
    d. all of the above

12. The category of agents associated with cumulative trauma is:
    a. biologic agents.
    b. chemical agents.
    c. ergonomic agents.
    d. physical agents.

13. The class of agents considered to be one of the most easily controlled is:
    a. biologic agents.
    b. ergonomic agents.
    c. physical agents.
    d. psychological agents.

14. Which of the following is a problem typically addressed by an employee assistance program?
    a. obesity
    b. smoking
    c. alcohol abuse
    d. lack of exercise

15. The Occupational Safety and Health Administration is:
    a. a part of the Centers for Disease Control.
    b. responsible for creating workplace safety and health regulations.
    c. a research agency that identifies the causes of work-related illnesses and injuries.
    d. a federal agency within the Department of Health and Human Services.

16. The National Institute for Occupational Safety and Health:
    a. examines potential hazards of new work technologies and practices.
    b. is a federal agency within the U.S. Department of Labor.
    c. develops and maintains a database of work-related deaths.
    d. sets standards that regulate workers' exposure to potentially toxic substances.

17. Rules for financial compensation of workers who suffer work-related health problems are set by:
    a. state laws.
    b. federal laws.
    c. company policies.
    d. the Department of Labor.

18. The focus of health promotion programs in the workplace is:
    a. awareness of workers' personal problems.
    b. treatment of illness and injury.
    c. safe work practices.
    d. healthy lifestyle habits.

19. One of the best methods an occupational health nurse can use in assessing workplace hazards is to:
    a. review incident reports.
    b. walk through the worksite.
    c. interview key employees.
    d. read the Standard Industrial Classification Code.

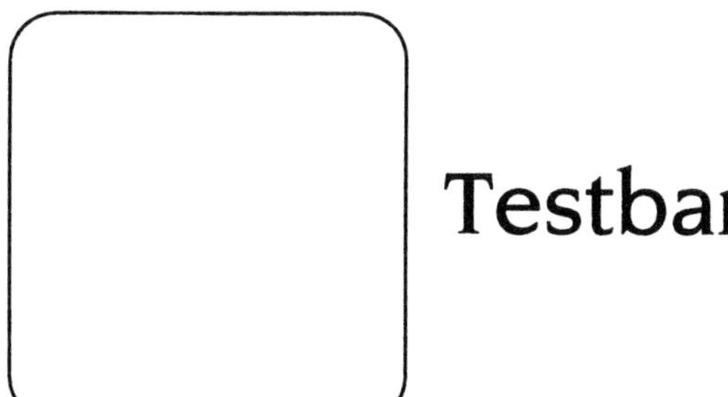

Testbank Answers

Chapter 1

1. d
2. d
3. d
4. c
5. d
6. b
7. a
8. b
9. c
10. b

Chapter 2

1. b
2. c
3. c
4. c
5. d
6. a
7. c
8. d
9. c
10. d

Chapter 3

1. d
2. a
3. a
4. b
5. b
6. a
7. b
8. c
9. a
10. b

Chapter 4

1. a
2. b
3. d
4. b
5. a
6. d
7. a
8. c
9. c
10. a
11. d
12. a
13. d
14. d
15. c

Chapter 5

1. b
2. d
3. c
4. b
5. d
6. a
7. c
8. a
9. c
10. c
11. a
12. b
13. a
14. a
15. a
16. c
17. b

Chapter 6

1. b
2. a
3. d
4. d
5. a
6. b
7. d
8. a
9. d
10. b
11. d
12. a
13. c
14. b
15. a
16. c
17. d

Chapter 7

1. c
2. a
3. d
4. b
5. c
6. a
7. c
8. d
9. d
10. c
11. a
12. d
13. a

Chapter 8

1. b
2. b
3. d
4. d
5. a
6. c
7. b
8. c
9. a
10. d
11. b
12. d
13. d
14. b

Chapter 9

1. c
2. d
3. a
4. c
5. a
6. d
7. c
8. b
9. d
10. a

Chapter 10

1. b
2. d
3. d
4. b
5. a
6. a
7. d
8. b
9. d
10. d
11. c
12. b
13. d

Chapter 11

1. b
2. c
3. b
4. c
5. b
6. a
7. a
8. b
9. c
10. c

11. c
12. b
13. d
14. d

Chapter 12

1. c
2. d
3. c
4. d
5. a
6. b
7. b
8. c
9. d
10. c

Chapter 13

1. d
2. a
3. c
4. c
5. c
6. d
7. b
8. a
9. c
10. d

Chapter 14

1. c
2. b
3. c
4. c
5. d
6. b
7. d
8. a
9. d
10. c
11. a
12. c

Chapter 15

1. b
2. d
3. c
4. d
5. a
6. d
7. c
8. d
9. a
10. a
11. c
12. a
13. d
14. d
15. b
16. b

Chapter 16

1. c
2. c
3. a
4. d
5. c
6. b
7. b
8. b
9. d
10. d
11. c

Chapter 17

1. a
2. c
3. c
4. a
5. b
6. a
7. d
8. c
9. b
10. d
11. a

Chapter 18

1. c
2. a
3. d
4. d
5. b
6. a
7. c
8. a
9. b
10. d

Chapter 19

1. b
2. b
3. d
4. c
5. b
6. b
7. d
8. c
9. d
10. d
11. c
12. a

Chapter 20

1. b
2. d
3. a
4. d
5. b
6. c
7. a
8. c
9. c
10. d
11. d
12. b
13. a
14. c
15. a
16. c

Chapter 21

1. a
2. b
3. c
4. b
5. c
6. c
7. a
8. d
9. c
10. b
11. b
12. c

Chapter 22

1. c
2. c
3. a
4. a
5. b
6. a
7. c
8. d
9. d
10. b

Chapter 23

1. a
2. c
3. d
4. c
5. b

6. b
7. d
8. c
9. b
10. c
11. d
12. a
13. d
14. a
15. d
16. a
17. d

Chapter 24

1. c
2. a
3. d
4. d
5. a
6. a
7. d
8. b
9. d
10. a
11. a
12. a
13. c
14. b
15. c

Chapter 25

1. d
2. c
3. d
4. b
5. d
6. a
7. d
8. c
9. c
10. a
11. d
12. b
13. d

Chapter 26

1. b
2. c
3. a
4. b
5. c
6. c
7. c
8. a
9. c
10. a
11. d

Chapter 27

1. a
2. c
3. c
4. b
5. d
6. b
7. a
8. d
9. b
10. c
11. d
12. b
13. d
14. b
15. c
16. d
17. a
18. d
19. d
20. a

Chapter 28

1. b
2. a
3. d
4. d
5. c
6. c
7. b
9. c
10. d
11. c
12. b
13. d
14. a
15. a
16. b

Chapter 29

1. a
2. c
3. a
4. d
5. c
6. d
7. c
8. b
9. b
10. a
11. d
12. d

Chapter 30

1. a
2. c
3. d
4. c
5. d
6. c
7. c
8. a
9. a
10. d
11. d
12. a
13. b
14. c
15. c
16. b
17. a

Chapter 31

1. c
2. d
3. a
4. d
5. b
6. d
7. b
8. a
9. d
10. c
11. c

Chapter 32

1. a
2. b
3. b
4. d
5. a
6. d
7. b
8. c
9. d
10. d
11. b
12. d

Chapter 33

1. a
2. d
3. a
4. b
5. c
6. b
7. c

8. b
9. d
10. b

Chapter 34

1. c
2. a
3. c
4. c
5. b
6. d
7. d
8. a
9. b
10. c
11. a
12. d
13. b

Chapter 35

1. d
2. c
3. a
4. c
5. a
6. a
7. b
8. a
9. c
10. d

Chapter 36

1. b
2. a
3. d
4. b
5. b
6. c
7. d
8. b
9. d
10. b

Chapter 37

1. b
2. d
3. a
4. b
5. b
6. a
7. b
8. d
9. c
10. b
11. a
12. a
13. d
14. b
15. a
16. c
17. d
18. c
19. d
20. a

Chapter 38

1. c
2. d
3. c
4, c
5. b
6. c
7. d
9. c
10. a
11. d
12. c
13. c
14. c
15. a
16. d

Chapter 39

1. d
2. b
3. c
4. b
5. b
6. c
7. b
8. d
9. c
10. a

Chapter 40

1. b
2. c
3. a
4. a
5. d
6. b
7. c
8. a
9. d
10. c
11. b
12. a

Chapter 41

1. a
2. d
3. b
4. c
5. b
6. a
7. c
8. d
9. a
10. a
11. c
12. b
13. d
14. a

Chapter 42

1. b
2. a
3. b
4. a
5. c
6. c
7. d
8. b
9. b
10. b

Chapter 43

1. b
2. a
3. c
4. d
5. a
6. b
7. d
8. c
9. c
10. a
11. b
12. c
13. b
14. c

Chapter 44

1. a
2. b
3. b
4. a
5. c
6. a
7. a
8. b

9. c
10. c

Chapter 45

1. d
2. b
3. a
4. d
5. c
6. d
7. b
8. a
9. c
10. c
11. c
12. c
13. c
14. c
15. b
16. a
17. a
18. d
19. b

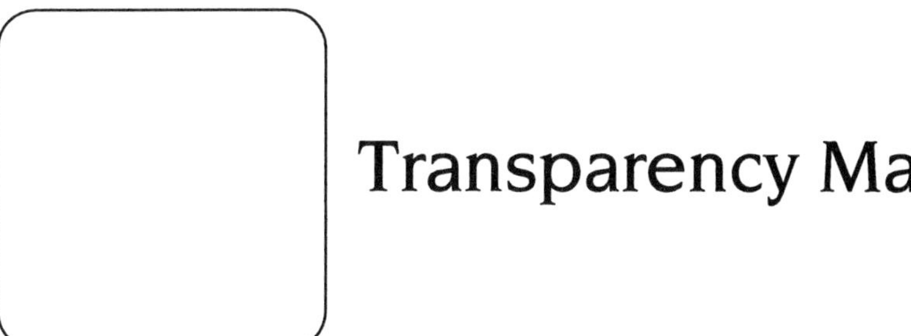

Transparency Masters

TM 1 Health services pyramid. (Figure 2-2)

TM 2 Arenas of practice. (Figure 2-4)

TM 3 Selected health care definitions.

TM 4 Characteristics of primary care and primary health care. (Table 3-2)

TM 5 Examples of federal regulatory mechanisms contributing to technology costs/control.

TM 6 Comparison of Medicare and Medicaid programs. (Table 5-11) (Modified from Medicaid/Medicare: *Which is which?* USDHHS Pub No 02129, Washington, DC, 1984; National Health Care Financing Administration: *Health*: *United States*, 1993, DHHS Pub No (PHS) 94-1232, Washington, DC, 1994.)

TM 7 Requirements of the patient self-determination act (PSDA). (From Omnibus Budget Reconciliation Act of 1990, sections 4206 and 4751, PL 101-508, Nov 5, 1990.)

TM 8 Client rights and professional responsibilities. (Figure 6-1)

TM 9 Early cultural awareness. (From Randall-David E: *Culturally competent HIV counseling and education*, McLean, Va, 1994, The Maternal and Child Health Clearinghouse.)

TM 10 Variations among selected cultural groups. (Table 7-4) (From Giger JN, Davidhizar RE: *Transcultural nursing*, 1995, Mosby; Spector RE: *Cultural diversity in health and illness*, ed 3, Norwalk, Conn, 1991, Appleton & Lange; Payne KT: In Taylor OL, editor: *Nature of communication disorders in culturally and linguistically diverse populations*, 1986, College Hill Press.)

TM 11 Components of an environmental exposure history.

TM 12 Summary of steps in formulating an environmental health nursing diagnosis. (Table 8-1)

TM 13 Key steps in the assessment process.

TM 14 How a bill becomes law. (Figure 9-2) (From Mason DJ, Talbott SW, Keavitt JK: *Policy and politics for nurses: action and change in the workplace, government, organizations, and community*, ed 2, Philadelphia, 1993, WB Saunders.)

TM 15 Tips for action. (From Mason DJ, Talbott SW, Keavitt JK: *Policy and politics for nurses: action and change in the workplace, government, organizations, and community*, ed 2, Philadelphia, 1993, WB Saunders.)

TM 16 Key terms to understanding frameworks for community health nursing. (Table 10-1) (From Kerlinger F: Foundations of behavioral research, ed 3, 1973, New York, Holt, Rinehart & Winston.)

TM 17 Standards of community health nursing practice. (American Nurses Association: *Standards of community health nursing*, Kansas City, 1986, The Association.)

TM 18 Categories of the Omaha intervention scheme.

TM 19 Examples of agent, host, and environmental factors in the epidemiologic triangle.

TM 20 Relation of the stages of disease to levels of prevention. (Table 11-3)

TM 21 Stages of the research process. (Selected stages of the research process are modified from Polit DF, Hungler BP: *Essentials of nursing research: methods, appraisal, and utilization*, Philadelphia, 1993, Lippincott.)

TM 22 Overview of six general educational theories. (Table 13-1) (Data from Driscoll MP: *Psychology of learning for instruction*, Boston, 1994, Allyn & Bacon; and Edwards L: In Edelman CL, Mandle CL, editors: *Health promotion throughout the lifespan*, St. Louis, 1990, Mosby.)

TM 23 Six principles that guide the educator. (From Knowles M: *The adult learner: a neglected species*, ed 4, Houston, 1990, Gulf.)

TM 24 Communication guidelines for educational interactions. (Modified from Damrosch S: *Nurs Clin North Am* 26(4):833-843, 1991.)

TM 25 Levels of application of preventive measures in the natural history of disease. (Figure 14-2) (From Leavell HR, Clark EG: *Preventive medicine for the doctor in his community: an epidemiological approach*, New York, 1965, McGraw-Hill.)

TM 26 A model of community health promotion. (Figure 14-3) (Laffrey SC, Kulbok PA: *An integrative model for community nursing*, 1995 [under review].)

TM 27 Eight essential conditions of community competence. (Table 15-2) (From Goeppinger J, Lassister PG, Wilcox B: *Nurs Outlook* 30(8):464-467, 1982.)

TM 28 Flow chart illustrating the nursing process with the community client. (Figure 15-1)

TM 29 Barriers to health care in rural environments.

TM 30 Characteristics of nursing practice in rural environments.

TM 31 Facilitator and barriers of the Healthy Cities Movement. (Table 17-1) (Flynn BC, Rider MS, Ray DW: *Health Education Quarterly* 18(3):331-347, 1991.)

TM 32 Contemporary nursing center model. (Figure 18-1)

TM 33 Key points in nursing center definitions.

TM 34 The nursing process and case management. (Table 19-1)

TM 35 Core components of case management. (Figure 19-1) (From Secord LJ: *Private case management for older persons and their families*, Excelsior, Minn, 1987 Interstudy.)

TM 36 Disaster preparedness responsibilities by agency. (Table 20-1) (From American Red Cross: *Disasters happen*, Washington, DC, 1993, American Red Cross. Used with the permission of the American Red Cross, Washington, DC, 1994.)

TM 37 Disaster response responsibilities by agency. (Table 20-2) (From American Red Cross: *Disasters happen*, Washington, DC, 1993, American Red Cross. Used with permission of the American Red Cross, Washington, DC, 1994.)

TM 38 Six steps in planning for program evaluation. (Figure 21-3)

TM 39 The evaluative process. (Figure 21-4)

TM 40 Model quality assurance program. (Figure 22-4)

TM 41 A group is a collection of interacting individuals who have a common purpose or purposes. (Figure 23-1)

TM 42 Influence of group norms on individual members. (Figure 23-3)

TM 43 Family health and community health: a systems perspective. (Figure 24-1) (Modified from Blum HL: *Expanding health care horizons from a general systems concept of health to a national health policy*, Oakland, Calif, 1976, Third Party Associates.)

TM 44 Family career of an individual. (Figure 24-2)

TM 45 Phases and activities of a home visit. (Table 25-3)

TM 46 Family assessment intervention model. (Figure 26-1) (From Mischke-Berkey KM, Warner P, Hanson SMH: In PJ Bomar, editor, *Nurses and family health promotion: concepts, assessment, and interventions*, Philadelphia, 1989, WB Saunders.)

TM 47 Guidelines for well-child care. (Table 27-1) (Modified for *American Academy of Pediatrics: Guidelines for health supervision.* II, Elk Grove Village, Ill, 1992, The Academy.)

TM 48 Assessment tools for children. (Table 27-6)

TM 49 Risk factors associated with breast cancer.

TM 50 Initiatives to improve maternal and infant health.

TM 51 Tasks of the young adult male.
Tasks of the middle adult male.

TM 52 Population of persons aged 65 and over: 1990 to 2050. (Figure 30-1) (From U.S. Senate Subcommittee on Aging, American Association of Retired Persons, Federal Council on Aging, U.S. Administration on Aging: *Aging American trends and projections*, DHHS Pub No (FCOA) 91-28001, Washington, DC, 1991, U.S. Department of Health and Human Services.)

TM 53 Major health problems in elders and community health nursing roles. (Table 30-4) (From Skipwith DH: The older adult. In Stanhope M, Lancaster J, editors: *Community health nursing: process and practice for promoting health*, ed 3, St. Louis, 1992, Mosby.)

TM 54 Potential effects of being physically compromised related to individuals, families, and and communities.

TM 55 Impediments to primary health care of the physically compromised. (Table 31-2) (Data from Gans BM, *Arch Phys Med Rehabil* 74(12-S):S-15-S-19; Nosek MA: *J Women's Health* 1(4).)

TM 56 Predisposing factors for vulnerability and potential outcomes of vulnerability. (Figure 32-2)

TM 57 The community health nurse as case manager for vulnerable populations. (Figure 32-4)

TM 58 The effects of poverty on the health of children.

TM 59 Health problems of homeless children.

TM 60 Guidelines for adoption counseling. (Modified from Brandsen CK: *A case for adoption*, Grand Rapids, Michigan, 1991, Bethany.)

TM 61 Guidelines for teen mother/newborn interactions.

TM 62 Characteristics of migratory streams. (Table 35-1)

TM 63 Legislation that influenced community mental health services. (Table 36-1)

TM 64 Problems and populations targeted in national health objectives for mental health. (Table 36-2) (Modified from *Healthy People* 2000: *national health promotion and disease prevention objectives*, Washington, DC, 1991, USDHHS, Public Health Service.)

TM 65 Federal drug control budget for 1994. (Figure 37-1)

TM 66 Community-based activities aimed at ATOD problem prevention.

TM 67 Behavioral indicators of potentially abusive parents.

TM 68 Indicators of actual or potential abuse.

TM 69 A multisystem approach to communicable disease control. (Table 39-3) (From Wenzel RP: In Last JM, and Wallace RB, editors: *Public Health and Preventive Medicine*, ed 13, Norwalk, 1992, Appleton and Lange.)

TM 70 Natural history of human immunodeficiency virus. (Figure 40-1)

TM 71 Relationship between nursing process and ANA standards of practice. (Table 41-3) (From American Nurses Association: *Standards of home health nursing practice*, Kansas City, MO, 1986, The Association.)

TM 72 Consultative intervention modes. (Table 43-1)

TM 73 The organization of the school health program. (Figure 44-1) (From School Health Programs, University of Colorado Health Science Center, 1989).

TM 74 Elements of the epidemiological triad applied to occupational health. (Figure 45-1)

TM 75 Use of the nursing process in the five functional roles of the occupational health nurse. (From Rogers B: In McCunnery RM, Brandt-Rauf PW: *A practical approach to occupational and environmental medicine*, Boston, 1994, Little, Brown, and Company.)

TM 1

Health services pyramid. (Figure 2-2)

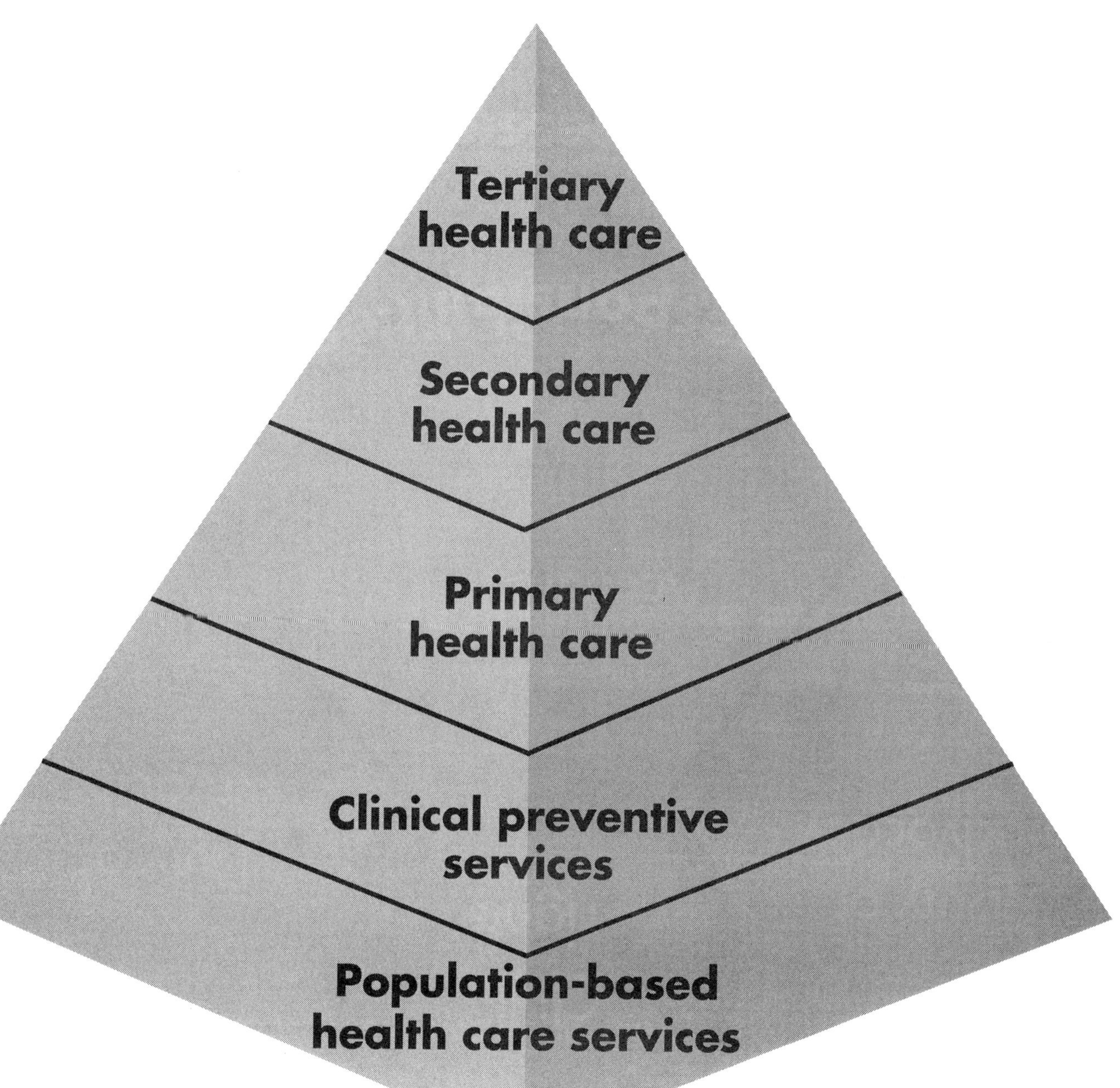

TM 2

Arenas of practice. (Figure 2-4)

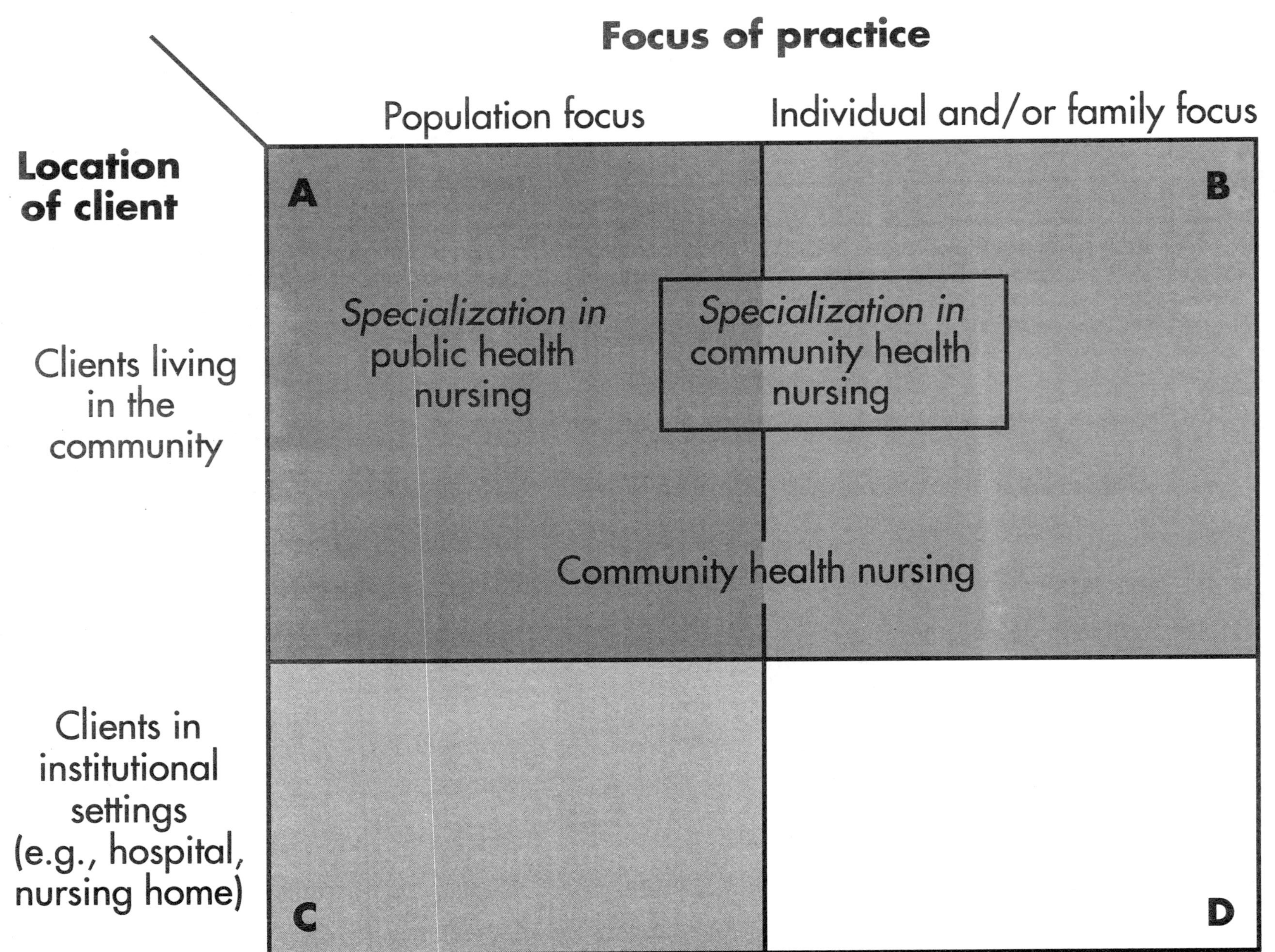

Stanhope/Lancaster: *Community Health Nursing*, ed 4

TM 3

Selected health care definitions.

Community-oriented primary care (COPC)—a community-responsive model of health care delivery that integrates aspects of both primary care and public health. It combines the care of individuals and families in the community with a focus on the community and its subgroups when services are planned, provided, and evaluated (Abramson, 1984).

Disease prevention—activities that have as their goal protecting people from the ill effects of actual or potential health threats.

Health—a state of complete physical, mental, and social well-being and not merely the absense of disease or infirmity (World Health Organization, 1986, p. 1).

Health promotion—activities that have as their goal developing human resources and behaviors that maintain or enhance well-being.

Primary care—personal health care services that provide for first contact, continuous, comprehensive, and coordinated care. Care is directed primarily at an individual's pathophysiological processes (Starfield, 1992).

Primary health care—essential care made universally accessible to individuals and families within a community, made available to them through their full participation, and provided at a cost that the community and country can afford (World Health Organization, 1978).

Primary prevention—actions designed to prevent a disease from occurring; reduces the probability of a specific illness occurring and includes active protection against unnecessary stressors or threats, that is, health promotion activities.

Public health—organized community efforts aimed at the prevention of disease and promotion of health. It links disciplines and rests on the scientific core of epidemiology (Institute of Medicine, 1988, p. 1).

Secondary prevention—early diagnosis and prompt treatment; includes activities such as screening for diseases, for example, hypertension, breast cancer, blindness, and deafness.

Tertiary prevention—treatment, care, and rehabilitation of people to prevent further progression of the disease (Pender, 1987).

TM 4

Characteristic of primary care and primary health care. (Table 3-2)

Primary care	Primary health care
Individual-focused	Community-focused
Preventive, rehabilitative, with emphasis on curative	Curative, rehabilitative, with emphasis on preventive
Care provided by generalist physicians, nurse practitioners, nurse midwives, and physician assistants with help of ancillary team members	Care provided by a wide variety of health care team members such as physicians, community health nurses, community outreach workers, nutritionists, sanitation experts
Professional dominance	Self-reliance

Stanhope/Lancaster: *Community Health Nursing*, ed 4

TM 5

Examples of federal regulatory mechanisms contributing to technology costs/control.

1906 Prescription drug regulation passes—Food, Drug, and Cosmetic Act; now Food and Drug Administration

1938 Manufacturers required to prove drug safety—Food, Drug, and Cosmetic Act

1952 Hill-Burton Act provides construction monies for new hospitals

1965 Amendments to Social Security Act providing Medicare and Medicaid result in increased use of technologies

1972 Social Security Act amendments extending coverage for end-stage renal disease provide payment for use of treatment technologies

1972 Social Security Act amendments provide for professional standards review organizations to review appropriateness of hospital care for Medicare and Medicaid recipients

1974 Health Planning and Resources Development Act introduces certificate-of-need authority to limit major health care expansion at local and state levels

1976 Medical devices amendments regulate safety and effectiveness of medical equipment, such as pacemakers

1978 Medicare End-Stage Renal Disease Amendment provides for home dialysis and for kidney transplantation

1978 Health Services Research, Health Statistics, and Health Care Technology Act establishes a national council on health care technology to develop standards for the use of medical technologies

1982 Tax Equity and Fiscal Responsibilities Act establishes prospective payment system for hospitalized Medicare patients by DRG category

1989 OBRA created a physician resource-based fee schedule to be implemented by 1992, with more emphasis on the "high tech" specialities of surgery

1989 OBRA created the Agency for Health Care Policy and Research to perform research on effectiveness of medical services, interventions, and technologies, including nursing

TM 6

Comparison of Medicare and Medicaid programs. (Table 5-11)

Feature	Medicare	Medicaid
Obtain information	Social Security Office	State welfare office
Recipients	Persons aged 65+ yr; disabled under 65 yr eligible after 2 yrs	Needy and low income, persons aged 65+ yr, blind, disabled, families with dependent children, some other children
Type of program	Insurance	Assistance
Government affiliation	Federal	Federal/state partnership
Availability	All states	All states
Hospital insurance	Financed by working persons; payroll contributions	Financed by federal and state government
Medical insurance	Monthly premiums paid by recipients (25%) and federal government (75%)	Federal and state government
Types of coverage	Inpatient and outpatient hospital care Posthospital skilled nursing facility Home health care Physician services Medical services and supplies Hospice care HMO Laboratory and radiological services	Inpatient and outpatient hospital care Skilled nursing facilities Home health care Physician services/dental services Other laboratory and x-ray services Screening, diagnosis, and treatment of children under 21 yr Family planning Health clinic services Supplements Medicare payments Services for mentally retarded persons Prescription drugs

Modified from Medicaid/Medicare: *Which is which?* USDHHS Pub No 02129, Washington, DC, 1984; National Health Care Financing Administration: *Health: United States*, 1993, DHHS Pub No (PHS) 94-1232, Washington, DC, 1994.

TM 7

Requirements of the Patient Self-Determination Act (PSDA).

- Provide written information to adult clients about their rights to make medical decisions, including the right to accept or refuse treatment and the right to formulate advance directives.
- Document in each client's record whether the client has previously executed an advance directive.
- Implement written policies regarding the various types of advance directives.
- Ensure compliance with state laws regarding medical treatment decisions and advance directives.
- Refrain from discriminating against individuals regarding their treatment decision specified in an advance directive.
- Provide education for staff and the community on issues and the law concerning advance directives.

From Omnibus Budget Reconciliation Act of 1990, sections 4206 and 4751, PL 101-508, Nov 5, 1990.

TM 8
Client rights and professional responsibilities. (Figure 6-1)

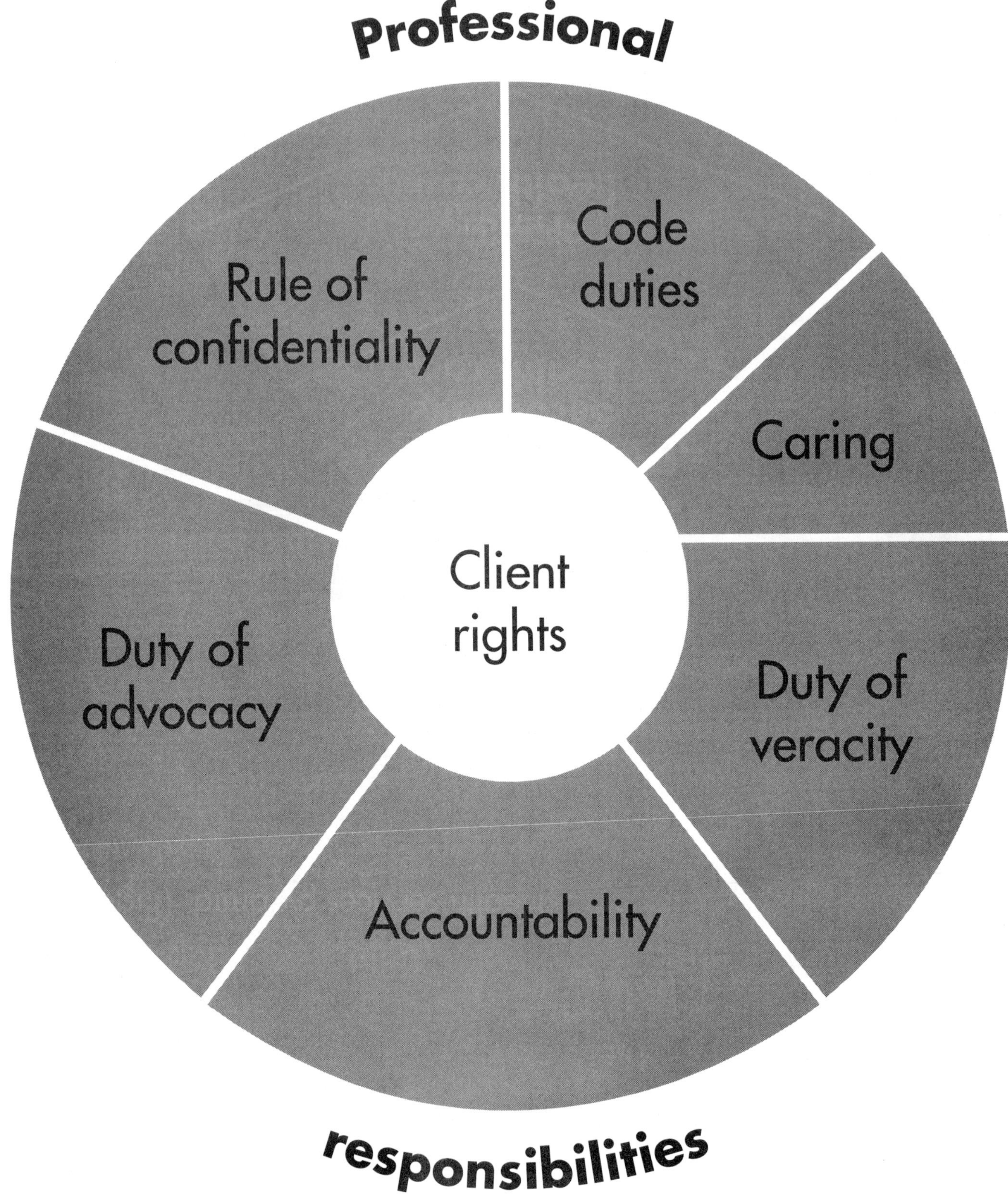

Stanhope/Lancaster: *Community Health Nursing*, ed 4

TM 9

Early cultural awareness.

Think about the first time you had contact with someone you realized was culturally different from you.
- Briefly describe the situation/event.
- How old were you?
- What were your feelings?
- What were your thoughts?

What did your parents and other significant adults say about those who were culturally different from your family?
- What adjectives were used?
- What attitudes were conveyed?

As you got older what messages did you get about minority groups from the larger community or culture?

As an adult how do others in the community talk about culturally different people?
- What adjectives were used?
- What attitudes were conveyed?
- How does this reinforce or contradict your earlier experience?

What parts of this cultural baggage make it difficult to work with clients from different cultural groups?

What parts of this cultural baggage facilitate your work with clients?

From Randall-David E: *Culturally competent* HIV *counseling and education*, McLean, Va, 1994, The Maternal and Child Health Clearinghouse.

TM 10

Variations among selected cultural groups. (Table 7-4)

	African-Americans	Asians	Hispanics	Native Americans
Verbal communication	Asking personal questions of some one that you have met for the first time is seen as improper and intrusive.	High respect for others, especially those in positions of authority.	Expression of negative feelings is considered impolite.	Speaks in a low tone of voice and expects that the listener will be attentive.
Non-verbal communication	Direct eye contact in conversation is often considered rude.	Direct eye contact among superiors may be considered disrespectful.	Avoidance of eye contact is usually a sign of attentiveness and respect.	Direct eye contact is often considered disrespectful.
Touch	Touching another's hair is often considered offensive.	It is not customary to shake hands with persons of the opposite sex.	Touching is often observed between two persons in conversation.	A light touch of the person's hand instead of a firm handshake is often used when greeting a person.
Family organization	Usually have close, extended family networks. Women play key roles in health care decisions.	Usually have close, extended family ties. Emphasis may be on family needs rather than individual needs.	Usually have close, extended family ties. All members of the family may be involved in health care decisions.	Usually have close, extended family ties. Emphasis tends to be on family rather than on individual needs.
Time	Often present oriented.	Often present oriented.	Often present oriented.	Often present oriented.
Perception of health	Harmony of mind, and spirit with nature.	When there is a balance between the "yin" and "yang" energy forces.	Balance and harmony among mind, body, spirit, and nature.	Harmony of mind, body, spirit, and emotions with nature.
Alternative healers	"Granny," "root doctor," voodoo priest, spiritualist.	Acupuncturist, acupressurist, herbalist.	Curandero, espiritualista, yerbero.	Medicine man, shaman.
Self-care practices	Poultices, herbs, oils, roots.	Hot and cold foods, herbs, teas, soups, cupping, burning, rubbing, pinching.	Hot and cold foods, herbs.	Herbs, corn meal, medicine bundle.
Biological variations	Sickle cell anemia, mongolian spots, keloid formation, inverted "T" waves, lactose intolerance, skin color.	Thalassemia, drug interactions, mongolian spots, lactose intolerance, skin color.	Mongolian spots, lactose intolerance, skin color.	Cleft uvula, lactose intolerance, skin color.

From Giger JN, Davidhizar RE: *Transcultural nursing*, ed 2, St Louis, 1995, Mosby; Spector RE: *Cultural diversity in health and illness*, ed 3, Norwalk, Conn, 1991, Appleton & Lange; Payne KT: In Taylor OL, editor: *Nature of Communication disorders in culturally and linguistically diverse populations*, San Diego, 1986, College Hill Press.

TM 11

Components of an environmental exposure history.

1. EXPOSURE

Location
Name of hazardous substance(s)
Form (solid, powder, liquid, vapor)
Route into body (inhalation, ingestion, dermal, injection)
Contact time (how long)
Contact frequency (how often)
Dose (amount)
Who knows, who needs to know about the exposure

2. ENVIRONMENT

A. Home

Water source (private well, city water)
Fertilizer use (farm)
Pesticide use
Home insulating, heating and cooling
Recent renovation/remodeling
Air pollution (indoor/outdoor)
Hobbies
Home cleaning agents
Proximity to heavy industry or hazardous waste site(s)

B. Work

Company
Job task
Names of hazardous substances worked with
Protective equipment recommended (is it used?)

3. HEALTH HISTORY

A. Host Factors

Health conditions currently experienced
Physical
Psychological/emotional
Chronic Conditons
Developmental
Children
Pregnancy
Lactating
Personal Habits
Smoking
Drinking
Hygiene

B. Cultural

Beliefs
Folk medicines
Dietary practices
Language barriers
Reading and writing skills

TM 12

Summary of steps in formulating an environmental health nursing diagnosis. (Table 8-1)

Step	Function	Question to answer
From the assessment	Identify target group or community aggregate who have been exposed and are at high risk for health effect (EXPOSURE ANALYSES)	Who in the community has been exposed?
1	Identify the unhealthful response or the risk for unhealthful response (TOXICOLOGICAL ANALYSES)	Is there a risk for injury or has an actual injury occurred?
2	Identify the related host and environmental factors	Host: What characteristics of the target group influence the risk for injury? Environment: What characteristics of the environment influence the risk for injury?
3	Identify any existing data that may substantiate the nursing diagnosis	Are there any epidemiological or other health outcome data that correlate injury risk with environmental contamination?

Stanhope/Lancaster: *Community Health Nursing*, ed 4

TM 13

Key steps in the assessment process.

- EXPOSURE ASSESSMENT. Determining what environmental exposures are occurring or are anticipated to occur for relevant populations.
- HAZARD IDENTIFICATION. Establishing whether the exposure causes the adverse effect.
- DOSE-RESPONSE ASSESSMENT. Relating dose to the toxicologic response.
- RISK CHARACTERIZATION. Determining the relationship among exposure, target dose, and adverse health consequences.

TM 14

How a bill becomes law. (Figure 9-2)

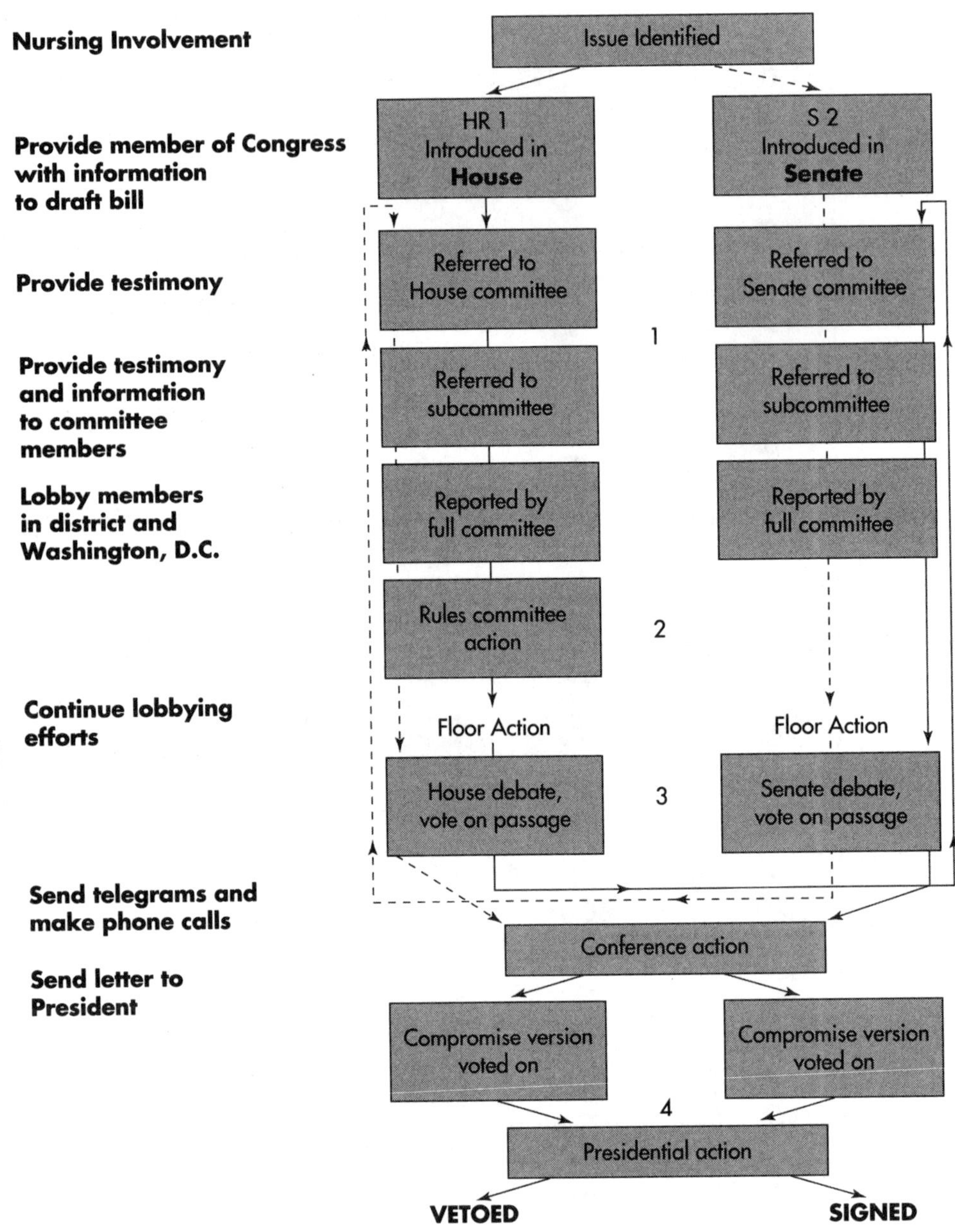

[1] A bill goes to full committee first, then to special subcommittees for hearings, debate, revisions, and approval. The same process occurs when it goes to full committee. It either dies in committee or proceeds to the next step.
[2] Only the House has a Rules Committee to set the "rule" for floor action and conditions for debate and amendments. In the Senate, the leadership schedules action.
[3] The bill is debated, amended, and passed or defeated. If passed, it goes to the other chamber and follows the same path. If each chamber passes a similar bill, both versions go to conference.
[4] The President may sign the bill into law, allow it to become law without his signature, or veto it and return it to Congress. To override the veto, both houses must approve the bill by a 2/3 majority vote.

From Mason DJ, Talbott SW, Keavitt JK: *Policy and politics for nurses: action and change in the workplace, government, organizations, and community*, ed 2, Philadelphia, 1993, WB Saunders.

TM 15

Tips for action.

- Get to know your legislators and the chair of your state board of nursing. Make sure you meet the governor and know the governor's chief executive aide (the person who really runs the show).
- Apply the problem-solving and negotiation skills you have developed in nursing to the process of making and implementing laws. They are the same skills you use to convince a diabetic patient to let you help him or her develop a care plan.
- Cultivate relationships with people who make the rules or pass the laws.
- Run for office.
- Develop a bipartisan nurse advisory council to assist your local legislator. (One state organized a statewide advisory group for a U.S. Senator. This group previewed U.S. health legislation for the Senator, and several nurses testified before the U.S. Senate Appropriations Subcommittee on Health and Human Services.)
- Spend an hour or two a week to upgrade your knowledge of political developments, health policy initiatives, legislators, and state government executives.
- Learn how health care funds are allocated through the political process.

From Mason DJ, Talbott SW, Keavitt JK: *Policy and politics for nurses: action and change in the workplace, government, organizations, and community*, ed 2, Philadelphia, 1993, WB Saunders.

TM 16

Key terms to understanding frameworks for community health nursing. (Table 10-1)

Term	Definition
Conceptual model	A set of concepts that provides a frame of reference for members of a discipline to guide their thinking, observations, and interpretations; propositions of a conceptual model are abstract and general.
Concepts	The building blocks of theory; they describe mental images of phenomena and can be concrete (chair) or abstract (body temperature).
Constructs	Concepts that describe phenomena that are not directly observable, such as society, intelligence, and age.
Propositions	Statements that describe the relationship between concepts; for example, "persons and their environment are in constant interaction" is a proposition.
Theory	A set of interrelated constructs (concepts), definitions, and propositions that present a systematic view of phenomena by specifying relationships among variables, with the purpose of explaining and predicting phenomena.

From Kerlinger F: *Foundations of behavioral research*, ed 3, 1973, New York, Holt, Rinehart & Winston.

Standards of community health nursing practice.

1. The nurse applies theoretical concepts as a basis for decisions in practice.
2. The nurse systematically collects data that are comprehensive and accurate.
3. The nurse analyzes data collected about the community, family, and individual to determine diagnoses.
4. At each level of prevention, the nurse develops plans that specify nursing actions unique to client needs.
5. The nurse, guided by the plan, intervenes to promote, maintain, or restore health; to prevent illness; and to effect rehabilitation.
6. The nurse evaluates responses of the community, family, and individual to interventions in order to determine progress toward goal achievement and to revise the data base, diagnoses, and plan.
7. The nurse participates in peer review and other means of evaluation to ensure the quality of nursing practice. The nurse assumes responsibility for professional development and contributes to the professional growth of others.
8. The nurse collaborates with other health care providers, professionals, and community representatives in assessing, planning, implementing, and evaluating programs for community health.
9. The nurse contributes to theory and practice in community health nursing through research.

American Nurses Association: *Standards of Community health nursing*, Kansas City, 1986, The Association.

TM 18

Categories of the Omaha Intervention Scheme.

I. Health Teaching, Guidance, and Counseling

Health teaching, guidance, and counseling are nursing activities that range from giving information, anticipating client problems, encouraging client action and responsibility for self-care and coping, to assisting with decision making and problem solving. The overlapping concepts occur on a continuum with the variation due to the client's self-direction capabilities.

II. Treatments and Procedures

Treatments and procedures are technical nursing activities directed toward preventing signs and symptoms, identifying risk factors and early signs and symptoms, and decreasing or alleviating signs and symptoms.

III. Case Management

Case management includes nursing activities of coordination, advocacy, and referral. These activities involve facilitating service delivery on behalf of the client, communicating with health and human service providers, promoting assertive client communication, and guiding the client toward use of appropriate community resources.

IV. Surveillance

Surveillance includes nursing activities of detection, measurement, critical analysis, and monitoring to indicate client status in relation to a given condition or phenomenon.

TM 19

Examples of agent, host, and environmental factors in the epidemiologic triangle.

AGENT

Infectious agents (bacteria, viruses, fungi, parasites)
Chemical agents (heavy metals, toxic chemicals, pesticides)
Physical agents (radiation, heat, cold, machinery)

HOST

Genetic susceptibility
Immutable characteristics (age and gender)
Acquired characteristics (immunologic status)
Life-style factors (diet and exercise)

ENVIRONMENT

Climate (temperature, rainfall)
Plant and animal life (may be agents or reservoirs or habitats for agents)
Human population distribution (crowding, social support)
Socioeconomic factors (education, resources, access to care)
Working conditions (levels of stress, noise, satisfaction)

Stanhope/Lancaster: *Community Health Nursing*, ed 4

TM 20

Relation of the stages of disease to levels of prevention. (Table 11-3)

STAGE OF DISEASE PROCESS		
Prepathogenesis →	Pathogenesis	Resolution
Susceptibility	→ Preclinical → Clinical	→ Death, disability, recovery
LEVELS OF PREVENTION		
Primary prevention	Secondary prevention	Tertiary prevention
EXAMPLES OF INTERVENTION		
Immunization Diet and exercise	Pap smear Screening for HIV	Physical therapy Surgery, medical treatment

Stanhope/Lancaster: *Community Health Nursing*, ed 4

TM 21

Stages of the research process.

ASSESSMENT/CONCEPTUAL STAGE

Identifying a problem for study
Initial review of related literature
Identifying the purpose of the research
Delineating the population to be studied

PLANNING/DESIGN STAGE

Formulating and delimiting the research problem
Continuing review of related literature
Selecting a conceptual framework
Selecting a research design and appropriate methodology
Designing the data collection plan
Finalizing and reviewing the research plan
Human subjects approval process
Pilot studies and revisions in design

IMPLEMENTATION/EMPIRICAL STAGE

Inviting potential participants to participate
Implementing data collection plan
Preparing data for analysis

EVALUATION/ANALYTICAL STAGE

Analyzing the data
Interpreting the results
Drawing conclusions

ACTION/DISSEMINATION STAGE

Communicating the research findings
Using the findings in practice
Informing health policy makers
Taking action for social change
Planning additional research

Selected stages of the research process are modified from Polit DF, Hungler BP: *Essentials of nursing research: methods, appraisal, and utilization*, Philadelphia, 1993, Lippincott.

TM 22

Overview of six general educational theories. (Table 13-1)

Theory	Focus	Method
Behavioral	Change behavior	Reinforcement/punishment
Social Learning	Change expectations and beliefs	Provide information
Cognitive	Change thought patterns	Variety of sensory input and repetition
Humanist	Use feelings and relationships	Self-determination of learners to do what is best for themselves
Developmental	Consider human developmental stage	Provide opportunities matching readiness to learn
Critical	Increase depth of knowledge	Ongoing dialogue and open inquiry

Data from Driscoll MP: *Psychology of learning for instruction*, Boston, 1994, Allyn & Bacon; and Edwards L: In Edelman CL, Mandle CL, editors: *Health promotion throughout the lifespan*, St Louis, 1990, Mosby.

TM 23

Six principles that guide the educator.

MESSAGE

Sending a clear message to the learner

FORMAT

Selecting the most appropriate learning format

ENVIRONMENT

Creating the best possible learning environment

EXPERIENCE

Organizing positive and meaningful learning experiences

PARTICIPATION

Engaging the learner in participatory learning

EVALUATION

Evaluating and giving objective feedback to the learner

From Knowles M: *The adult learner: a neglected species*, ed 4, Houston, 1990, Gulf.

TM 24

Communication guidelines for educational interactions.

- Begin strongly—people remember the first point.
- Use a clear, direct, and succinct style—this helps the learner to remain focused.
- Use the active voice—for example, the educator may say, "We will discuss relaxation techniques," instead of "Relaxation techniques will be discussed."
- Accentuate the positive—for example, the educator may say, "The majority of individuals are able to lose weight with a well-balanced diet and exercise," instead of "A few people have not been able to lose weight with a well-balanced diet and exercise."
- Use vivid communication, not statistics or jargon—specific case histories are often more meaningful than general, nonspecific terms or dry statistics.
- Refer to trustworthy sources—for example, "the surgeon general" is a more credible source than "some people."
- Base strategies on a knowledge of the audience—be aware of the perceptions and perspectives of the audience.
- Make points explicitly—be direct, and give clear instructions.
- End strongly—the last point made is likely to be remembered.

Modified from Damrosch S: *Nurs Clin North Am* 26(4):833-843, 1991.

TM 25

Levels of application of preventive measures in the natural history of disease. (Figure 14-2)

The Natural History of Any Disease of Man

Prepathogenesis period		Period of pathogenesis		
Health promotion	**Specific protection**	**Early diagnosis and prompt treatment**	**Disability limitation**	**Rehabilitation**
Health education Good standard of nutrition adjusted to developmental phases of life Attention to personality development Provision of adequate housing, recreation, and agreeable working conditions Marriage counseling and sex education Genetics Periodic selective examinations	Use of specific immunizations Attention to personal hygiene Use of environmental sanitation Protection against occupational hazards Protection from accidents Use of specific nutrients Protection from carcinogens Avoidance of all allergens	Case-finding measures, individual and mass Screening surveys Selective examinations Objectives: To cure and prevent disease processes To prevent the spread of communicable diseases To prevent complications and sequelae To shorten period of disability	Adequate treatment to arrest the disease process and to prevent further complications and sequelae Provision of facilities to limit disability and to prevent death	Provision of hospital and community facilities for retraining and education for maximum use of remaining capacities Education of the public and industry to utilize the rehabilitated As full employment as possible Selective placement Work therapy in hospitals Use of sheltered colony
Primary prevention		**Secondary prevention**		**Tertiary prevention**
Levels of application of preventive measures				

From Leavell HR, Clark EG: *Preventive medicine for the doctor in his community: an epidemiological approach*, New York, 1965, McGraw-Hill.

TM 26

A model of community health promotion. (Figure 14-3)

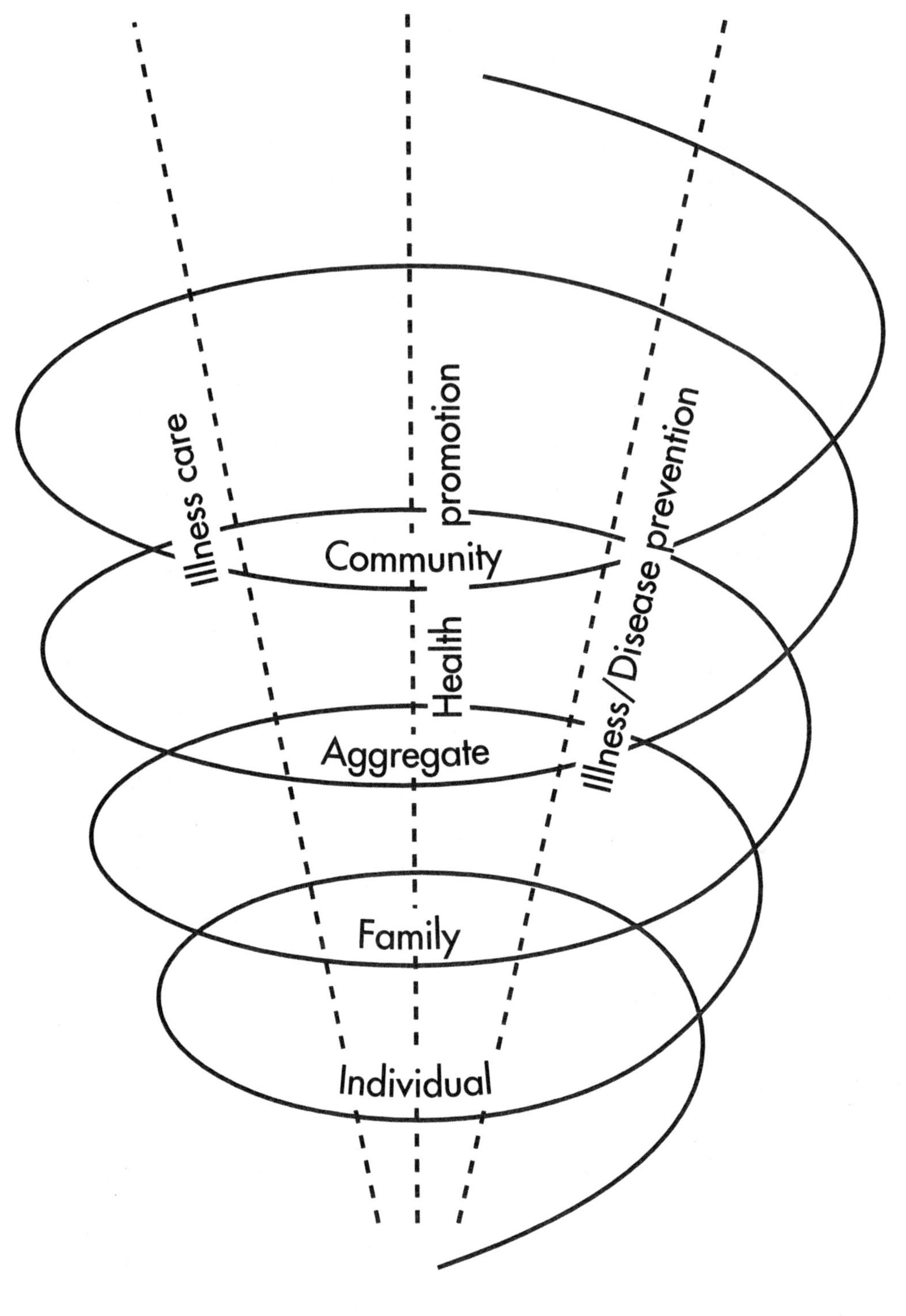

From Laffrey SC, Kulbok PA: *An integrative model for community nursing*, 1995 (under review).

TM 27

Eight essential conditions of community competence. (Table 15-2)

Condition	Definition
Commitment	The affective and cognitive attachment to a community "that is worthy of substantial effort to sustain and enhance" (Cottrell, 1976, p. 198)
Self-other awareness and clarity of situational definitions	The lucid and realistic perception of one's own and the other's community components, identities, and positions on issues
Articulateness	The technical aspects of formulating and stating one's views in relation to the other's views
Effective communication	The accurate transmission of information, based on the development of common meaning among the communicators
Conflict containment and accommodation	The inventive and effective assimilation and management of true, or realistically, perceived differences
Participation	Active, community-oriented involvement
Management of relations with larger society	Adeptness at recognizing, obtaining, and using external resources and supports and, when necessary stimulating the creation and use of alternative or supplementary resources
Machinery for facilitating participant interaction and decision-making	Flexible and responsible procedures, formal and informal, facilitates interaction and decision-making

From Goeppinger J, Lassiter PG, Wilcox B: *Nurs Outlook* 30(8):464-467, 1982.

TM 28

Flow chart illustrating the nursing process with the community client. (Figure 15-1)

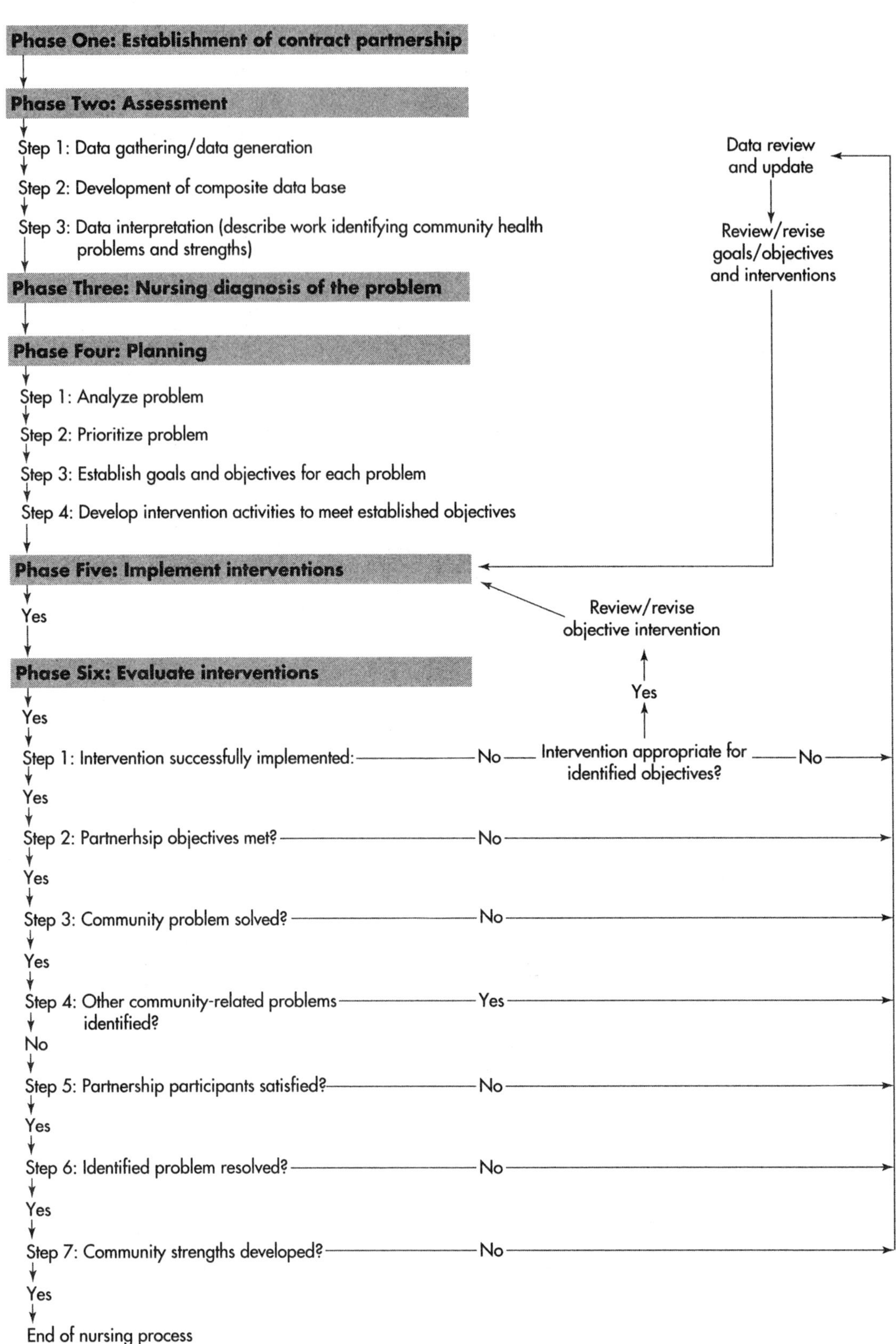

TM 29

Barriers to health care in rural environments.

- Great distances to obtain services
- Lack of personal transportation
- Unavailable public transportation
- Lack of telephone services
- Unavailable outreach services
- Inequitable reimbursement policies for providers
- Unpredictable weather conditions
- Inability to pay for care
- Lack of "know how" to procure entitlements/services
- Providers' attitudes and knowledge levels about rural populations

TM 30

Characteristics of nursing practice in rural environments.

Variety/diversity in clinical experiences
Broader/expanding scope of practice
Generalist skills
Flexibility/creativity in delivering care
Sparse resources (materials, professionals, equipment, fiscal)
Professional/personal isolation
Greater independence
More autonomy
Role overlap with other disciplines
Slower paced
Lack of anonymity
Increased opportunity for informal interactions with patients/co-workers
Opportunity for client follow-up upon discharge in informal community settings
Discharge planning allows for integration of formal with informal resources
Care for clients across the lifespan
Exposed to clients with a full range of conditions/diagnoses
Status in the community; viewed as an occupation of prestige
Viewed as a professional "role model"
Opportunity for community involvement and informal health education

TM 31

Facilitators and barriers of the Healthy Cities Movement. (Table 17-1)

Facilitators	Barriers
Overt and covert political support	Lack of support by local officials
Smaller cities	Lack of broad-based representation on Healthy City Committee
Broad-based representation on Healthy City Committee	Larger cities
Committee action	
Technical support	
Positive media response	

From Flynn BC, Rider MS, Ray DW: *Health Education Quarterly* 18(3):331-347, 1991.

TM 32

Contemporary nursing center model. (Figure 18-1)

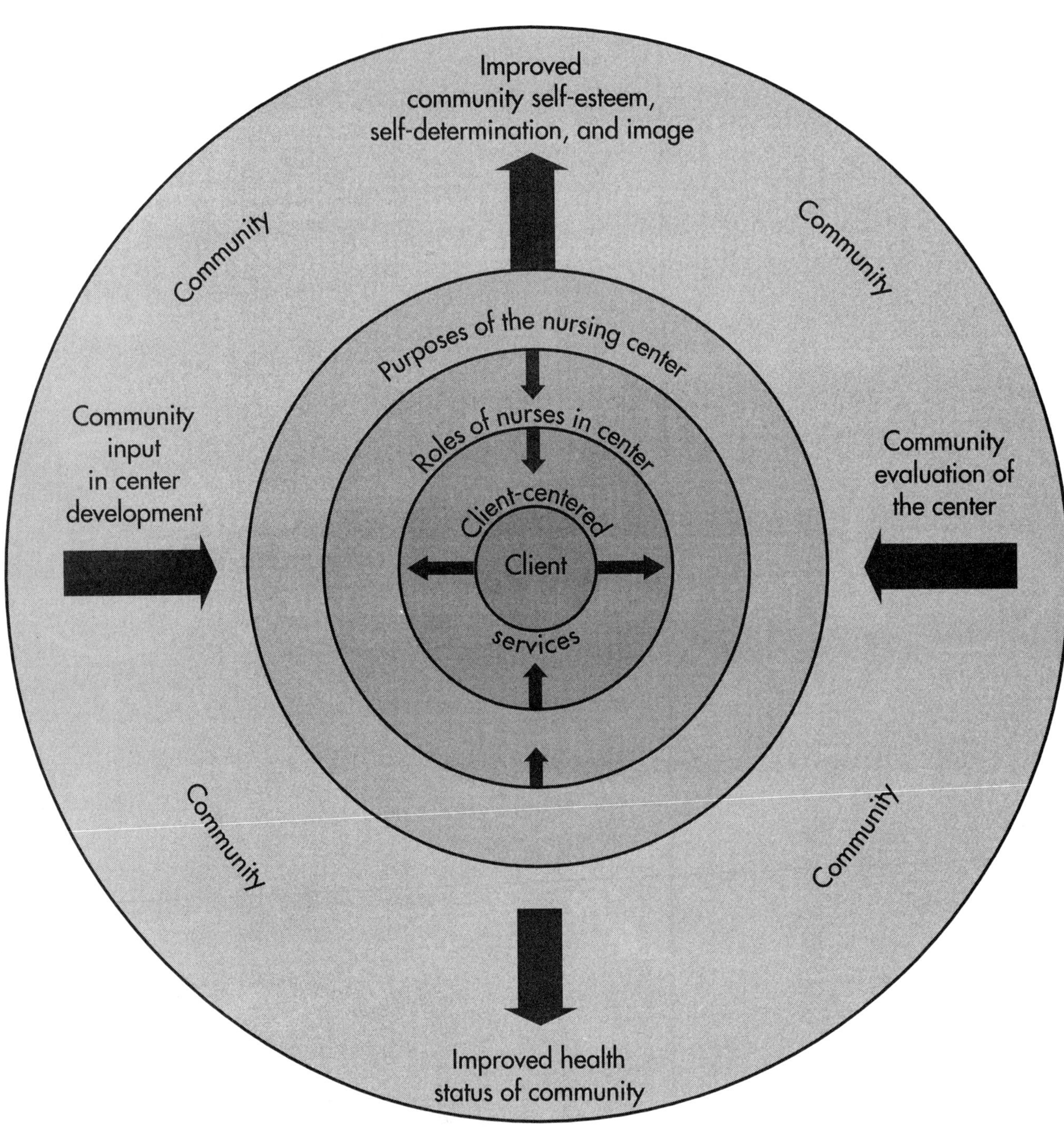

TM 33

Key points in nursing center definition.

An organization where:

- The client has direct access to nursing services.
- Nurses diagnose, treat, and promote health and optimal functioning.
- Services are client centered.
- Services are reimbursed.
- Accountability and responsibility for client care remain with the nurse.
- Overall accountability for the center remains with the nurse executive.

TM 34

The nursing process and case management. (Table 19-1)

Nursing process	Case management process	Activities
Assessment	Case finding; identification of incentives for the target population; screening and intake; determination of eligibility; assessment	Develop networks with target population; disseminate written materials; seek referrals; apply screening tools according to program goals and objectives; use written and on-site screens; apply comprehensive assessment methods (physical, social, emotional, cognitive, economic, and self-care capacity); perform interdisciplinary, family, and client conferences.
Diagnosis	Identification of the problem	Determine conclusion based on assessment; use interdisciplinary team.
Planning/outcome	Problem prioritizing; planning to address care needs	Validate and prioritize problems with all participants; develop activities, timeframes, and options; gain client's consent to implement; have client choose options.
Implementation	Advocation of clients' interests; arrangement of delivery of service; monitoring of clients during service	Contact providers; negotiate services and price; coordinate service delivery; monitor for changes in client or service status.
Evaluation	Reassessment	Examine outcomes against goals; examine needs against service; examine costs; examine satisfaction of client, providers, and case manager.

Stanhope/Lancaster: *Community Health Nursing*, ed 4

TM 35

Core components of case management. (Figure 19-1)

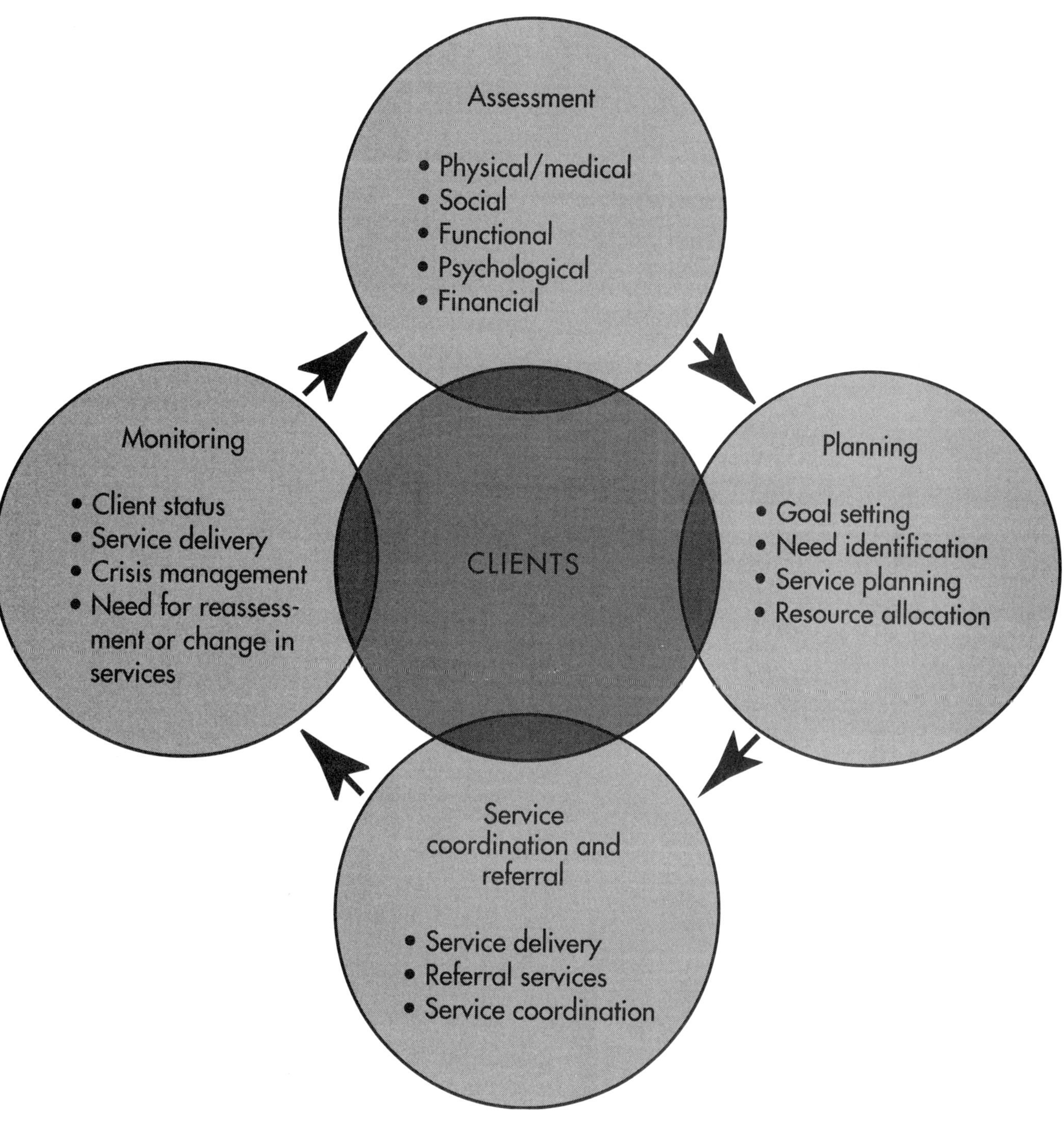

From Secord LJ: *Private case management for older persons and their families*, Excelsior, Minn, 1987, Interstudy.

TM 36

Disaster preparedness responsibilities by agency. (Table 20-1)

American Red Cross	Other voluntary organizations	Business and labor organizations	Local government
Participates with government in developing and testing community disaster plan. Designates persons to serve as representatives at government emergency operations centers and command posts. Develops and tests local Red Cross disaster plans. Identifies and trains personnel for disaster response. Collaborates with other voluntary agencies in developing and maintaining a local Voluntary Organizations Active in Disaster group to promote cooperation and coordinate resources and people for disaster work. Works with business and labor organizations to identify resources and people for disaster work. Educates the public about hazards and ways to avoid, prepare for, and cope with their effects. Acquires material resources needed to ensure effective response.	Collaborates in developing and maintaining a local Voluntary Organizations Active in Disaster group to identify roles, resources, and plans for disasters. Identifies and train personnel for disaster response. Identifies community issues and special populations for consideration in disaster preparedness. Makes plans to continue to serve regular clients after a disaster. Identifies facilities, resources, and people to serve in time of disaster. Educates specific client groups on disaster preparedness.	Develops disaster plans for business locations and integrate their plans with the community disaster plan. Develops procedures to facilitate continuity of operations in time of disaster. Develops plans for assisting business employees after a disaster. Identifies union and business facilities, resources, and people who may be able to support community disaster plans. Provides volunteers, financial contributions, and in-kind gifts to Red Cross and other voluntary organizations to support disaster preparedness. Educates employees and union members about disaster preparedness.	Coordinates the development of the community plan and conducts evaluation exercises. Trains staff to carry out the plan. Passes legislation to mitigate the effects of potential disasters. Designs measures to warn the population of disaster threats. Conducts building safety inspections. Develops procedures to facilitate continuity of public safety operations in time of disaster. Identifies public facilities, resources, and public employees for disaster work. Educates the public about disaster threats in the community and safety procedures.

From American Red Cross: *Disasters happen*, Washington, DC, 1993, American Red Cross. Used with the permission of the American Red Cross, Washington, DC, 1994.

TM 37

Disaster response responsibilities by agency. (Table 20-2)

American Red Cross	Other voluntary organizations	Business and labor organizations	Local government
Operates shelters.	Provides services that are identified in predisaster planning.	Takes action to protect employees and ensure the safety of the facility.	Provides for coordination of the overall relief effort.
Provides feeding services.	Provides regular services to ongoing client groups.	Advises public safety forces of hazardous conditions.	Advises the public on safety measures such as evacuation.
Provides individual and family assistance to meet immediate emergency needs. Services include providing the means to purchase groceries, clothing, and household items.	Identifies unanticipated needs and provide resources to meet those needs.	Identifies resources such as union halls, generators, and heavy equipment that are available to support the disaster response.	Provides public health services.
Provides disaster health services, including mental health support.	Acts as advocates for their client groups.	Provides volunteers, financial contributions, and gifts of goods and services to the relief effort.	Provides fire and police protection to the affected area.
Handles inquiries from concerned family members outside the area.	Coordinates services with all other groups involved with the disaster response.		Inspects facilities for safety and health codes.
Coordinates relief activities with other agencies, business, labor, and government.	Seeks and accept donations from those wanting to help.		Provides ongoing social services for the community.
Informs the public of services available.			Repairs public buildings, sewage and water systems, streets, and highways.
Seeks and accepts contributions from those wanting to help.			

From American Red Cross: *Disasters happen*, Washington, DC, 1993, American Red Cross. Used with permission of the American Red Cross, Washington, DC, 1994.

TM 38

Six steps in planning for program evaluation. (Figure 21-3)

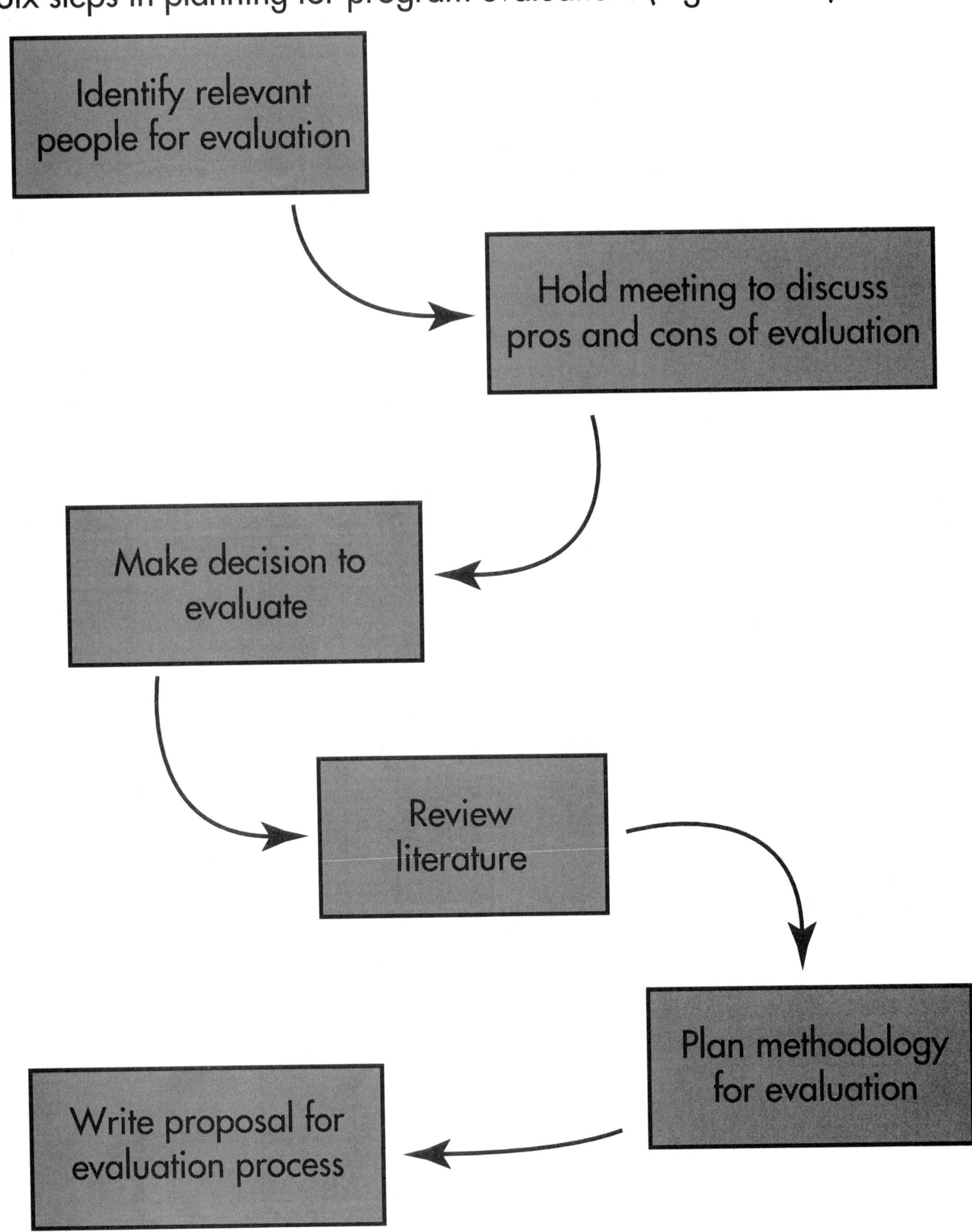

Stanhope/Lancaster: *Community Health Nursing*, ed 4

TM 39

The evaluative process. (Figure 21-4)

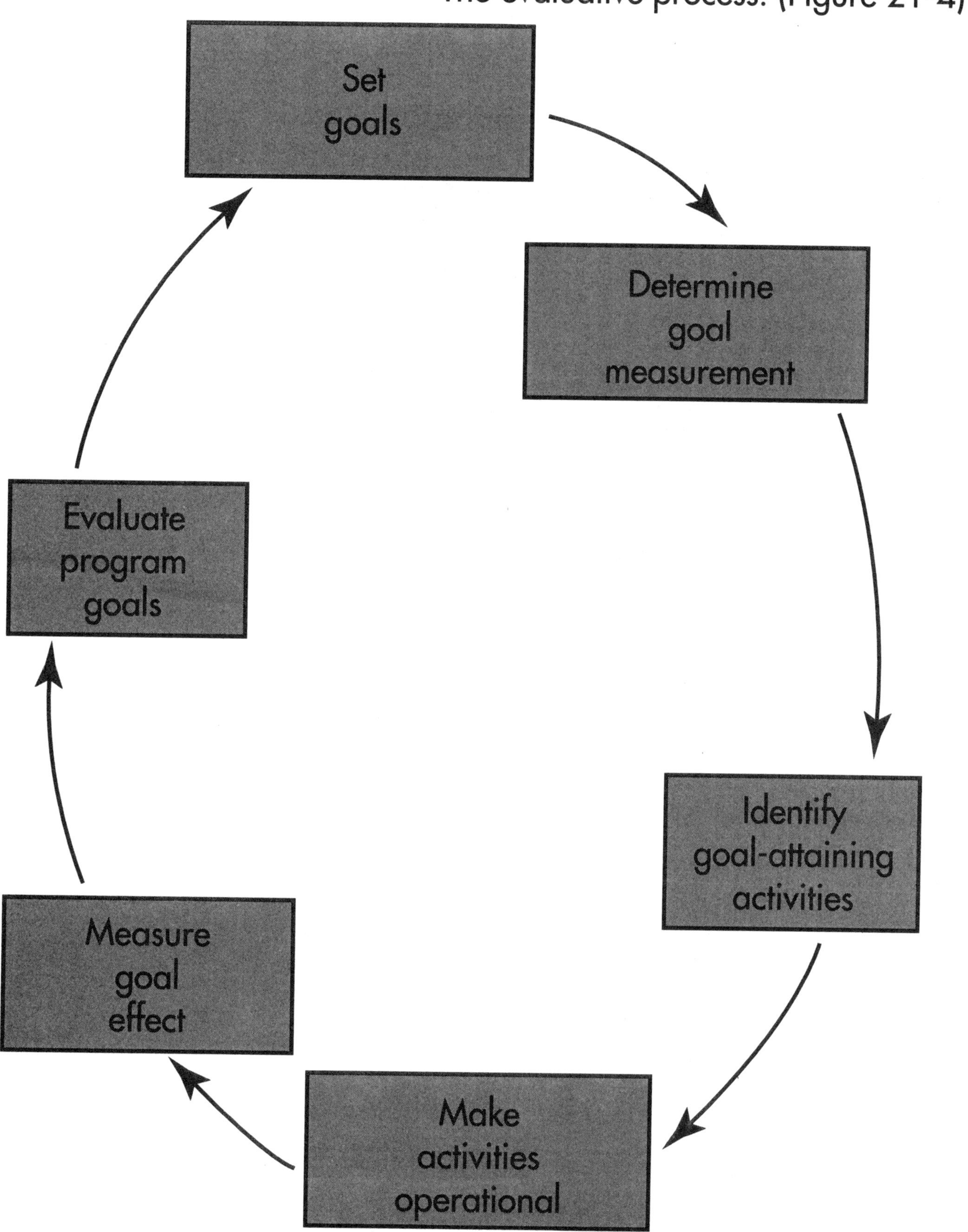

TM 40
Model quality assurance program. (Figure 22-4)

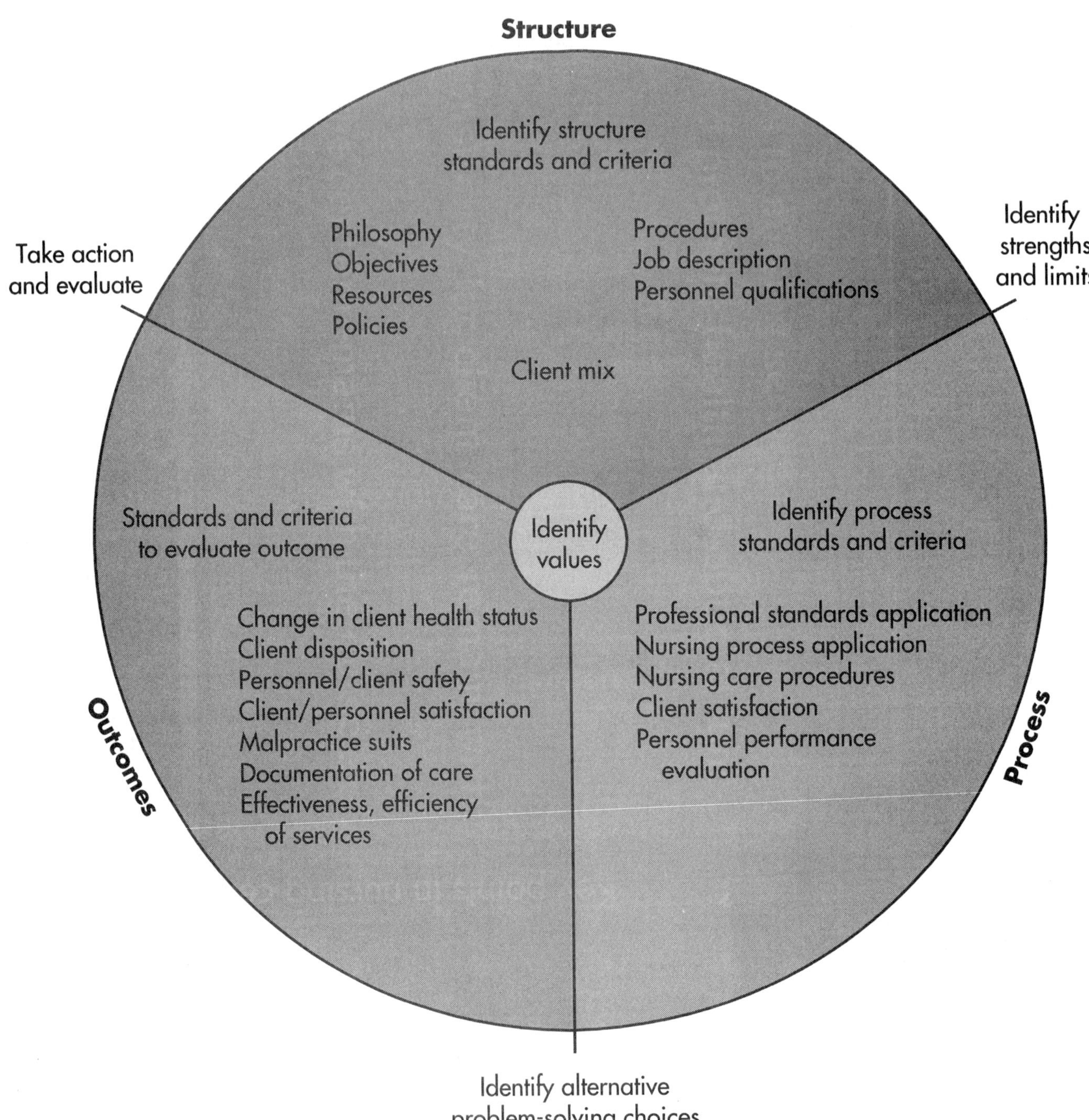

TM 41

A group is a collection of interacting individuals who have a common purpose or purposes. (Figure 23-1)

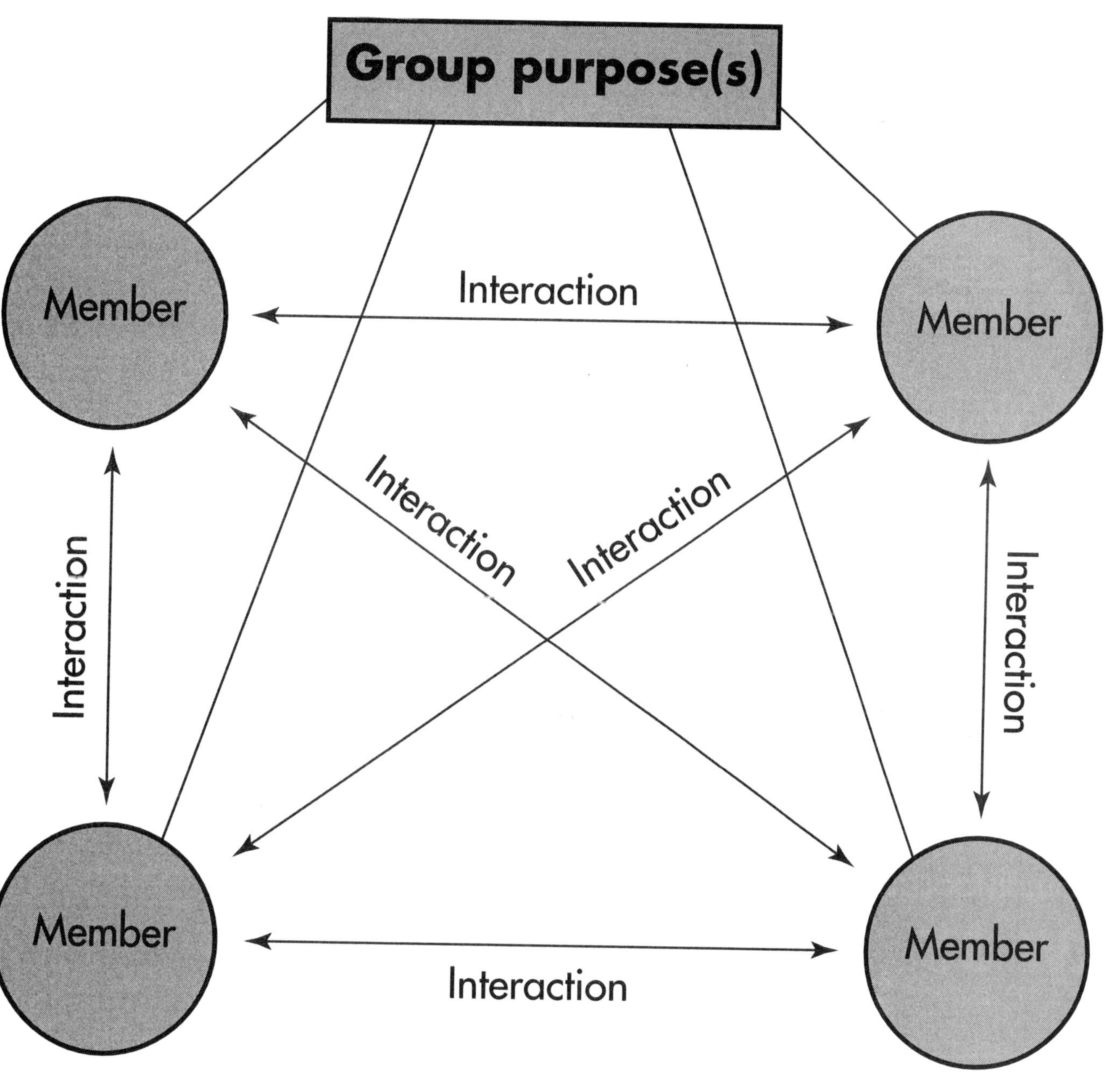

TM 42

Influence of group norms on individual members. (Figure 23-3)

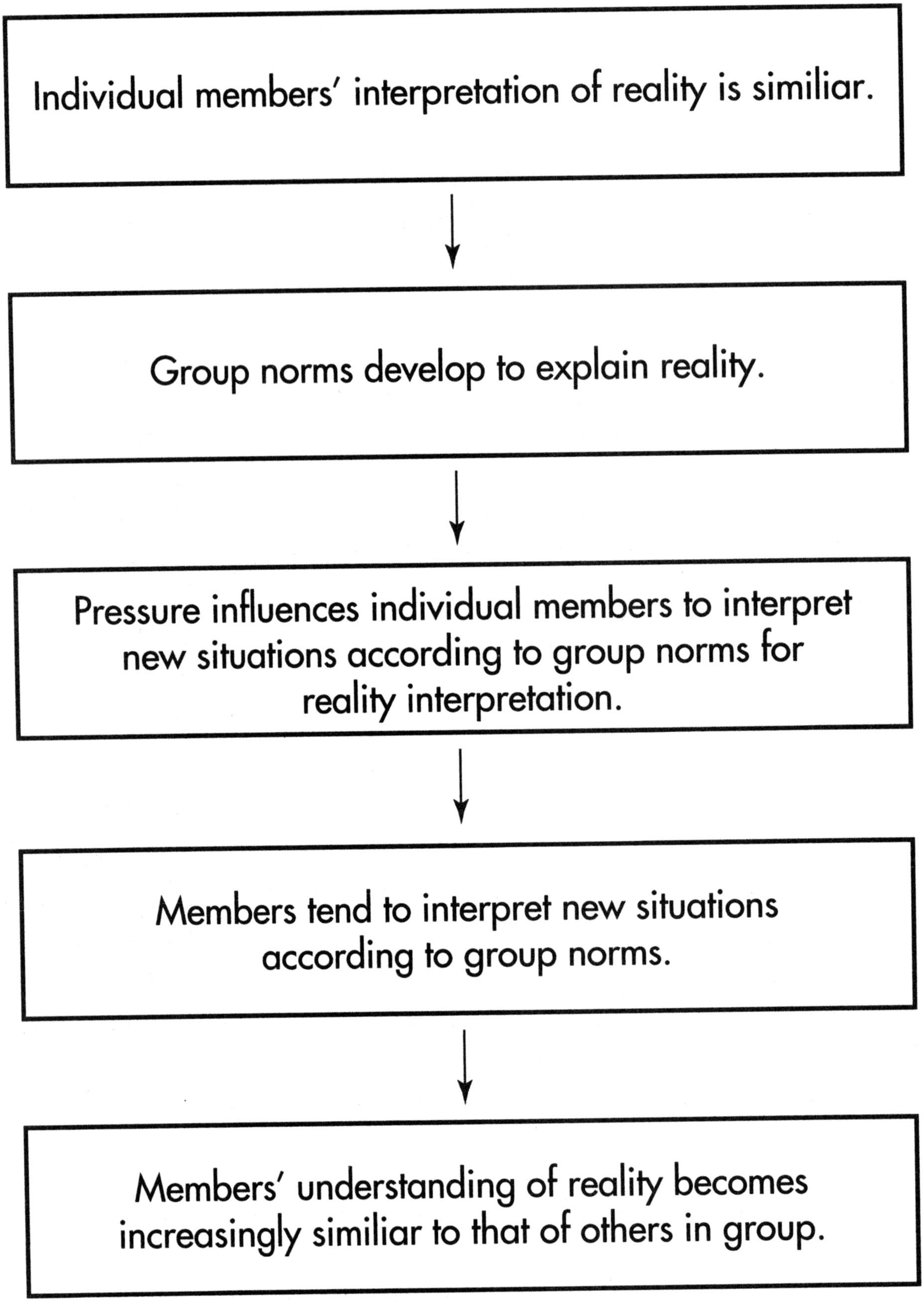

Individual members' interpretation of reality is similiar.

↓

Group norms develop to explain reality.

↓

Pressure influences individual members to interpret new situations according to group norms for reality interpretation.

↓

Members tend to interpret new situations according to group norms.

↓

Members' understanding of reality becomes increasingly similiar to that of others in group.

TM 43

Family health and community health: a systems perspective. (Figure 24-1)

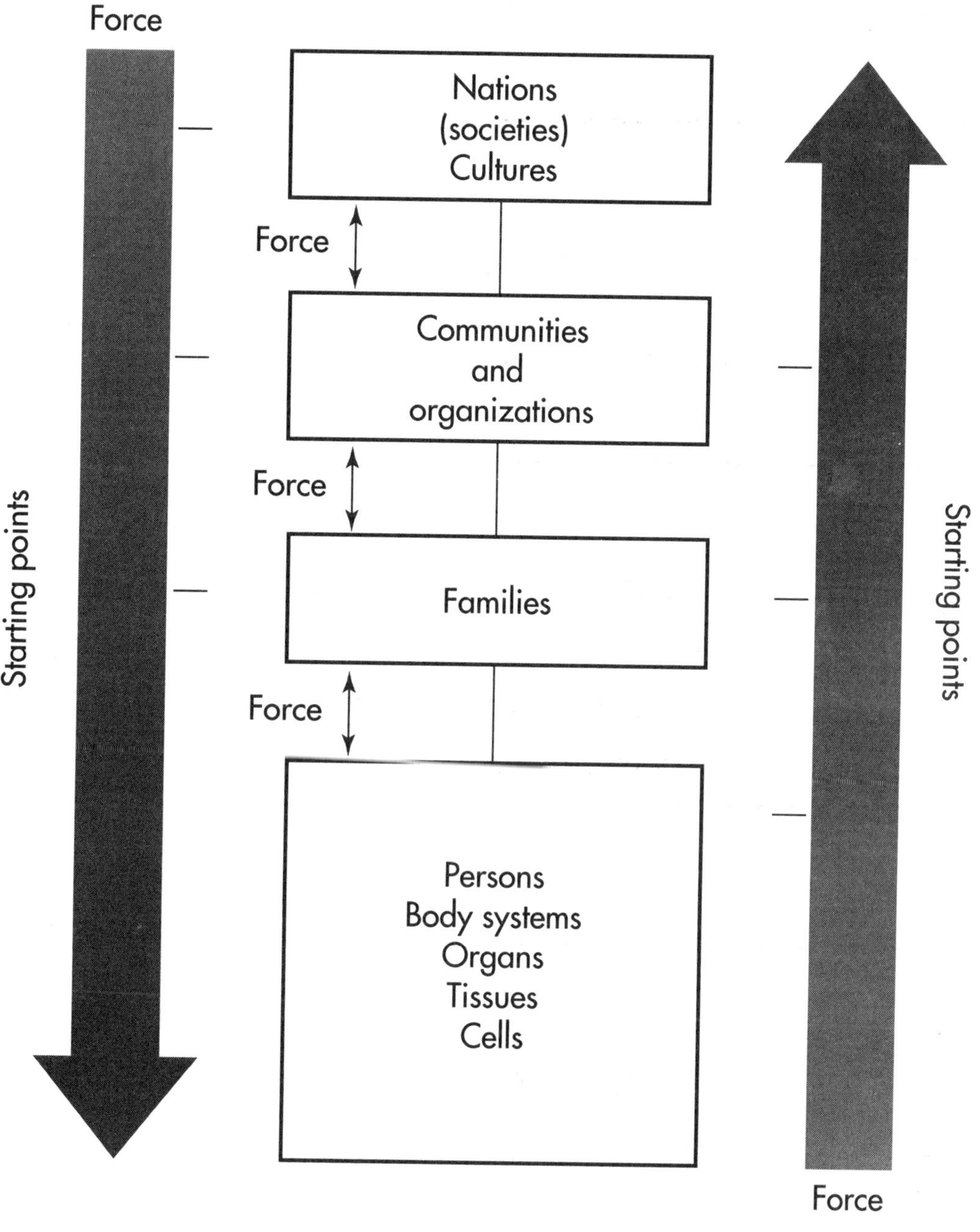

Modified from Blum HL: *Expanding health care horizons from a general systems concept of health to a national health policy*, Oakland, Calif, 1976, Third Party Associates.

TM 44

Family career of an individual. (Figure 24-2)

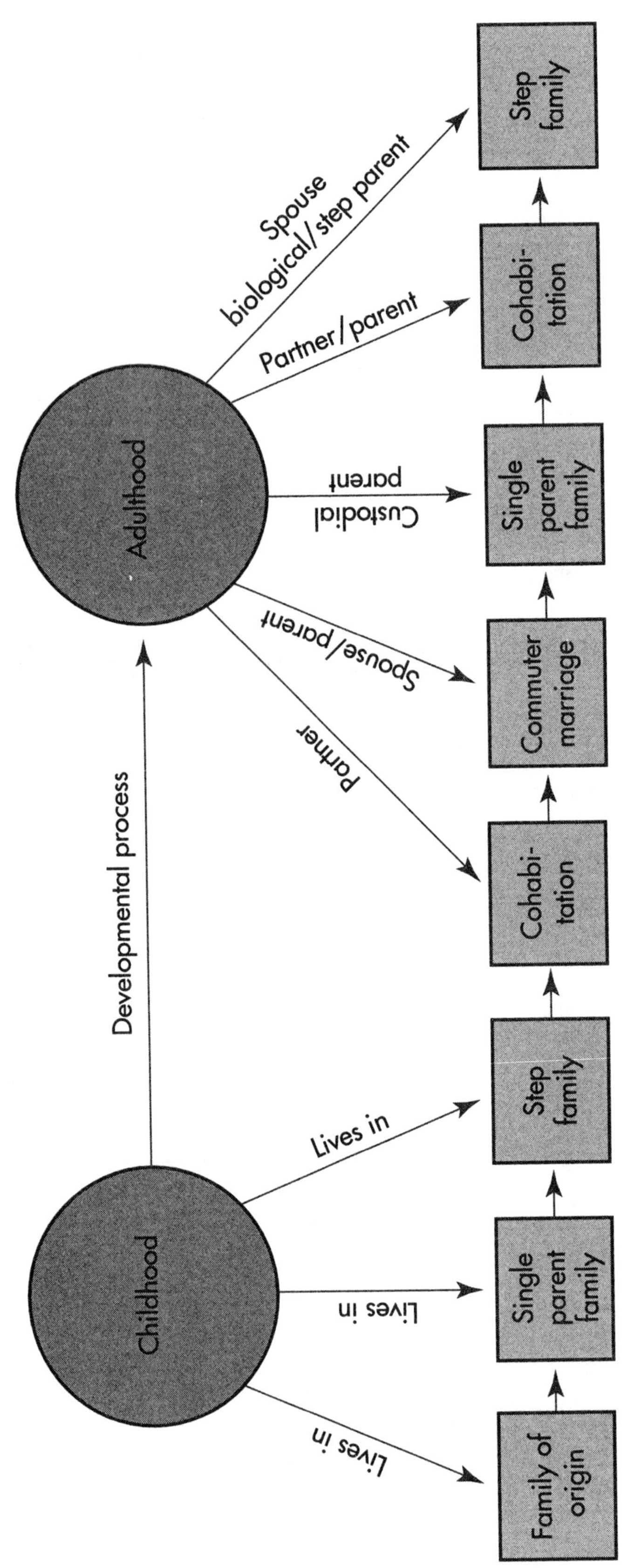

Stanhope/Lancaster: *Community Health Nursing*, ed 4

TM 45

Phases and activities of a home visit. (Table 25-3)

Phase	Activity
I Initiation Phase	Clarify source of referral for visit Clarify purpose for home visit Share information on reason and purpose of home visit with family
II Previsit Phase	Initiate contact with family Establish shared perception of purpose with family Determine family's willingness for home visit Schedule home visit Review referral and/or family record
III In-Home Phase	Introduction of self and professional identity Social interaction to establish rapport Establish nurse-client relationship Implement nursing process
IV Termination Phase	Review visit with family Plan for future visits
V Postvisit Phase	Record visit Plan for next visit

TM 46

Family assessment intervention model. (Figure 26-1)

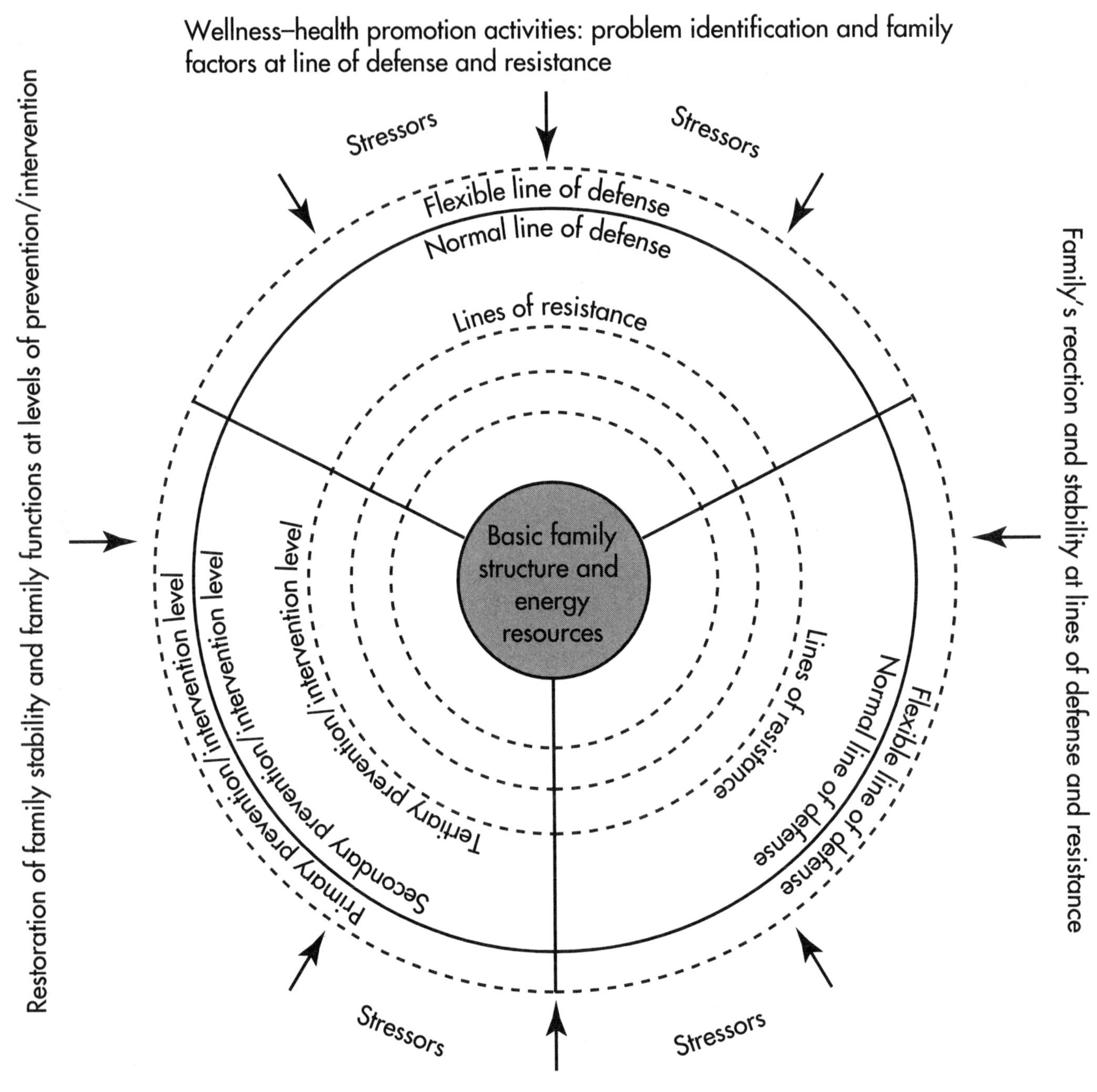

From Mischke-Berkey KM, Warner P, Hanson SMH: In PJ Bomar, editor, *Nurses and family health promotion: concepts, assessment, and interventions*, Philadelphia, 1989, WB Saunders.

TM 47

Guidelines for well-child care. (Table 27-1)

	Age												
	Months							Years					
	2	4	6	9	12	15	18	2	3	4-6	8-10	12-14	16-18
Physical examination	•	•	•	•	•	•	•	•	•	•	•	•	•
Height/weight	•	•	•	•	•	•	•	•	•	•	•	•	•
Head circumference	•	•	•	•	•	•	•						
Blood pressure									•	•	•	•	•
Vision	S	S	S	S	S	S	S	S	S	•	•	•	•
Hearing	S	S	S	S	S	S	S	S	S	•	•	•	•
Developmental	•	•	•	•	•	•	•	•	•	•	•	•	•
Hematocrit/hemoglobin				•						•		•	
Urinalysis										•		•	
Tuberculosis skin test					•					•		•	
Lead level					•					•			
Anticipatory guidance:													
Feeding/nutrition	•	•	•	•	•	•	•	•	•	•	•	•	•
Growth/development	•	•	•	•	•	•	•	•	•	•	•	•	•
Behavior	•	•	•	•	•	•	•	•	•	•	•	•	•
Safety/poisons/injury	•	•	•	•	•	•	•	•	•	•	•	•	•
Sexual behaviors											a	a	a
Substance abuse											a	a	a
Physical activity										a	a	a	a

Modified from *American Academy of Pediatrics: Guidelines for health supervision*. II, Elk Grove Village, Ill, 1992, The Academy.
S, Subjectively determined by behavioral observations; ***blank***, formal assessment as determined by history; *a*, as appropriate for age.

TM 48

Assessment tools for children. (Table 27-6)

Test	Focus	Ages	Summary
Denver II	Developmental screen	Birth to 6 years	Screening of gross motor, fine motor, adaptive/language, and personal/social skills
Revised Denver Prescreening Developmental Questionnaire	Developmental screen	3 months to 6 years	Parent questionnaire; short form of the Denver to identify children who need further testing
Developmental Profile II	Developmental screen	Birth to 9 years	Structured interview with parent; screens physical/motor, self-help, social, academic, and communication skills
Preschool Readiness Experimental Screening Scale	Preschool readiness	4 to 5 years	Addresses school-related skills and maturation
Early Language Milestone Scale	Speech and language screening	Birth to 36 months	Screening tool for general speech/language development; includes visual, auditory receptive, and auditory expressive areas; combines history, direct testing, and observation
Denver Articulation Screening Examination	Speech and language screening	2 to 6 years	Word imitation to screen articulation and intelligibility of speech
Brazelton Neonatal Behavioral Assessment Scale	Infant behavior, state, and temperament patterns	Birth to 1 month	Assessment of reflexes and behavioral responses; tests for state and individual characteristics to identify abnormalities and provides parent education
Infant Temperament Questionnaire	Temperament	1 to 12 months	Child's temperamental characteristics identified based on parental responses; assess the following aspects of temperament: activity, rhythmicity, adaptability, approach, sensory threshold, intensity, mood, distractibility, and persistence
Toddler Development Scale		1 to 3 years	
Behavioral Style Questionnaire		3 to 7 years	
Middle Childhood Questionnaire		8 to 12 years	

TM 49

Risk factors associated with breast cancer.

MAJOR RISK FACTORS

Over 50 years old

Family history (mother, sister, or daughter)

Previous breast cancer

MODEST RISK FACTORS

First pregnancy after 30 years of age

Nulliparity

Menarche before 12 years old

Menopause after 55 years old

Proliferative atypical breast hyperplasia

History of ovarian or endometrial cancer

Obesity after menopause

High socioeconomic status

Stanhope/Lancaster: *Community Health Nursing*, ed 4

TM 50

Initiatives to improve maternal and infant health.

- Providing family planning services for all women who want to use them.
- Providing preconceptional and interconceptional counseling.
- Providing maternity benefits for all pregnant women.
- Improving accessibility of health care services for pregnant women by the provision of an adequate number of strategically located clinics, transportation, and child care facilities.
- Removing barriers to prenatal care, including negative provider attitudes, lack of continuity in care, and unnecessary waiting for care.
- Protecting childbearing women from occupational hazards.
- Extending the Special Supplemental Food Program for Women, Infants, and Children (WIC) to all pregnant and breast-feeding women.
- Implementing programs to help pregnant women decrease smoking and use of drugs and alcohol.
- Providing special follow-up of all high-risk women after delivery.
- Granting parental leave for employed parents.

Stanhope/Lancaster: *Community Health Nursing*, ed 4

TM 51

Tasks of the young adult male. (*Top*)
Tasks of the middle adult male. (*Bottom*)

1. Develops an intimate relationship with another
2. Chooses a mate
3. Establishes a husband or father role or both
4. Manages a household independent of his parents' home and care
5. Develops a career or vocation
6. Continues development of a social structure
7. Develops a community role focusing on citizenship
8. Develops a life-style suitable to his philosophy on life

1. Promotes a deep relationship with the spouse
2. Nurtures and shares in the growth of children and the next generation
3. Adjusts to physical changes
4. Reassesses self and career goals
5. Achieves desired goals in life and career
6. Builds acceptable leisure activities
7. Copes with the empty nest syndrome

TM 52

Population of persons aged 65 and over: 1990 to 2050. (Figure 30-1)

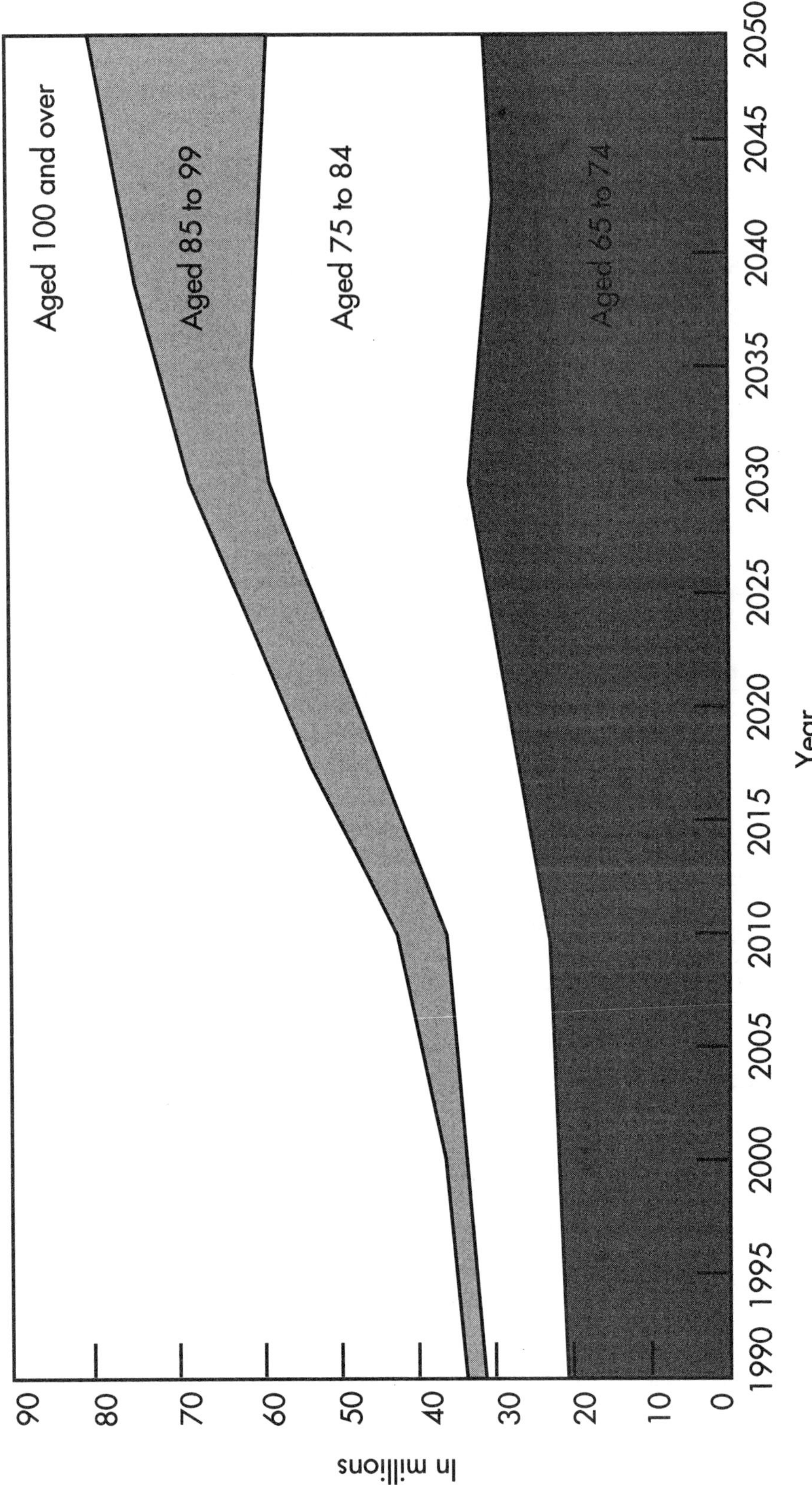

From U.S. Senate Subcommittee on Aging, American Association of Retired Persons, Federal Council on Aging, U.S. Administration on Aging: *Aging America: trends and projections*, DHHS Pub No (FCOA) 91-28001, Washington, DC, 1991, U.S. Department of Health and Human Services.

TM 53

Major health problems in elders and community health nursing roles. (Table 30-4)

Problem	Community health nursing roles
Hypertension	Monitor blood pressure and weight; educate about nutrition and antihypertensive drugs; teach stress management techniques; promote an optimal balance between rest and activity; establish blood pressure screening programs; assess client's current life-style and promote life-style changes; promote dietary modifications by using techniques such as a diet diary.
Cancer	Obtain health history; promote monthly breast self-examinations and yearly Pap smears and mammograms for older women; promote regular physical examinations; encourage smokers to stop smoking; correct misconceptions about processes of aging; provide emotional support and quality care during diagnostic and treatment procedures.
Arthritis	Help adult avoid the false hope and expense of arthritis quackery; educate adult about management of activities, correct body mechanics, availability of mechanical appliances, and adequate rest; promote stress management; counsel and assist the family to improve communication, role negotiation, and use of community resources.
Visual impairment (e.g., loss of visual acuity, eyelid disorders, opacity of the lens)	Provide support in a well-lighted, glare-free environment; use printed aids with large, well-spaced letters; assist adult with cleaning eyeglasses; help make arrangements for vision examinations and obtain necessary prostheses; teach adult to be cautious of fraudulent advertisements.
Hearing impairment (e.g., presbycusis)	Speak with clarity at a moderate volume and pace and face audience when performing health teaching; help make arrangements for hearing examination and obtain necessary prostheses; teach adult to be cautious of fraudulent advertisements.
Confusional states	Provide complete assessment; correct underlying causes of disease (if possible); provide for a protective environment; promote activities that reinforce reality; assist with adequate personal hygiene, nutrition, and hydration; provide emotional support to the family; recommend applicable community resources such as adult day care, home health aides, and homemaker services.
Alzheimer's disease	Maintain optimal functioning, protection, and safety; foster human dignity; demonstrate to the primary family caregiver techniques to dress, feed, and toilet adult; provide frequent encouragement and emotional support to caregiver; act as an advocate for client when dealing with respite care and support groups; ensure that clients's rights are protected; provide support to maintain family members' physical and mental health; maintain family stability; recommend financial services if needed.
Dental problems	Perform oral assessment and refer as necessary; emphasize regular brushing and flossing, proper nutrition, and dental examinations; encourage clients with dentures to wear and take care of them; allay fears about dentist; help provide access to financial services (if necessary) and access to dental care facilities.
Drug use and abuse	Obtain drug history; educate adult about safe storage, risks of drug, drug-drug, and drug-food interactions, and general information about drug (e.g., drug name, purpose, side effects, dosage); instruct adult about presorting technique (using small container with one dose of drug that are labeled with specific administration times).
Substance abuse	Arrange and monitor detoxification if appropriate; counsel adults about substance abuse; promote stress management to avoid need for drugs or alcohol; encourage adult to use self-help groups such as Alcoholics Anonymous and Al-Anon; educate public about dangers of substance abuse.

From Skipwith DH: In Stanhope M, Lancaster J, editors: *Community health nursing: process and practice for promoting health*, ed 3, St Louis, 1992, Mosby.

TM 54

Potential effects of being physically compromised related to individuals, families, and communities.

PERSON

Related health problems (e.g., nutrition, oral health, hygiene, limited activity and stamina)

↓ Self-concept/self esteem

↓ Life expectancy and risk for infection and secondary injury

Developmental tasks; change in role expectations

FAMILY

Stress on family unit

Need for ↑ use of external resources

in role expectations

↓ options in use of any discretionary income

Social stigma

COMMUNITY

Need/demand to reallocate resources

Discomfort or fear due to lack of knowledge of disability

Need to comply with legislation

Services provided by health department, health care providers

↑ need for other services beyond medical diagnosis (e.g., transportation, etc.)

Stanhope/Lancaster: *Community Health Nursing*, ed 4

TM 55

Impediments to primary health care of the physically compromised. (Table 31-2)

Issues	Examples
1. Transportation	1. May not be able to drive; limited flexibility in public/private transporation; may need specially equipped van
2. Access to clinic/office	2. Entrances, halls, restrooms may all be inadequate. Exam tables, scales, life equipment unavailable or inappropriate. Increased time needed for disabled client's visit.
3. Inadequate care from primary care providers	3. Limited or no training in primary care needs/health promotion of those with disabilities; lack of understanding reasons that those with disabilities often delay treatment until at crisis levels; limited ability to distinguish between progress in a disability and different, new health problems.
4. Information given to clients	4. Often unavailable or available only to few specialists; may not have been given basic health information in school; most have never received comprehensive rehabilitation.
5. Finances	5. Health maintenance/health promotion costly: good food, someone to obtain and prepare it; exercise: transporation, fees of facilities and assistant with exercise.
6. Personal assistance	6. Needed by some with disabilities for most basic health activities, hygiene, laundry, etc.

Data from Gans BM: *Arch Phys Med Rehabil* 74 (12-S): S-15-S-19; Nosek MA: J *Womens Health* 1(4).

TM 56

Predisposing factors for vulnerability and potential outcomes of vulnerability. (Figure 32-2)

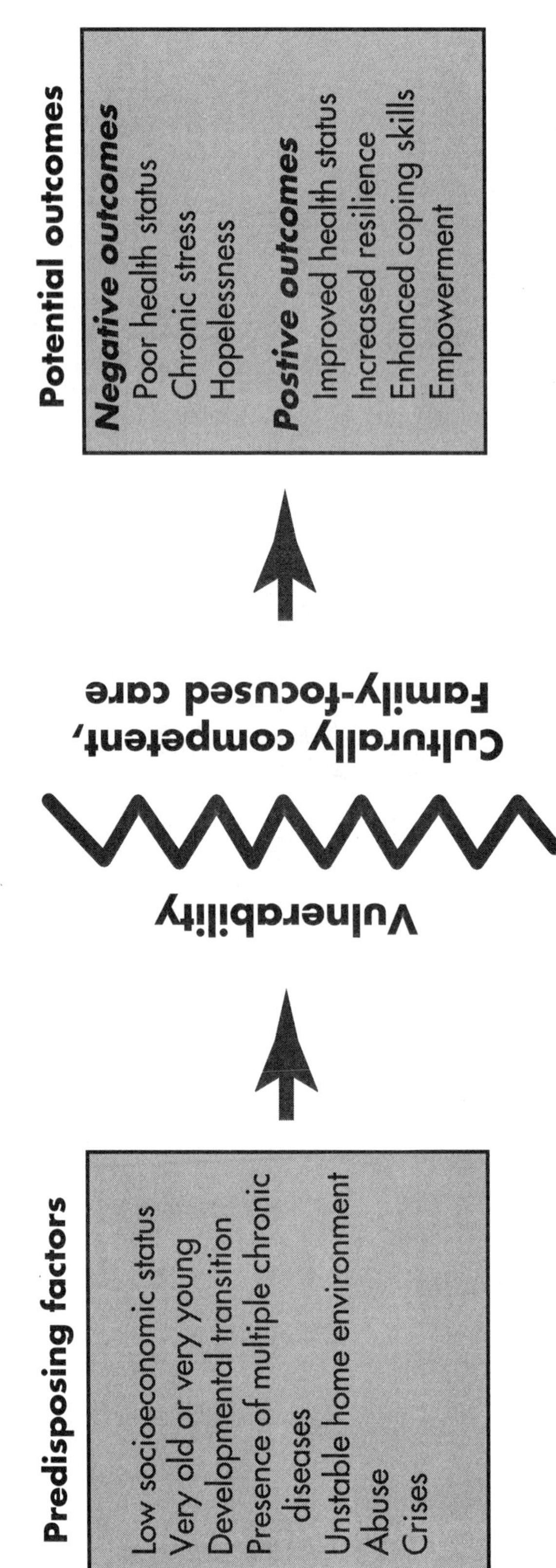

Stanhope/Lancaster: *Community Health Nursing*, ed 4

TM 57

The community health nurse as case manager for vulnerable populations. (Figure 32-4)

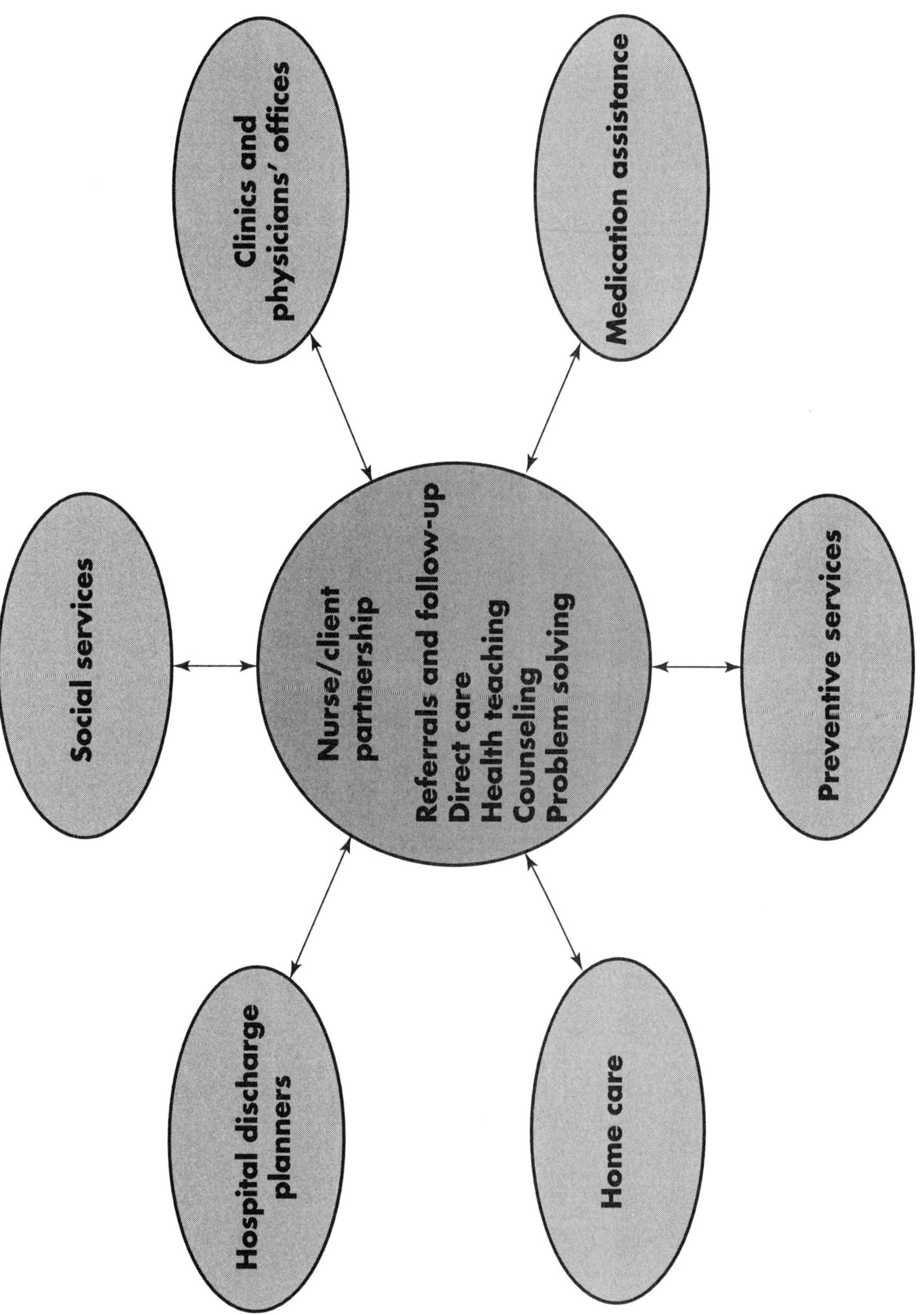

Stanhope/Lancaster: *Community Health Nursing*, ed 4

TM 58

The effects of poverty on the health of children.

- Higher rates of prematurity, low birth weight, and birth defects
- Higher infant mortality rates
- Increased incidence of chronic disease
- Increased incidence of traumatic death and injuries
- Increased incidence of nutritional deficits
- Increased incidence of growth retardation and developmental delays
- Increased incidence of iron deficiency anemia
- Increased incidence of elevated lead levels
- Increased incidence of infections
- Increased incidence of delayed immunizations
- Increased risk for homelessness
- Decreased opportunities for education, income, and occupation

Stanhope/Lancaster: *Community Health Nursing*, ed 4

TM 59

Health problems of homeless children.

PHYSICAL HEALTH PROBLEMS

Scabies
Lice
Dermatologic infections
Dental problems
Chronic cardiovascular problems
Neurological disorders
Anemia
Asthma
Bronchitis
Incomplete immunization status
Inadequate nutrition

SOCIAL AND DEVELOPMENTAL PROBLEMS

Developmental problems
Behavioral problems
School-related problems
  Erratic attendance
  Failure
Anxiety and depression

TM 60

Guidelines for adoption counseling.

1. Assess your own thoughts and feelings on adoption. Do not impose your opinion on the decision-making process of teen mothers.
2. Be knowledgeable about state laws, local resources, and various types of adoption services.
3. Choose language sensitively. For example:
   a. Avoid saying "giving away a child" or "putting up for adoption." It is more appropriate and positive to say "releasing a child for adoption," "placing for adoption," or "making an adoption plan."
   b. Avoid saying "unwanted child" or "unwanted pregnancy." A more appropriate term may be "unplanned pregnancy."
   c. Avoid saying "natural parents" or "natural child," since the adopted parents would then seem to be "unnatural." The terms "biological parents" and "adopted parents" are more appropriate.
4. Assess when a discussion of adoption is appropriate. It can be helpful to begin with information on adoption, then explore feelings and concerns over time. Individuals will vary in how much they may have already considered adoption, and this will influence the counseling session.
5. Assess the relationship between the pregnant teen and her partner and what role she expects him to play. Discuss the reality of this.
6. It may be helpful for a pregnant teen to talk with other teens who have been pregnant, are raising a child, have released a child for adoption, or have been adopted themselves.
7. A young woman can be encouraged to begin writing letters to her baby. These can be saved or given to the child when released to the adoptive family.

Modified from Brandsen CK: A *case for adoption*, Grand Rapids, Michigan, 1991, Bethany.

TM 61

Guidelines for teen mother/newborn interactions.

1. Make eye contact with your baby. Position your face 8 to 10 inches from your baby's face and smile.
2. Talk to your baby often. Use simple sentences, but try to avoid baby talk. Allow time for your baby to "answer." This will help your baby acquire language and communication skills.
3. Babies often enjoy when you sing to them, and this may help soothe them during a difficult time or help them fall asleep. Experiment with different songs and melodies to see which your baby seems to like.
4. Babies at this age cannot be spoiled. Instead, when babies are held and cuddled, they feel secure and loved.
5. Babies cry for many reasons and for no reason at all. If your baby has a clean diaper, has recently been fed and is safe and secure, he or she may just need to cry for a few minutes. What works to calm your baby may be different from other babies you have known. You can try rocking, gentle reassuring words, soft music, or quiet.
6. Make feeding times pleasant for both of you. Do not prop the bottle in your baby's mouth. Instead, you should sit comfortably, hold your baby in your arms, and offer the bottle or breast.
7. When babies are awake, they love to play. They enjoy taking walks and looking at brightly colored objects or pictures and toys that make noises, such as rattles and musical toys.

TM 62

Characteristics of migratory streams. (Table 35-1)

Migrant stream	Primary residence	Member's origin	Characteristics
East Coast	Southern Florida	Mexican-American, Mexican, Central American, Puerto Rican, and less often, American black, Haitian, and Appalachian white	Headed by a "crew leader," who is paid directly by the grower and redistributes the money to the pickers minus cost of meals and transportation
Midwest	Southern Texas (largest population in the nation)	Mexican-American, Mexican, and more recently Southeast Asian	Families, friends, and single males live together in "colonies," which are not required to have water, sewer, or electricity services. The "truckero" usually transports personal possessions of the workers, who follow in car caravans.
West Coast	Southern California	Mexican-American, Mexican, and a small percentage of American black, nonHispanic white, Southeast Asian, and Central American (many Southeast Asian workers quickly settle in the area and leave the migrant stream)	Individual families and single males often travel independently in cars, trucks, and vans. West Coast housing is known as "the best of the best and the worst of the worst," meaning the work and general living conditions vary widely.

Stanhope/Lancaster: *Community Health Nursing*, ed 4

TM 63

Legislation that influenced community mental health services. (Table 36-1)

Year	Legislation	Focus
1955	Mental Health Study Act	Resulted in Joint Commission on Mental Illness and Health that recommended transformation of state hospital systems and establishment of community mental health clinics
1963	Community Mental Health Centers Act	Marked beginning of community mental health centers concept and led to deinstitutionalization of large psychiatric hospitals
1975	Developmental Disabilities Act	Addressed the rights and treatment of people with developmental disabilities and provided foundation for similar action for individuals with mental disorders
1977	President's Commission on Mental Health	Reinforced importance of community-based services, protection of human rights, and national health insurance for mentally ill persons
1978	Omnibus Reconciliation Act	Rescinded much of the 1977 commission's provisions and shifted funds for all health programs from federal to state governments
1986	Protection and Advocacy for Mentally Ill Individuals Act	Legislated advocacy programs for mentally ill persons
1990	Americans with Disabilities Act	Prohibited discrimination and promoted employment opportunities for people with disabilities, including mental disorders

TM 64

Problems and populations targeted in national health objectives for mental health. (Table 36-2)

Problem	Target population
Persistent mental disorders	Children Adolescents Adults
Adverse health effects from stress	Adults
Injurious suicide attempts	Adolescents
Suicide	Adolescents Adult and elderly men Native Americans and Alaska natives in reservation states
Maltreatment	Children and youth aged 18 yr and younger
Assault injuries	Children aged 12 yr and older Adults
Physical abuse	Women
Rape and attempted rape	Women and adolescents aged 12 yr and older
Homicide	Children aged 3 yr and younger Spouses African-American men and women Hispanic-American men Native Americans and Alaska natives in reservation states

Modified from *Healthy People* 2000: *national health promotion and disease prevention objectives*, Washington, DC, 1991, USDHHS, Public Health Service.

TM 65

Federal drug control budget for 1994. (Figure 37-1)

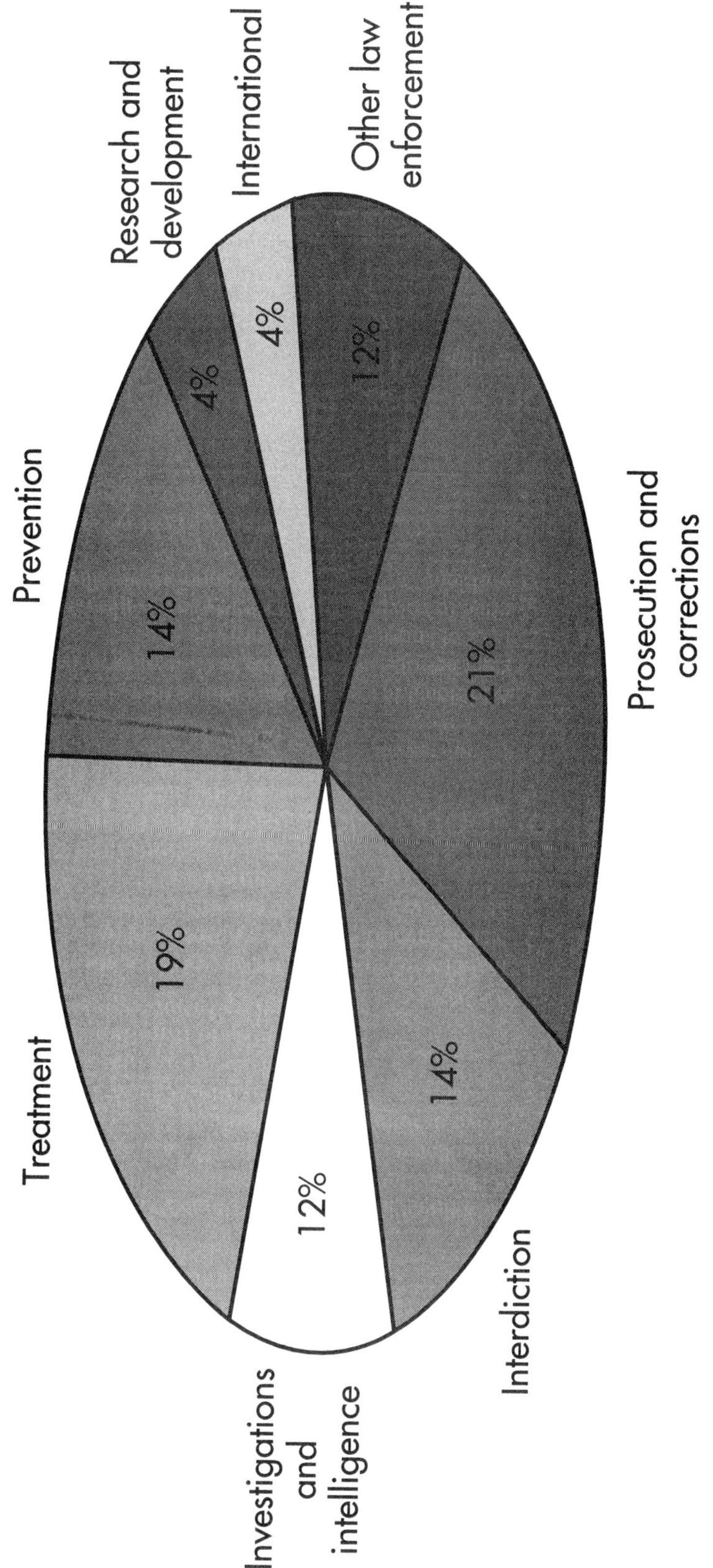

Stanhope/Lancaster: *Community Health Nursing*, ed 4

TM 66

Community-based activities aimed at ATOD problem prevention.

Increased involvement and pride in school activities

Student assistant programs

Students Against Drunk Driving (SADD)

Parent awareness and action groups (e.g., MADD)

Increased availability of recreation facilities

Parental commitment to nondrinking parties

Active involvement of religious institutions in conveying nonuse messages and providing activities associated with nonuse

Curtailment of media messages that glamorize drug and alcohol use

Support and reinforcement for antidrug peer pressure

General health screenings, including ATOD use

Collaboration among community leaders to solve problems related to crime, housing, jobs, and access to health care

TM 67

Behavioral indicators of potentially abusive parents.

The following characteristics in couples expecting a child constitute warning signs of actual or potential abuse.

1. Denial of the reality of the pregnancy, as evidenced by a refusal to talk about the impending birth or to think of a name for the child
2. An obvious concern or fear that the baby will not meet some predetermined standard: sex, hair color, temperament, or resemblance to family members
3. Failure to follow through on the desire for or seeking of an abortion
4. An initial decision to place the child for adoption and a change of mind
5. Rejection of the mother by the father of the baby
6. Family experiencing stress and numerous crises so that the birth of a child may be the "straw that broke the camel's back"
7. Initial and unresolved negative feelings about having a child
8. Lack of support for the new parents
9. Isolation from friends, neighbors, or family
10. Parental evidence of poor impulse control or fear of losing control
11. Contradictory history
12. Appearance of detachment
13. Appearance of misusing drugs or alcohol
14. Shopping for hospitals or health care providers
15. Unrealistic expectations of the child
16. Abuse of mother by father, especially during pregnancy
17. Child is not biological offspring of male stepfather or mother's current boyfriend

TM 68

Indicators of actual or potential abuse.

1. An unexplained injury
   a. Skin: burns, old or recent scars, ecchymosis, soft tissue swelling, human bites
   b. Fractures: recent or ones that have healed
   c. Subdural hematomas
   d. Trauma to genitalia
   e. Whiplash (caused by shaking small children)
2. Dehydration or malnourishment without obvious cause
3. Provision of inappropriate food or drugs (alcohol, tobacco, medication prescribed for someone else, foods not appropriate for the child's age)
4. Evidence of general poor care: poor hygiene, dirty clothes, unkempt hair, dirty nails
5. Unusually fearful of nurse and others
6. Considered to be a "bad" child
7. Inappropriately dressed for the season or weather conditions
8. Reports or shows evidence of sexual abuse
9. Injuries not mentioned in history
10. Seems to need to take care of the parent and speak for the parent
11. Maternal depression
12. Maladjustment of older siblings

TM 69

A multisystem approach to communicable disease control. (Table 39-3)

Goal	Example
Improve host resistance to infectious agents and other environmental hazards	Improved hygiene, nutrition, and physical fitness; increased immunization coverage; provision of chemoprophylaxis and chemotherapy; stress control and improved mental health
Improve safety of the environment	Improved sanitation, provision of safe water and clean air; proper cooking and storage of food; appropriate control of vectors and animal reservoir hosts
Improve public health systems	Increased access to health care; adequate health education; improved surveillance systems
Facilitate social and political changes to ensure better health for all people	Individual, organizational, and community action; legislation

From Wenzel RP: In Last JM, and Wallace RB, editors: *Public health and preventive medicine*, ed 13, Norwalk, 1992, Appleton and Lange.

TM 70

Natural history of human immunodeficiency virus. (Figure 40-1)

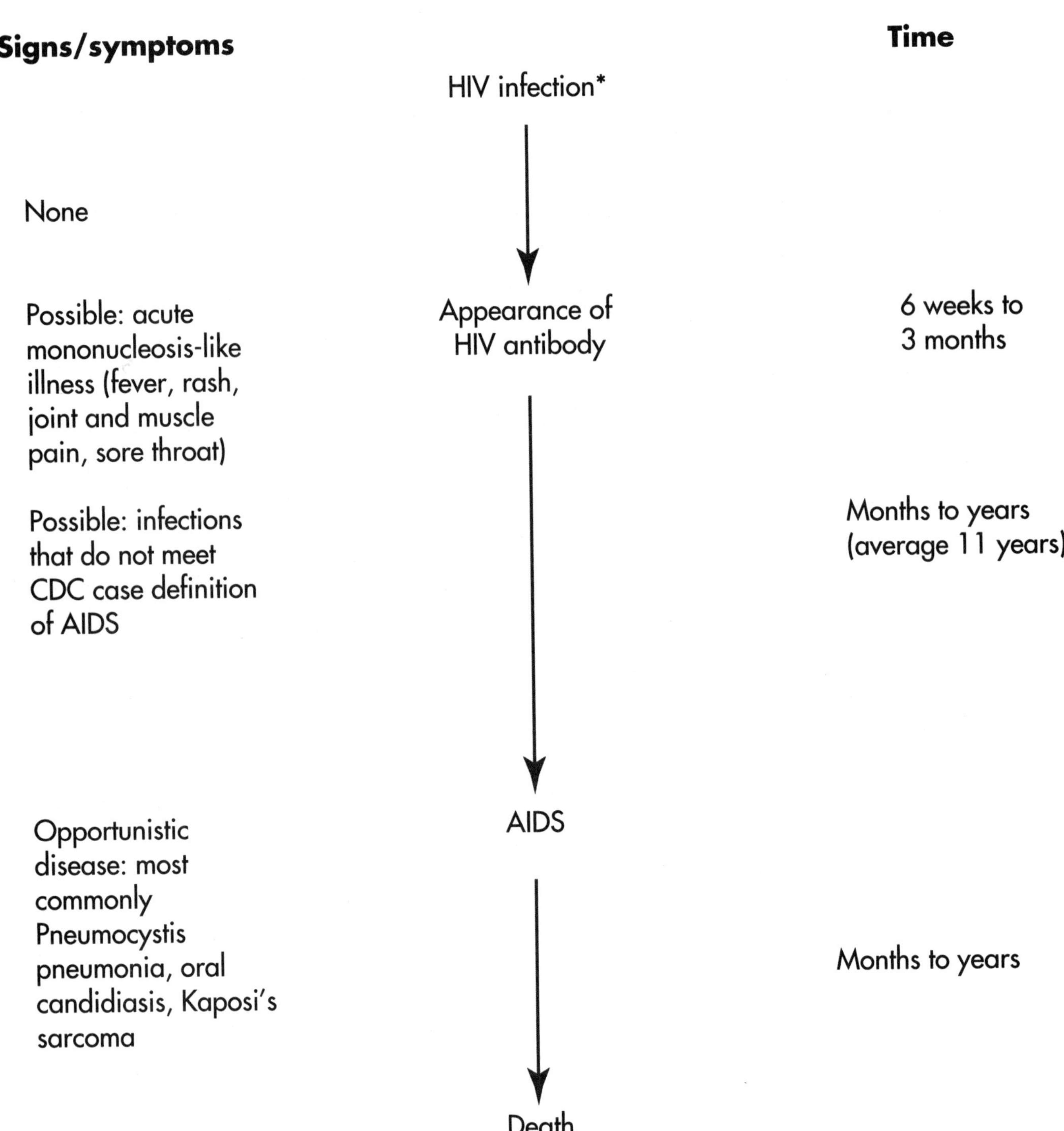

*Incubation period varies between individuals and may last from several months to several years

TM 71

Relationship between nursing process and ANA standards of practice. (Table 41-3)

Nursing process	Standard		Description
Assess	I.	Organization	All home health services are planned, organized, and directed by a master's-prepared professional nurse with experience in community health and administration.
	II.	Theory	The nurse applies theoretical concepts as a basis for decisions in practice.
	III.	Data Collection	The nurse continuously collects and records data that are comprehensive, accurate, and systematic.
	IV.	Diagnosis	The nurse uses health assessment data to determine nursing diagnoses.
Plan	V.	Planning	The nurse develops care plans that establish goals. The care plan is based on nursing diagnoses and incorporates therapeutic, preventive, and rehabilitative nursing actions.
Implement	VI.	Intervention	The nurse, guided by the care plan, intervenes to provide comfort, to restore, improve, and promote health, to prevent complications and sequelae of illness, and to effect rehabilitation.
Evaluate	VII.	Evaluation	The nurse continually evaluates the client's and family's responses to interventions in order to determine progress toward goal attainment and to revise the data base, nursing diagnoses, and plan of care.
	VIII.	Continuity of Care	The nurse is responsible for the client's appropriate and uninterrupted care along the health care continuum, and therefore uses discharge planning, case management, and coordination of community resources.
	IX.	Interdisciplinary Collaboration	The nurse initiates and maintains a liaison relationship with all appropriate health care providers to assure that all efforts effectively complement one another.
	X.	Professional Development	The nurse assumes responsibility for professional development and contributes to the professional growth of others.
	XI.	Research	The nurse participates in research activities that contribute to the profession's continuing development of knowledge of home health care.
	XII.	Ethics	The nurse uses the code for nurses established by the American Nurses Association as a guide for ethical decision-making in practice.

From American Nurses Association: *Standards of home health nursing practice*, Kansas City, Mo, 1986, The Association.

TM 72

Consultative intervention modes. (Table 43-1)

Intervention mode	Definition	Problem example	Consultant actions
Acceptance	Consultant urges client to share feelings to move to more objective problem solving.	1. Low morale 2. Feelings of powerlessness to change a situation	1. Attempt to understand the client's feelings about the situation. 2. Listen actively. 3. Encourage the client to talk. 4. Try to clarify the client's feelings and help the client to accept those feelings. 5. Refrain from agreeing or disagreeing with the client's situation. 6. Encourage the client to explore ways of dealing with the problems. 7. Listen for more data to reveal the total scope of the problem.
Catalytic	Consultant broadens client's knowledge of problem by offering new data or clarifying existing data.	1. Standards are violated or changed 2. Inability to meet goals or objectives	1. Set a nonauthoritarian tone for the interaction by beginning the intervention with social conversation. 2. Ask the client to describe the situation and use the description as a basis for the interaction. 3. Suggest data-gathering techniques that may provide new information of interest to the client. 4. Provide support to the client as the client attempts to accurately perceive the problem. 5. Avoid specific suggestions. 6. Encourage the client to make decisions about problem resolution.
Confrontation	Consultant presents clients with indisputable facts.	1. Additional insight needed 2. Unwillingness to solve problem	1. Continually question clients about their description of the situation. 2. Present data and logic to test clients' chosen courses of action. 3. Challenge clients' chosen courses of action. 4. Probe for motives and causes of present situation. 5. Provide own thoughts about situation without personally attacking client's values.
Prescriptive	Consultant tells client how to solve problem.	1. Inability to cope 2. Needs immediate answer	1. Probe for data about the client's situation. 2. Act authoritatively. 3. Control by telling the client how the problem is to be perceived. 4. Tell the client the best solutions. 5. Remind the client if he/she is procrastinating in implementing actions. 6. Offer praise if the client does what the consultant suggests.
Theory-Principles	Consultant teaches how to solve problem using theories or principles.	1. Additional insight needed 2. Lack of knowledge to solve problem	1. Introduce theories for problem-solving to the client. 2. Use techniques to assist the client to internalize theories. 3. Provide strategies for practical application of the theories, such as problem situations or critiques of application. 4. Offer support when the theory is applied in the actual problem situation.

TM 73

The organization of the school health program. (Figure 44-1)

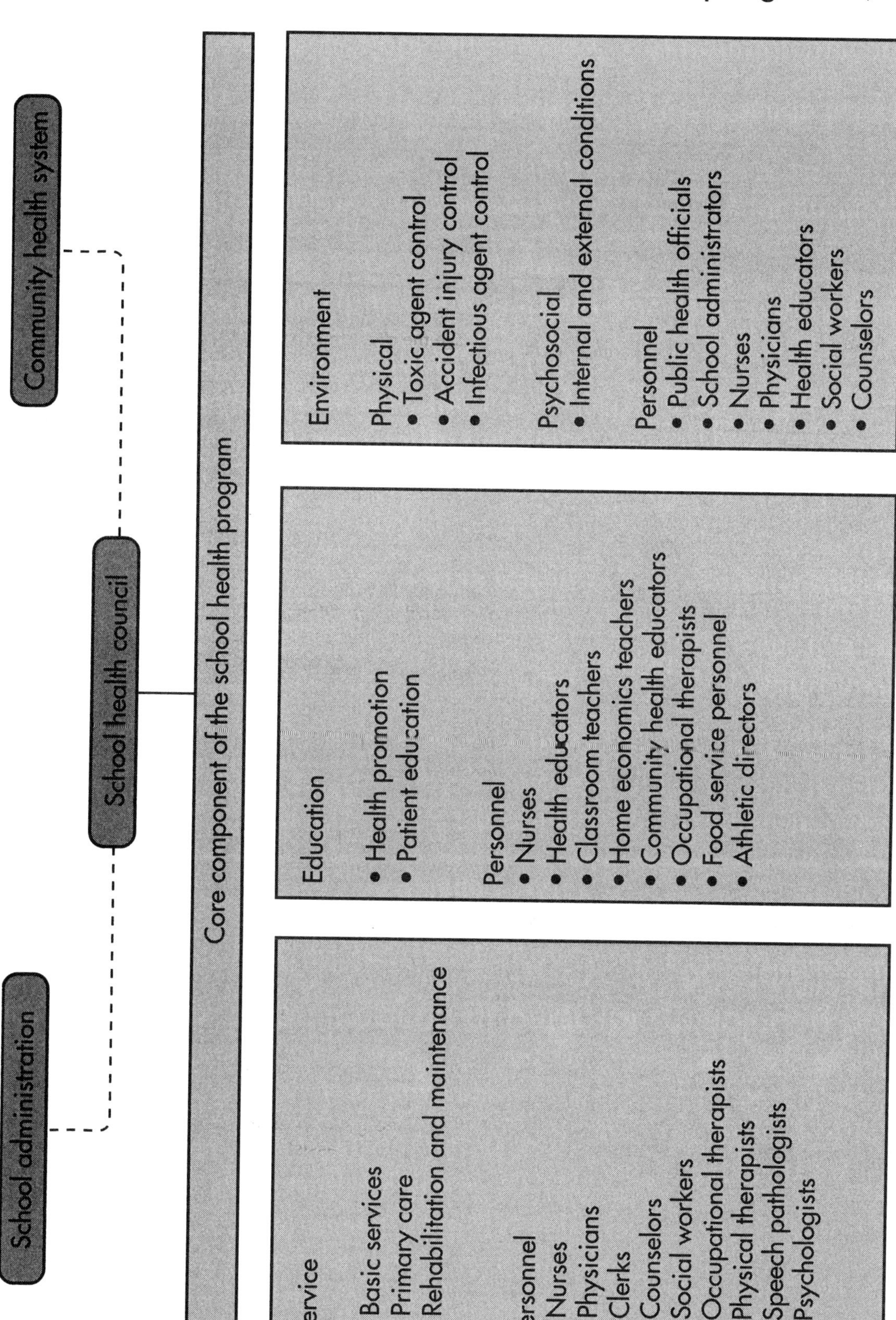

From School Health Programs, University of Colorado Health Science Center, 1989.

TM 74

Elements of the epidemiological triad applied to occupational health. (Figure 45-1)

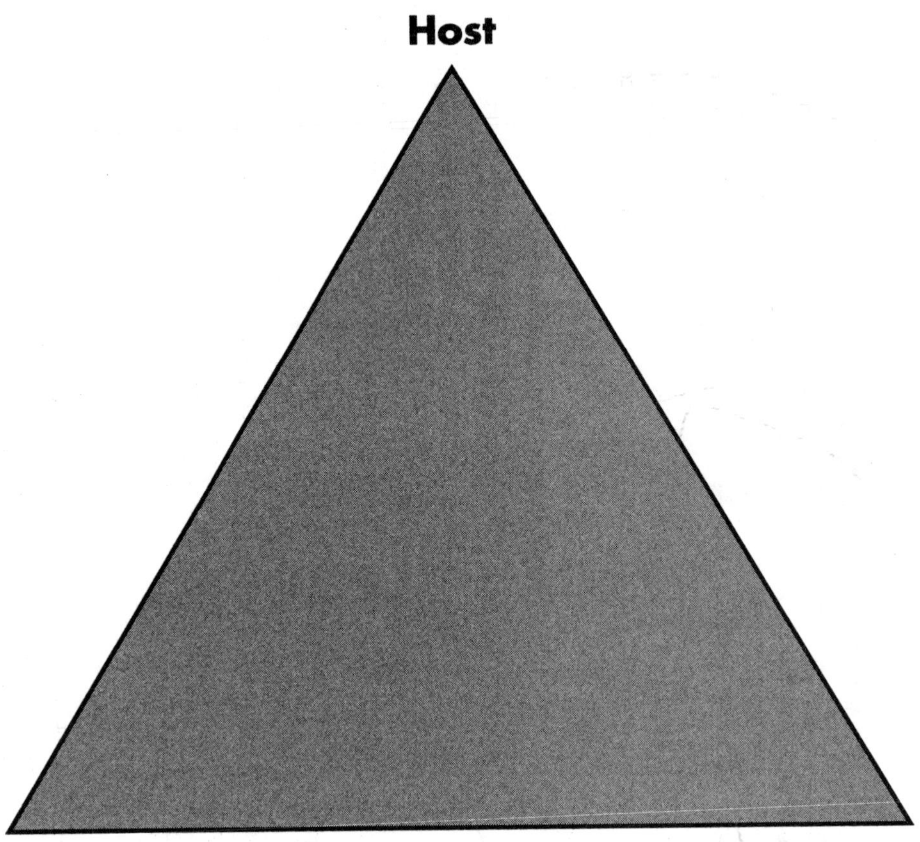

Stanhope/Lancaster: *Community Health Nursing*, ed 4

TM 75

Use of the nursing process in the five functional roles of the occupational health nurse.

NURSE CLINICIAN/PRACTITIONER

- Assesses the work environment for actual or potential health hazards.
- Collects data about the health status of the worker through an occupational health history, physical assessment, and appropriate laboratory measurements.
- Develops a nursing diagnosis to formulate a plan of nursing care in collaboration with the employee and other health care professionals.
- Records health data and maintains accurate employee health records.
- Provides counseling for worker health problems, health promotion, and disease prevention interventions (e.g., immunization, respiratory protection, hypertension screening, hearing conservation programs).
- Develops liaison relationships with community health care providers and organizations for worker health enhancement (e.g., referral to private providers and non-profit and governmental agencies).

NURSE ADMINISTRATOR

- Assesses the health needs of the workforce to help plan and develop cost-effective health services.
- Defines goals and objectives for the occupational health nursing service.
- Determines resources, such as facilities, staff, and operating expenses necessary to accomplish unit goals and develops an appropriate, realistic budget, as well as develops policies and procedures aimed at fostering goal attainment and work performance.
- Provides nursing leadership in the management and evaluation of human and operational resources, such as opportunities for enhancement of professional growth and quality management.

NURSE EDUCATOR

- Assesses the needs of the workforce with respect to health information and educational interventions.
- Develops, implements, and evaluates health promotion and education programs and materials.
- Acts as a liaison to community agencies in establishing networks for health education and promotion resources.
- Provides current information to all workers regarding health issues, trends, and factors that influence health behaviors and impact on health outcomes.

NURSE RESEARCHER

- Identifies issues to be considered through an occupational health and safety research effort.
- Participates with others in the conduction of research.
- Disseminates research findings.
- Incorporates research findings into the delivery of occupational health nursing services.

NURSE CONSULTANT

- Provides advice about the scope and development of occupational health services and programs, considering regulatory and other trends in health care.
- Serves as a resource to management on occupational health nursing issues.
- Serves as a resource for information and professional networking.

From Rogers B: In McCunnery RM, Brandt-Rauf PW: A *practical approach to occupational and environmental medicine*, Boston, 1994, Little, Brown, and Company.

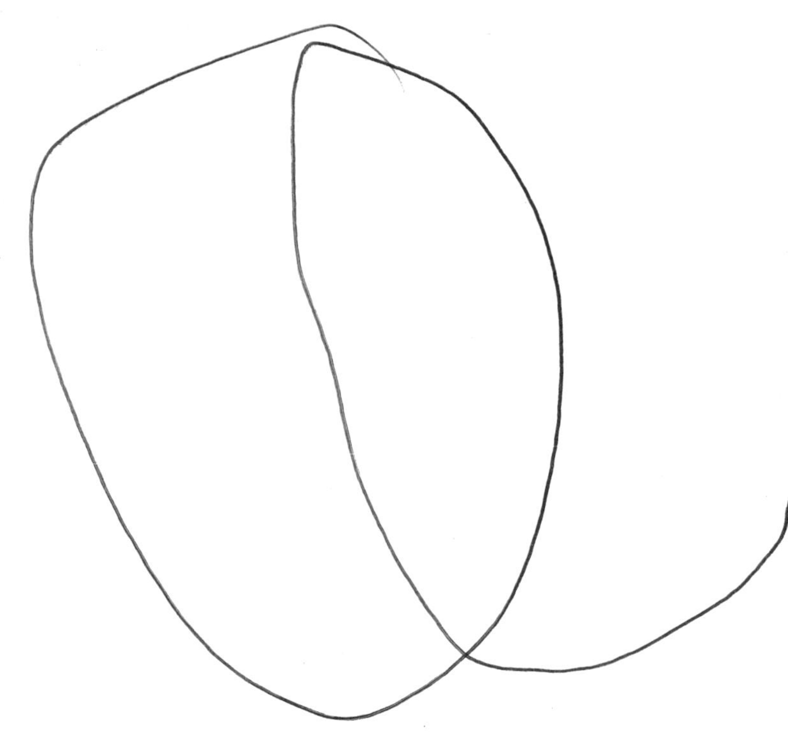